Study Guide
Linton

Medical-Surgical Nursing

Eighth Edition

Study Guide
Linton

Medical-Surgical Nursing

Eighth Edition

Brittany Hunter, DNP, RN, CMSRN

Dallas College
Dallas, Texas

ELSEVIER

Elsevier
3251 Riverport Lane
St. Louis, Missouri 63043

Study Guide
Medical-Surgical Nursing, 8th Edition

ISBN: 978-0-323-82672-3

Notice

Practitioners and researchers must always rely on their own experience and knowledge in evaluating and using any information, methods, compounds or experiments described herein. Because of rapid advances in the medical sciences, in particular, independent verification of diagnoses and drug dosages should be made. To the fullest extent of the law, no responsibility is assumed by Elsevier, authors, editors or contributors for any injury and/or damage to persons or property as a matter of products liability, negligence or otherwise, or from any use or operation of any methods, products, instructions, or ideas contained in the material herein.

Senior Content Strategist: Nancy O'Brien/Brandi Graham
Senior Content Development Manager: Lisa Newton
Content Development Specialist: Andrew Schubert
Publishing Services Manager: Deepthi Unni
Project Manager: Sindhuraj Thulasingam
Designer: Renee Duenow

Printed in India

Last digit is the print number: 9 8 7 6 5 4 3 2 1

Working together
to grow libraries in
developing countries

www.elsevier.com • www.bookaid.org

This book is dedicated to the healthcare heroes who have worked tirelessly to save the lives of others throughout the Covid-19 pandemic. Thank you for your service.

Preface

TO THE STUDENT

Welcome to the eighth edition of the Study Guide for *Medical-Surgical Nursing*. This Study Guide is a companion to the textbook *Medical-Surgical Nursing* by Adrianne Dill Linton and Mary Ann Matteson and is designed to help reinforce the material studied in the textbook and learned in class. It uses medical terminology originally introduced in the textbook. Each chapter in the Study Guide corresponds to a chapter in the textbook and contains questions and activities related to the chapter content. Some questions are easy and require simple recall; other exercises are more difficult and are designed to help you apply, analyze, and synthesize basic concepts. This requires you to view previously learned content and encourages you to integrate it with new content. Some of the questions encourage you to think critically and integrate a variety of concepts. By answering many different types of questions, you will establish a solid base of knowledge in medical-surgical nursing. Because the practice of licensed practical/vocational nurses has increased in long-term care and community-based settings, many questions require application of content in these settings.

It is recommended that you work through all the exercises in every chapter. For some of you, working in groups may be valuable and make the learning process more enjoyable. Student-to-student interaction often encourages active learning.

This new edition brings a focus on preparation for the Next-Generation NCLEX-PN® examination. The Next-Generation NCLEX-PN® examination uses real-world case studies to reflect the kinds of critical decisions nurses have to make in a variety of health-care settings. These types of questions assists in evaluating clinical judgment. The beginning of each chapter lists the related NCLEX categories that are covered in that chapter. There are questions in every chapter related to the NCLEX client needs categories and subcategories.

The Answer Key and many other helpful resources are provided on your Evolve site (http://evolve.elsevier.com/Linton/medsurg/), including a fluid and electrolyte tutorial and interactive NCLEX questions.

ORGANIZATION

The Study Guide chapters are divided into four parts: Part I, Mastering the Basics; Part II, Putting It All Together; Part III, Challenge Yourself! Getting Ready for NCLEX; and Part IV, Next-Generation NCLEX® Examination-Style Questions.

Part I, Mastering the Basics, contains matching, multiple-response, labeling, diagram reading, and fill-in-the-blank questions related to major content areas in the corresponding textbook chapter. These exercises help you instill medical-surgical nursing knowledge. The questions in Part I are at the basic knowledge and comprehension levels.

Part II, Putting It All Together, contains multiple-choice and multiple-response questions that integrate the chapter content. Most of the questions in Part II are at the comprehension and application levels, and are related to basic pathophysiology and basic nursing content.

Part III, Challenge Yourself! Getting Ready for NCLEX contains multiple-choice, multiple-response, case studies, fill-in-the-blank calculations, ordering, and prioritizing questions that are related to the NCLEX client needs and integrated processes content. Because the practice of practical/vocational nursing involves application of knowledge, skills, and abilities, the majority of questions in Part III are written at the application or analysis levels of cognitive ability and are related to nursing application content.

Part IV, Next-Generation NCLEX® Examination-Style Questions contains single-episode case studies and patient scenarios with one Next-Generation NCLEX-PN® style question per scenario for selected chapters. Question types include bowtie, trend, multiple choice, matrix multiple choice, multiple response – select all that apply, drop-down cloze, drop-down table, drag-and-drop cloze, drop-down rationale, drag-and-drop rationale, and highlight text. These styles of questions are written to assess clinical judgment skills related to nursing application content.

Acknowledgments

Sincere thanks and appreciation go to the many individuals who have contributed to the publication of this Study Guide.

I would like to thank the team at Elsevier: Senior Content Strategist Brandi Graham, Senior Content Development Manager Lisa Newton, Content Development Specialist Andrew Schubert, Deepthi Unni, and Sindhuraj Thulasingam for their continuous support and expert professional guidance. I also would like to thank Andrew Schubert for keeping me on schedule with manuscript submission and for his accessibility and encouragement throughout this process.

I especially want to thank my husband, Ja'Michael, who provided continuous support throughout this process. Your words of encouragement and willingness to listen pushed me to complete this project. I would like to also take the time to thank the various nurses that I have worked with along the way, who provided inspiration and insight on what it feels like to be a bedside nurse in the current healthcare environment.

Lastly, very special thanks go to the vocational nursing students. I want to thank all of the nursing students at Central Texas College and Dallas College, who have trusted me to assist them in preparing them for the NCLEX examination and entering the workforce. I appreciate your thought-provoking questions and enthusiasm to learn. Your willingness to seek learning opportunities made me a better professor. I am extremely honored to have been a part of your journey.

Contents

Illustration Credits

Chapter 5

p. x: From Black JM, Hawks JH: *Medical-surgical nursing: clinical management for positive outcomes*, 8th ed. St. Louis: Saunders; 2009.

p. x: From Monahan FD, Drake DT, Neighbors M, editors: *Medical-surgical nursing: foundations for clinical practice*, 2nd ed. Philadelphia: Saunders; 1998.

Chapter 15

MyPlate My Wins. DG Tip Sheet No. 1. https://www.choosemyplate.gov/ten-tips-choose-myplate. Retrieved July 20, 2017.

p. x: Courtesy of U.S. Food and Drug Administration.

Chapter 17

p. x: From Ignatavicius DD, Workman ML, Mishler MA: *Medical-surgical nursing across the health care continuum*, 3rd ed. Philadelphia: Saunders; 1999.

p. x: From Ignatavicius DD & Workman ML: *Medical-surgical nursing: patient-centered collaborative care*, 8th ed. St. Louis: Saunders; 2016.

Chapter 18

p. x: From Black JM, Hawks JH: *Medical-surgical nursing: clinical management for positive outcomes*, 8th ed. St. Louis: Saunders-Elsevier; 2009.

p. x: From Lewis SM, Bucher L, Heitkemper MM, Harding MM: *Medical-surgical nursing: assessment and management of clinical problems*, 10th ed. St. Louis: Elsevier; 2017.

Chapter 22

p. x: From Patton KT, Thibodeau GA: *The human body in health & disease*, 7th ed. St. Louis: Elsevier; 2018.

p. x: From Ignatavicius DD, Workman ML: *Medical-surgical nursing: patient-centered collaborative care*, 6th ed. St. Louis: Saunders; 2010.

Chapter 25

p. x: From McCance KL, Huether SE: *Understanding pathophysiology*, 6th ed. St. Louis: Mosby; 2013.

Chapter 26

p. x: From Lewis SM, Dirksen SR, Heitkemper MM, et al: *Medical-surgical nursing: assessment and management of clinical problems*, 8th ed. St. Louis: Mosby; 2011.

Chapter 31

p.x: From Thibodeau GA, Patton, KT: *Anatomy and physiology*, 8th ed. St. Louis: Mosby; 2013.

Chapter 33

p. x (both figures): From Herlihy B: *The human body in health and illness*, 4th ed. St. Louis: Saunders; 2011.

Chapter 34

p. x: From Monahan FD, Drake DT, Neighbors M, editors: *Medical-surgical nursing: foundations for clinical practice*, 2nd ed. Philadelphia: Saunders; 1998.

Chapter 37

p. x: From Thibodeau GA, Patton KT: *The human body in health and disease*, 6th ed. St. Louis: Mosby; 2014.

Chapter 40

p. x: From Lewis SM, Heitkemper MM, Dirksen SR: *Medical-surgical nursing: assessment and management of clinical problems*, 5th ed. St. Louis: Mosby; 2000.

Chapter 41

p. x: From Patton KT, Thibodeau GA: *Human body in health & disease*, 7th ed. St. Louis: Elsevier; 2018.

Chapter 45

p. x: Redrawn from Polaski AK, Tatro SE. *Luckmann's core principles and practice of medical-surgical nursing*, Philadelphia: Saunders; 1996.

p. x: From Ignatavicius DD, Workman ML. *Medical-surgical nursing: patient-centered collaborative care*, 8th ed. St. Louis: Saunders; 2016.

p. x: From Lewis SM, Heitkemper MM, Dirksen SR, et al. *Medical-surgical nursing: assessment and management of clinical problems*, 7th ed. St. Louis: Mosby; 2007.

p. x: From Black JM, Hawks JH. *Medical-surgical nursing: clinical management for positive outcomes*, 8th ed. St. Louis: Saunders; 2009.

Chapter 47

p. x: From Patton KT, Thibodeau GA. *The human body in health & disease*, 7th ed. St. Louis: Elsevier; 2018.

Chapter 51

p. x: From Patton KT, Thibodeau GA. *Human body in health & disease*, 7th ed. St. Louis: Elsevier; 2018.

Chapter 52

p. x: From Monahan FD, Drake DT, Neighbors M, editors. *Medical-surgical nursing: foundations for clinical practice*, 2nd ed. Philadelphia: Saunders; 1998.

Chapter 53

p. x: From Seidel HM, Ball JW, Dains JE, et al. *Mosby's guide to physical examination*, 7th ed. St. Louis: Mosby; 2010.

Chapter 56

p. x: From Proctor D, et al: *Kinn's the medical assistant: an applied learning approach*, 13th ed. St. Louis: Elsevier; 2017.

p. x: From Patton KT, Thibodeau GA: *Human body in health & disease*, 7th ed. St. Louis: Elsevier; 2018.

Aspects of Medical-Surgical Nursing

chapter

1

Go to http://evolve.elsevier.com/Linton/medsurg/ for additional activities and exercises.

NCLEX CATEGORIES

Safe and Effective Care Environment:
Coordinated Care

PART I: MASTERING THE BASICS

A. Key Terms
Match the definition in the numbered column with the most appropriate term in the lettered column.

1. _____ Professional negligence that results in injury or death of patient

2. _____ Belief that one's culture and values are superior to others

3. _____ A civil wrong against a person or property

4. _____ Addresses ethical questions related to health care

5. _____ Focuses on the day-to-day operations of the team

6. _____ Creates a vision, which along with unifying goals sets a mission for the team to work toward

A. Bioethics
B. Ethnocentrism
C. Leadership
D. Malpractice
E. Management
F. Tort

B. Roles
Choose the most appropriate answer or select all that apply.

1. Which are roles of the LPN/LVN medical-surgical nurse? Select all that apply.
   1. Caregiver
   2. Case manager
   3. Care coordinator
   4. Staff educator
   5. Administrator/manager

2. How are the roles that an LPN/LVN can assume officially determined?
   1. Each health care institution identifies roles based on needs and staffing
   2. Specified by each state's nurse practice act
   3. U.S. legislation specifies roles for all health care workers
   4. Education, setting, specialized training, and/or certification of the LPN/LVN
   5. NAPNES' *Standards of Practice and Educational Competencies of Graduates of Practical/Vocational Nursing Programs*

PART II: PUTTING IT ALL TOGETHER

C. Multiple Choice/Multiple Response
Choose the most appropriate answer or select all that apply.

1. Which are essential knowledge and skills required of an LPN/LVN? Select all that apply.
   1. Prescribing drugs
   2. Managing care
   3. Caring interventions
   4. Health status assessment
   5. Diagnosis
   6. Communication

2. What professional organization defines the standards for nursing practice and educational competencies for nurses practicing in medical-surgical settings?
   1. National League of Nursing
   2. The Academy of Medical-Surgical Nurses (AMSN)
   3. American Medical Association
   4. National Institutes of Health

Match the descriptions in the numbered column with the correct ethical principle in the lettered column.

3. _____   Respecting the rights of individuals
4. _____   Acting in the best interests of the patient
5. _____   Being truthful and honest
6. _____   Protecting patient privacy
7. _____   Considering fairness, equity, and appropriateness
8. _____   Doing no harm

A. Autonomy
B. Beneficence
C. Justice
D. Nonmaleficence
E. Confidentiality
F. Veracity

9. Which are examples of negligence in nursing care that could result in lawsuits against the hospital and the nurse? Select all that apply.
   1. Failure to document
   2. Failure to monitor a patient
   3. Failure to administer prescribed drugs due to perceived allergic reactions
   4. Failure to ensure patient safety, particularly for those at risk for injury
   5. Failure to respond immediately to all patient requests
   6. Failure to respond to or carry out orders

10. What is a medical-surgical nurse's best protection against negligence or malpractice?
    1. Adhere to the standards of practice.
    2. Never be alone with a patient.
    3. Record all patient interactions with a cell phone.
    4. Ask permission from the managing nurse prior to performing any duties.

Identify whether each of the characteristics listed below is more associated with leadership or management responsibilities.

11. _____   Broader, more future-oriented
12. _____   Develops vision
13. _____   Focuses on day-to-day operations
14. _____   Creates mission for team
15. _____   Local focus
16. _____   Task-oriented

A. Leadership
B. Management

17. Which are characteristics of effective leaders? Select all that apply.
    1. Communicates effectively
    2. Elevates conflict to a higher authority
    3. Uses authoritative approach in decision-making
    4. Proactive and flexible
    5. Delegates work appropriately
    6. Knowledgeable and competent in delivery of care

18. What must nurses consider when delegating work to team members? Select all that apply.
    1. Whether the state nurse practice act allows LPN/LVNs to delegate authority
    2. Knowledge of patient preferences
    3. Knowledge of capability required for delegated tasks
    4. Loyalty of staff to leadership
    5. Outcome documentation
    6. Knowledge of staff preferences for assignments

19. Nurses are responsible not only for their actions but also for the actions of staff to whom they delegate work, including accurate documentation. What is the principle associated with this responsibility?
    1. Coordination of care
    2. Authoritativeness
    3. Accountability
    4. Conflict resolution

PART III: CHALLENGE YOURSELF!

D. Getting Ready for NCLEX
Choose the most appropriate answer or select all that apply.

1. A patient refuses to continue with chemotherapy even though she is aware that without it she will probably not recover. Why is the nurse unable to force the patient to pursue chemotherapy?
   1. The patient has threatened a lawsuit if treatment is continued.
   2. Only the patient's physician can require her to continue treatment.
   3. The ethical principle of autonomy allows a patient to make his or her own decisions regarding care.
   4. The ethical principle of beneficence requires the nurse to do no harm, and the nurse believes that the treatment could be harmful.

2. A patient is admitted to the hospital. The nurse interviews the patient and his family, and takes routine vital signs. The nurse also reviews the patient's chart to identify further information. This is a demonstration of which standard competency?
   1. Diagnosis
   2. Assessment
   3. Accountability
   4. Safety

3. After moving to another state, a nurse wants to identify which roles he can perform before applying for a job. Where would he find the information?
   1. Academy of Medical-Surgical Nurses
   2. Each health care institution documents the roles that can be assumed by LPN/LVNs
   3. State's nurse practice act
   4. NAPNES' Standards of Practice and Educational Competencies of Graduates of Practical/Vocational Nursing Programs

4. What are some types of knowledge the nurse requires to guide the nursing assessment of a patient? Select all that apply.
   1. Related pathophysiology
   2. Insurance
   3. Complications
   4. Nursing interventions
   5. Expected patient responses
   6. Complementary medical alternatives

5. Why are ethical dilemmas complicated? Select all that apply.
   1. Situations may conflict with a nurse's moral beliefs.
   2. Ethics are a formal process to explore proper conduct.
   3. Ethics do not provide a single correct answer to a dilemma.
   4. Individuals involved in the dilemma usually hold strong opinions.
   5. In medical situations, there is insufficient time to process the dilemma.

6. Which situations can lead to a tort against a nurse? Select all that apply.
   1. A nurse tells friends something unusual about a patient that she noted in the patient's chart.
   2. A patient refuses medication, but the nurse forces her to take it for the patient's own good.
   3. A patient refuses a blood transfusion on religious grounds.
   4. In a staff meeting, a nurse repeats a rumor about a patient's personal life.
   5. A patient prone to falls keeps getting out of bed, so the nurse places an alarm on the bed to alert staff.
   6. A stranger asks for details regarding a patient, and the nurse refers him to the patient or her family.

7. A prescription states a patient must receive medication exactly at 6:00 PM; however, the nurse was on break and did not ensure other team members were aware of the prescription. The patient's condition worsened. What is the legal term describing this act of professional negligence?
   1. Malfeasance
   2. Malpractice
   3. Dereliction
   4. Liability

8. A nurse wants to prepare a patient report utilizing SBAR, which she knows is a systematic method of communication. To ensure the report is thorough, what types of information does she need? Select all that apply.
   1. Situation of the patient
   2. Barriers to providing treatment
   3. Assessment of patient
   4. Reasons why report is needed
   5. Background leading up to the situation
   6. Recommendations for moving forward

Choose the most appropriate answer for questions 9–12 regarding the following scenario. A nurse is attending classes on Saturday to earn her gerontology certificate, but she has just been informed that she must now work every other Saturday.

9. On the first Saturday the nurse reports to work, she is unwilling to speak to her colleagues except as needed. What stage of conflict is portrayed in this example?
   1. Frustration
   2. Conceptualization
   3. Action
   4. Outcome

10. On the next Saturday, she calls in sick. She continues calling in each Saturday she is scheduled to work. What stage of conflict is portrayed in this example?
    1. Frustration
    2. Conceptualization
    3. Action
    4. Outcome

11. The nurse's supervisor calls a conference and informs her that she must come in on Saturdays or she will be dismissed. What stage of conflict is portrayed in this example?
    1. Frustration
    2. Conceptualization
    3. Action
    4. Outcome

12. Before registering for the certificate program, the nurse had informed her supervisor, who seemed supportive; therefore, she believed her class time would be protected. Due to changes in staff, the supervisor considered sharing the workload to take precedence over personal goals, and the supervisor's perception of the conversation was that the workplace takes priority. What stage of conflict is portrayed in this example?
    1. Frustration
    2. Conceptualization
    3. Action
    4. Outcomes

Medical-Surgical Practice Settings

Go to http://evolve.elsevier.com/Linton/medsurg/ for additional activities and exercises.

NCLEX CATEGORIES

Safe and Effective Care Environment:
Coordinated Care, Safety and Infection Control

Psychosocial Integrity

Physiological Integrity: Basic Care and Comfort, Physiological Adaptation

PART I: MASTERING THE BASICS

A. Key Terms
Match the definition in the numbered column with the most appropriate term in the lettered column.

1. _____ Measurable loss of function, usually delineated to indicate a diminished capacity for work
2. _____ Restore maximal function after illness or injury
3. _____ Physical or psychological disturbance in functioning
4. _____ Inability to perform one or more normal daily activities because of mental or physical disability
5. _____ Long-term residential care that provides basic room, board, and supervision

A. Impairment
B. Handicap
C. Disability
D. Rehabilitation
E. Domiciliary Care

B. Disability Terms
Match the definition in the numbered column with the most appropriate term in the lettered column.

1. _____ Severe limitations in one or more activities of daily living (ADLs); unable to work
2. _____ Slight limitation in one or more ADLs; usually able to work
3. _____ Total disability characterized by near complete dependence on others for assistance with ADLs; unable to work
4. _____ Moderate limitation in one or more ADLs; able to work but workplace may need modifications

A. Level I
B. Level II
C. Level III
D. Level IV

PART II: PUTTING IT ALL TOGETHER

C. Multiple Choice/Multiple Response
Choose the most appropriate answer or select all that apply.

1. Which basic criteria for home health care must be met to receive Medicare reimbursement? Select all that apply.
   1. Patient care must be continuous for 24 hours per day.
   2. The patient needs intermittent skilled nursing care.
   3. The patient needs meals to be delivered at home.
   4. The patient must be homebound.
   5. The health care provider prescribes skilled nursing care for a specific condition.
   6. The patient must be bedridden.

2. Which are four of the most common intravenous therapies that can be given in a home health setting? Select four that apply.
   1. Hydration
   2. Chemotherapy
   3. Blood transfusion
   4. Antibiotics
   5. Platelet infusion
   6. Pain control

3. Which are examples of places where long-term care is provided? Select all that apply.
   1. Personal homes
   2. Board and care homes
   3. Hospitals
   4. Nursing homes
   5. Assisted-living centers
   6. Acute care facilities

4. Care delivered in a long-term care residential facility is based upon what three principles? Select three that apply.
   1. Maintenance of autonomy
   2. Prevention of illness
   3. Maintenance of function
   4. Treatment of disease
   5. Promotion of independence

5. What are positive responses to institutionalization of residents in long-term care facilities? Select all that apply.
   1. Increased depersonalization
   2. Improved nutrition
   3. Management of medical problems
   4. Surgical treatment of fractures
   5. Improved socialization
   6. Social withdrawal

6. By providing clear documentation of functional losses and goals for care, the nurse is meeting the Medicare criterion of:
   1. skilled care.
   2. reasonable and necessary care.
   3. homebound patient care.
   4. intermittent care.

7. What is the LPN/LVN's role in skilled observation and assessment of patients in home settings?
   1. Develop a plan of care.
   2. Implement a teaching plan.
   3. Perform focused assessments.
   4. Observe early signs and symptoms of illness.

PART III: CHALLENGE YOURSELF!

D. Getting Ready for NCLEX

Choose the most appropriate answer or select all that apply.

1. A patient is being transferred from an acute care hospital to a rehabilitation facility. The focus of rehabilitation is to:
   1. restore maximum possible functioning.
   2. function independently.
   3. assist with ADLs.
   4. eliminate impairment.

2. People born without arms can perform ADLs by using their feet and assistive devices. What are these people said to have?
   1. A disability
   2. A handicap
   3. Paralysis
   4. Impairment

3. How is an individual with an injured back who has a diminished capacity for work classified?
   1. Handicapped
   2. Impaired
   3. Disabled
   4. Dependent

4. The nurse is working in a rehabilitation center taking care of a poststroke patient. Which safety interventions play a role in preventing a secondary disability for this patient who is at risk for falls and fractures? Select all that apply.
   1. Use of walker
   2. Passive range-of-motion exercises
   3. Exercise three times a day for 30 minutes
   4. Modifications of the environment
   5. Teach patient to change positions every two hours
   6. Keep the side rails up

5. A patient was hospitalized with a stroke and is being transferred to a rehabilitation facility. Which is a goal of rehabilitation?
   1. Teach disabled individuals to take care of themselves.
   2. Return disabled individuals to maximum state of functioning.
   3. Perform skilled nursing procedures for patients.
   4. Respond promptly to patient requests for assistance with care.

6. Which requires the home health LPN/LVN to call the RN case manager? Select all that apply.
   1. Changes in vital signs
   2. Changes in weight
   3. Wound parameter changes
   4. Signs of patient abuse or neglect
   5. Presence of family member caretakers
   6. Report of what the patient ate for breakfast

7. Which is an example of a safety measure a nurse provides to prevent a secondary disability?
   1. Perform dressing changes for a postoperative patient.
   2. Provide walker for poststroke patient.
   3. Teach patient with diabetes how to draw up insulin in a syringe.
   4. Administer pain medications to a patient who has had a hip replacement.

8. Which nursing intervention is an example of the principle of maintenance of autonomy in long-term residential care?
   1. Place a urinal near the bed for immobile, incontinent patients.
   2. Allow nursing home residents to assist in establishing care goals.
   3. Explore factors that may be responsible for the patient's incontinence.
   4. Set specific goals for each resident that encourage independence.

9. What is the focus of traditional community health nursing? Select all that apply.
   1. Making home health care visits to house-bound individuals
   2. Public health education for communities
   3. Screening for disease detection
   4. Providing services for people outside the acute care setting

10. Which examples of secondary disabilities in a patient with a stroke should the nurse plan to prevent? Select all that apply.
    1. Eye infection
    2. Pneumonia
    3. Paralysis
    4. Pressure ulcers
    5. Limb contractures
    6. Urinary incontinence

11. Which skilled nursing procedure is reimbursed by Medicare?
    1. Unsterile dressing changes
    2. Enema administration
    3. Foley catheter insertion
    4. Injecting insulin

12. A patient rings the call bell. What is the first action the nurse should take to prevent the patient feeling indignity?
    1. Knock on the patient's door before entering.
    2. Talk with the patient about events inside and outside the long-term care facility.
    3. Simplify language and activities for the patient and avoid baby talk.
    4. Give the patient some flexibility and measure of control in daily activities.

13. A patient in a long-term care facility exhibits new behaviors that include staying in bed most of the day, expressing difficulty walking, and losing conversational skills. Which effect of institutionalization is this patient exhibiting?
    1. Social withdrawal
    2. Indignity
    3. Regression
    4. Depersonalization

14. A 72-year-old patient who has had a recent stroke has been transferred to a rehabilitation facility. The nurse notices an unused walker in the corner of the room. What referral needs to be made to improve his mobility?
    1. Physical therapist may need to increase strengthening exercises and gait training
    2. Social worker to address the patient's fears
    3. Speech therapist to improve communication
    4. Occupational therapist to help the patient improve fine motor skills

15. What can the nurse do to maintain autonomy of the patient in a long-term care setting?
    1. Focus care on restoring and preserving function.
    2. Allow the patient to decide the time of his bath.
    3. Select specific goals for the patient.
    4. Knock on the patient's door before entering the room.

16. The nurse is making a home health visit to see a patient who is recovering from a stroke. In addition to giving direct care to the patient, the most important role is to:
    1. assess the home for safety problems.
    2. make arrangements for a daily bath for this patient.
    3. make referrals to community support groups.
    4. teach the patient and family to care for themselves.

17. The home health nurse is collecting data from a patient for the plan of care. Data collected by the nurse that may detect heart failure problems early in this patient include:
    1. confusion and elevated blood sugar.
    2. weight gain and ankle edema.
    3. shortness of breath and urinary retention.
    4. jaundice and dyspepsia.

18. The nurse is working in a home health setting. The health care provider authorized a plan of care that is used by the nurse to develop a nursing care plan. Which must be included in the provider's authorized plan of care? Select all that apply.
    1. Plans for discharge from home care
    2. Results of mental status examination
    3. Plans for daily visits from home health personnel
    4. Rehabilitation potential
    5. Safety measures to protect against injury

Medical-Surgical Patients: Individuals, Families, and Communities

Go to http://evolve.elsevier.com/Linton/medsurg/ for additional activities and exercises.

NCLEX CATEGORIES

Psychosocial Integrity

PART I: MASTERING THE BASICS

A. Key Terms

Match the definition in the numbered column with the most appropriate term in the lettered column. Answers may be used more than once.

1. _____ Minimize complications of an illness or injury to return a patient to health

2. _____ Inability to express feelings and thoughts in a manner that can be understood by others

3. _____ Health promotion and practices that prevent injury or illness

4. _____ Clear transmission of messages in which both the sender and the receiver are active participants

5. _____ Help the patient to manage long-term care of a change in his or her health

A. Dysfunctional communication
B. Functional communication
C. Primary prevention
D. Secondary prevention
E. Tertiary prevention

B. Culture

1. What are the three basic characteristics of all cultures? Select the three that apply.
   1. Culture is often identified by symbols.
   2. Culture is based on ethnic background.
   3. Culture is shared among a group or a family.
   4. Culture is learned from family or cultural leaders.
   5. Culture is based on religious background.
   6. Culture is based on health literacy.

2. Order the proper sequence of the three phases of culture shock associated with hospitalization.
   A. _____ Patient becomes disenchanted with the whole situation, frustrated, and withdraws.
   B. _____ Patient begins to adapt to new environment and is able to maintain a sense of humor.
   C. _____ Patient asks questions regarding the hospital routine and the hospital's expectations of the patient.

3. Which are true regarding ethnic and cultural groups? Select all that apply.
   1. Languages among cultural and ethnic groups can vary.
   2. Nonverbal language is strictly an American concept.
   3. Institutions receiving federal funds are required to provide translators for non-English speakers and those who are hard of hearing.
   4. Individuals within certain cultures may turn to folk healers if their physical and psychosocial needs are not met by western medicine.
   5. It is safe to assume that all individuals within a particular ethnic or cultural group share the same beliefs.
   6. Culture impacts many aspects of family life.

C. Developmental Stages
Choose the most appropriate answer or select all that apply.

1. Which of the following describes middle adulthood? Select all that apply.
   1. Focus on marriage, childbearing, and work
   2. "Sandwich" generation
   3. Redirection of energy and talents to new roles and activities
   4. Earn most of their money
   5. Retirement
   6. Establish career goals

2. Which of the following describes young adulthood? Select all that apply.
   1. Settling down to job and raising a family
   2. Decreased short-term memory
   3. Pay the most taxes
   4. Establish career goals
   5. Develop satisfying leisure activities
   6. Establish meaningful social relationships

3. Which of the following relate to older adulthood? Select all that apply.
   1. Guidance of grown children
   2. Home and time management
   3. They are a very heterogeneous group
   4. Help growing and grown children to become happy, responsible adults
   5. Frequently have limited formal education
   6. Many who engage in exercise continue to function well

Match the health developmental task in the numbered column with the developmental stage in the lettered column.

4. _____   Generativity versus stagnation
5. _____   Intimacy versus isolation
6. _____   Ego integrity versus despair
A. Young adulthood
B. Middle adulthood
C. Older adulthood

D. Age-Related Health Problems
Choose the most appropriate answer or select all that apply.

1. Which health problems are related to middle adulthood? Select all that apply.
   1. Benign or malignant prostate enlargement
   2. Bone mass begins to decrease
   3. Vehicular accidents and suicide
   4. Injuries frequently causing absence from work among men
   5. Stress related to managing a household
   6. Perimenopausal period
   7. Stress related to caregiving role for older parents

2. Which are the most common health problems in older adults? Select all that apply.
   1. Presbyopia
   2. Heart disease
   3. Obesity
   4. Arthritis
   5. Diabetes
   6. Cancer

PART II: PUTTING IT ALL TOGETHER

E. Multiple Choice
Choose the most appropriate answer.

1. What cultural information does the nurse need to collect from a patient? Select all that apply.
   1. Food practices
   2. Family roles
   3. Religious beliefs
   4. Health literacy

2. Why is it important to provide culturally sensitive care to all patients?
   1. It is legally required by all health care institutions.
   2. Patients not treated according to their beliefs may bring in folk healers.
   3. Can reduce stress and decrease recovery time.
   4. To be politically correct.

3. Which ethnic group responds better to diuretics for treatment of hypertension than other groups?
   1. African Americans
   2. Latinos
   3. Native Americans
   4. Caucasians

4. Adapting nursing care to the cultural differences of patients is called:
   1. holistic care.
   2. complementary care.
   3. awareness and cultural competency.
   4. cultural diversity.

5. Establishing financial independence is a developmental task of the:
   1. middle adult.
   2. older adult.
   3. young adult.
   4. adolescent.

6. The nurse is assisting with an education program for young adults on health care needs. Topics that should be discussed include which of the following?
   1. Family planning
   2. Cancer screenings
   3. Diabetes Management
   4. Perimenopausal management

7. In what age group are unintentional injuries one of the top 10 causes of death?
   1. 15–25
   2. 30–45
   3. 45–60
   4. 65 and above

8. How is family identified/defined for each patient?
   1. Blood relations or through marriage or adoption
   2. Identified by the patient
   3. Through power of attorney
   4. Varies by state

9. Which are internal family coping mechanisms? Select all that apply.
   1. Family group reliance
   2. Role flexibility
   3. Maintaining a normal life
   4. Seeking support

PART III: CHALLENGE YOURSELF!

F. Getting Ready for NCLEX
Choose the most appropriate answer or select all that apply.

1. In western culture, most people believe illness is treatable. What are some beliefs about illness held by other cultures? Select all that apply
   1. Illness is a punishment for sins.
   2. Illness is related to western medicine
   3. Illness is beyond one's control.
   4. Illness is a metaphysical concept.

2. The nurse is admitting a new patient to the hospital. The patient expresses fear about being in the hospital. What are the three stages of culture shock associated with hospitalization? Select three that apply.
   1. Asking questions
   2. Denial
   3. Adaptation
   4. Bargaining
   5. Being disenchanted
   6. Generalization

3. A 62-year-old patient in the hospital states that he does not like to take baths routinely and is very modest about disrobing in front of strangers. Which are appropriate responses of the nurse? Select all that apply.
   1. Explain to the patient that baths will be taken every morning before noon.
   2. Knock before entering the room.
   3. Ask permission before touching the patient.
   4. Reassure the patient that it is all right to disrobe in the hospital, as you will pull the curtain to provide privacy.
   5. Ask permission from the patient to assist with personal hygiene.
   6. Explain the importance of personal hygiene for all patients in the hospital.

4. The nurse is teaching a community group about the importance of immunizations. Which of the following are barriers to teaching about health promotion to people with low literacy levels and economical disadvantages? Select all that apply.
   1. Clients have difficulty reading the materials presented
   2. Clients live in crowded housing conditions
   3. Clients have inadequate diets
   4. Clients have access to online resources

5. The nurse is on a home health visit to see a 56-year-old female patient who had ankle surgery 2 weeks ago. Her family is supportive and is learning to assist with her care at home. Which of the following does the nurse recognizes as the most important influence on family interaction?
   1. Self-esteem of each member
   2. Family income
   3. Family size
   4. Type of family configuration

6. The nurse is talking with an 82-year-old male patient and his wife and daughter in a long-term care facility. The patient is newly admitted and his family is concerned about how he will adjust to the new environment. Which are ways for the nurse to collect data about the wife and daughter and their coping strategies? Select all that apply.
   1. Determine stressors being experienced.
   2. Assess family communication patterns.
   3. Find out what kinds of coping strategies are used.
   4. Explore each family member's religious views.
   5. Attach meaning to the experience.

7. The nurse is providing home hospice care for a 68-year-old female patient with cancer. She is surrounded by her husband and children. What are the most important strategy for assisting this family to cope? Select all that apply.
   1. Encourage all family members to be involved in the process.
   2. Work with the most influential member of the family.
   3. Support new coping strategies instead of using old coping strategies that have worked in the past.
   4. Reinforce coping styles that have been helpful in the past.

8. When taking care of a patient in the hospital, how can the nurse best assist the patient and family?
   1. Decide roles for the family members.
   2. Focus care on the patient and have the family members wait in the family room.
   3. Determine whether the family members are supportive of or detrimental to the patient's recovery process.
   4. Provide information only to the patient because of confidentiality.

9. The nurse is collecting data from a newly admitted older adult patient. The nurse observes that the patient is having difficulty adjusting to the physical, psychological, and sociologic changes that may occur with aging. The patient is probably at risk for:
   1. isolation.
   2. stagnation.
   3. generativity.
   4. despair.

10. To collect data about the developmental tasks of young adulthood, the nurse asks:
    1. whether the patient has meaningful intimate relationships.
    2. what the patient does for leisure or recreation.
    3. what the patient does each day.
    4. what signs of depression the patient has.

11. Which health screening tests should begin in young adulthood? Select all that apply.
    1. Routine glucose testing
    2. Mammograms
    3. Pap smears
    4. Routine cholesterol
    5. Routine blood pressure screens

12. The nurse is teaching a community group of middle-aged people about health promotion. Which intervention is directed toward reducing the incidence of type 2 diabetes mellitus among middle-aged adults?
    1. Maintain ideal weight.
    2. Recognize and modify stressors.
    3. Increase physical activity.
    4. Limit alcohol intake.

Health, Illness, Stress, and Coping

chapter 4

Go to http://evolve.elsevier.com/Linton/medsurg/ for additional activities and exercises.

NCLEX CATEGORIES

Health Promotion and Maintenance

Psychosocial Integrity

PART I: MASTERING THE BASICS

A. Maslow's Hierarchy
List the five levels of human needs in order of priority from Maslow's hierarchy.

1. _____
2. _____
3. _____
4. _____
5. _____

Match the need in the numbered column with the correct item in the lettered column.

6. _____ Oxygen, fluid, nutrition, temperature, elimination, shelter, rest, and sex

7. _____ Protection from harm, freedom from anxiety and fear

8. _____ Feeling loved by family and friends, and accepted by peers and community

9. _____ Feeling good about oneself and feeling that others hold one in high regard

10. _____ Self-fulfillment; able to problem-solve, accept criticism from others, and eager to acquire new knowledge; self-confidence; maturity

A. Self-esteem
B. Safety and security
C. Physiologic
D. Self-actualization
E. Love and belonging

11. Which components of nursing care are related to physiologic needs of Maslow's Hierarchy of Human Needs? Select all that apply.
    1. Breathe normally.
    2. Work so that there is a sense of accomplishment.
    3. Worship according to one's faith.
    4. Eat and drink adequately.
    5. Eliminate body wastes.
    6. Avoid dangers in the environment.

B. Health, Disease, Coping, and Illness
Match the descriptions in the numbered column with the correct terms in the lettered column. Answers may be used more than once.

1. _____ The ability to express the full range of one's physical and mental potential within one's environment

2. _____ Includes personal, interpersonal, and cultural perceptions of and reactions to a disease

3. _____ Can be recognized by objective findings such as fever or presence of bacteria

4. _____ Regarded as a disruption of biologic and/or psychological functions

5. _____ Deviation from a state of health

A. Health
B. Illness
C. Disease

6. Which are factors influence the effect of illness on the family? Select all that apply.
   1. Seriousness of disease
   2. Duration of disease
   3. Balance of work and recreation
   4. Adequate nutrition of the family
   5. Social and cultural customs of the family

Match the descriptions in the numbered column with the correct terms in the lettered column. Answers may be used more than once.

7. _____   Rapid onset and short duration
8. _____   Patient free of acute symptoms
9. _____   Permanent change in health status
10. _____   Recurrence of acute symptoms
11. _____   Requires long-term rehabilitation or treatment
12. _____   Appendicitis
13. _____   Urinary tract infection
14. _____   Diabetes mellitus

A. Acute illness
B. Chronic illness
C. Remission
D. Exacerbation

15. What characteristics impact an individual's ability to cope with illness? Select all that apply.
    1. Age
    2. Self-concept
    3. Educational level
    4. Family
    5. Employment
    6. Spirituality
    7. Community resources
    8. Weight

C. Cultural Considerations

1. Which considerations help patients cope with illness? Select all that apply.
   1. Ensuring patient comprehends the care facility's cultural framework
   2. Recognizing how the nurse's own values may differ from his or her patients'
   3. Developing a care plan that reduces patient stress
   4. Explaining to the patient that each patient is treated the same regardless of cultural differences

Match the descriptions in the numbered column with the correct terms in the lettered column. Answers may be used more than once.

2. _____   Stress and fear due to changes in body image
3. _____   Mechanisms, adaptive or maladaptive, that address the consequences of illness
4. _____   Belief that illness is a punishment from God
5. _____   Reaction to life changes due to illness
6. _____   Vague, sometimes intense, sense of impending doom
7. _____   Response to a real or perceived threat
8. _____   Emotional response to loss
9. _____   Involuntary separation from cherished relationships, abilities, or hopes
10. _____   Mechanism through which grief is processed

A. Spirituality
B. Self-concept
C. Emotions
D. Stress
E. Fear
F. Anxiety
G. Loss
H. Grief
I. Mourning

PART II: PUTTING IT ALL TOGETHER

D. Multiple Choice/Multiple Response
Choose the most appropriate answer or select all that apply.

1. What are some factors that impact coping mechanisms to stressors? Select all that apply.
   1. Family
   2. Values
   3. Culture
   4. Boredom
   5. Community

2. An individual may express anger when faced with which feelings?
   1. Denial
   2. Helplessness
   3. Monotony
   4. Conflicted

3. Which is an example of a physiologic stressor?
   1. Excessive noise
   2. Grieving loss of spouse
   3. Inadequate financial resources
   4. Diagnosis of cancer

4. Which is an example of an emotional stressor?
   1. Chronic pain
   2. Winning the lottery
   3. Sunburn
   4. Running a marathon

5. What is an individual's emotional or physiologic response to stressors called?
   1. Homeostasis
   2. Development
   3. Adaptation
   4. Disease

6. Teaching relaxation techniques to a patient usually does not work under which condition?
   1. Cultural biases
   2. Inability to concentrate due to pain
   3. Lack of self-control
   4. Deeply religious

7. Coping strategies such as journaling and aromatherapy directed toward maintaining or enhancing well-being as a protection against illness are related to:
   1. health adaptation.
   2. health promotion.
   3. prevention of illness.
   4. homeostasis measures.

8. Which is a symptom of maladaptive coping?
   1. Unemployment
   2. Sensory deprivation
   3. Feeling of powerlessness
   4. Ethnic difference

9. Which are examples of methods to relieve stress that focus the patient's mind inward? Select all that apply.
   1. Massage
   2. Surgery
   3. Guided imagery
   4. Meditation
   5. Generic drugs
   6. Biofeedback

10. Which are focus areas of *Healthy People 2020*? Select all that apply.
    1. Cancer
    2. Thyroid disorders
    3. Diabetes
    4. Infectious disease
    5. Autoimmune disorders
    6. Access to quality health services

11. Which populations are focus areas of *Healthy People 2020*? Select all that apply.
    1. Adolescents
    2. Pregnant women
    3. People with disabilities
    4. Health care workers
    5. LGBT

12. What does the fight-or-flight reaction to stress enable?
    1. Initial stress
    2. Resistance
    3. Exhaustion
    4. Physiologic

13. Which are examples of self-actualization according to Maslow? Select all that apply.
    1. Has rich emotional experiences
    2. Self-mastery
    3. Desire to help others
    4. Ability to direct one's own life
    5. Feeling loved by one's family
    6. Feeling confident about oneself

14. Which statements describe stress? Select all that apply.
    1. Health is related to the ability to adjust to stressors.
    2. Internal stressors are less important than external stressors.
    3. Stressors are related to negative occurrences only.
    4. Stress is vital for growth and development.
    5. Resolving mild stress can lead to improved self-esteem.
    6. At any given moment, we are all adapting to stress.

PART III: CHALLENGE YOURSELF!

E. Getting Ready for NCLEX
Choose the most appropriate answer or select all that apply.

1. Nursing interventions to increase adaptability in older adults should be geared toward helping them to:
   1. use past successful coping mechanisms to deal with new stressors.
   2. assess their strengths and weaknesses in dealing with new stressors.
   3. develop new coping mechanisms to deal with new stressors.
   4. learn new methods of dealing with stressors.

2. A coworker asks the nurse questions about taking care of a chronically ill patient. The nurse responds that tasks for chronically ill individuals include:
   1. reversing changes in the course of the illness.
   2. preventing and managing crises.
   3. curing the chronic disease.
   4. decreasing social interactions.

3. The nurse is caring for a patient who has just been given a complex diagnosis that can impact his future quality of life. The patient asks for more details about his condition. How should the nurse respond? Select all that apply.
   1. Instruct the patient to discuss the condition with the health care provider.
   2. Provide patient access to the Internet.
   3. Go over the basics about his condition.
   4. Answer patient questions about his diagnosis.
   5. Allow patient to express his fears and concerns.

4. What observations of a patient newly admitted to the hospital enabled the nurse to identify that he is struggling with the stress of his illness? Select all that apply.
   1. Inability to perform self-care
   2. Blaming himself for his disease
   3. Discusses ways to manage illness upon release from the hospital
   4. Does not talk when his family is present
   5. Makes attempts to remain physically active
   6. Attempts to perform self-grooming routine on a daily basis

5. Which question will the nurse ask the patient to help determine the external coping strategies of the patient?
   1. "What is your worst possible stressor, and how does this present stress compare with the worst?"
   2. "What ways have you coped with stress in the past that have been successful for you?"
   3. "What kinds of things do you do when you are stressed? Do you eat more or less?"
   4. "Whom do you turn to when you are feeling stressed?"

6. A patient is having trouble adapting to the stressors of hospitalization. Which observation indicates evidence of inability to adapt?
   1. Patient experiences a sense of control.
   2. Patient is expressing anger at his health care team.
   3. Patient experiences increased self-awareness.
   4. Patient believes that the creative process is healing.

7. To help a patient increase adaptability to illness, the nurse collects data about the internal coping strategies of the patient. The best question for the nurse to ask this patient about internal coping strategies is:
   1. "Do you eat more or less when you are stressed?"
   2. "To whom do you turn when you are feeling stressed?"
   3. "Do you talk with others, or do you keep things inside?"
   4. "Do you contact your health care provider when you have a problem?"

8. When older patients experience new stress, the best nursing intervention is to:
   1. explore the patient's limitations and find ways to decrease the limitations.
   2. discuss reducing alcohol intake and smoking.
   3. help the patient use past successful coping mechanisms.
   4. encourage patients to seek support from outside social agencies.

9. The patient is a 45-year-old male who has been admitted to the hospital with pneumonia. As the nurse is conducting the admission interview, she finds out the following. Which findings indicate safety and security needs of the patient? Select all that apply.
   1. He has recently separated from his wife and three children.
   2. He is afraid to jog due to crime in his neighborhood.
   3. He states that he feels like he will never amount to anything.
   4. His parents live 300 miles away and he has few close friends in town.
   5. He states he fears he will lose his job if he is in the hospital too long.
   6. He states he feels alone a lot.

10. A patient with diabetes mellitus is experiencing psychological stress in the hospital. Which is a psychological stressor?
    1. Chronic pain
    2. Starvation
    3. Running a marathon
    4. Inadequate financial resources

Immunity, Inflammation, and Infection

chapter

5

Go to http://evolve.elsevier.com/Linton/medsurg/ for additional activities and exercises.

NCLEX CATEGORIES

Safe and Effective Care Environment:
Coordinated Care, Safety, and Infection Control

Health Promotion and Maintenance

Physiological Integrity: Reduction of Risk
Potential, Physiological Adaptation

PART I: MASTERING THE BASICS

A. Key Terms

Match the definition in the numbered column with the most appropriate term in the lettered column.

1. _____ An antigen that causes a hypersensitive reaction

2. _____ A protein that is created in response to a specific antigen

3. _____ A substance, usually a protein, that is capable of stimulating a response from the immune system

4. _____ Microorganisms that are resistant to one or more classes of antimicrobial agents

A. Allergen
B. Antibody
C. Antigen
D. Multidrug-resistant organisms (MDROs)

Match the definition in the numbered column with the most appropriate term in the lettered column.

5. _____ Limiting the spread of microorganisms; often called *clean technique*

6. _____ Elimination of microorganisms from any object that comes in contact with the patient; often called *sterile technique*

7. _____ Cellular changes that signal the body's response to injury or infection

8. _____ Hospital-acquired infections (infections that were not present at the time of admission)

9. _____ Presence of an infectious organism on a body surface or an object

10. _____ Process involving the invasion of body tissues by microorganisms, the multiplication of invading organisms, and subsequent damage of tissue

11. _____ A condition in which the body is unable to distinguish self from nonself, causing the immune system to react and destroy its own tissues

12. _____ Illness caused by infectious organisms or their toxins that can be transmitted, either directly or indirectly, from one person to another

13. _____ Condition in which the immune system is unable to defend the body against organisms

14. _____ Resistance to or protection from a disease

A. Autoimmunity
B. Communicable disease
C. Contamination
D. Immunity
E. Immunodeficiency
F. Infection
G. Inflammation
H. Medical asepsis
I. Health care–associated infection
J. Surgical asepsis

B. Infection

Choose the most appropriate answer or select all that apply.

1. Which are infectious agents? Select all that apply.
   1. Helminths
   2. Protozoa
   3. Macrophages
   4. Fungi
   5. Allergens
   6. Viruses

2. Which are observable signs (objective data) of infection? Select all that apply.
   1. Redness
   2. Pus
   3. Pain
   4. Swelling
   5. Discoloration
   6. Heat

3. Place the six factors in the chain of infection in sequence. (Note: Begin by numbering causative agent as 1.)
   A. _____ Portal of entry
   B. _____ Reservoir
   C. _____ Susceptible host
   D. _____ Mode of transfer
   E. _____ Portal of exit
   F. _____ Causative agent

4. Which classifications of medications often place patients at risk for infection? Select all that apply.
   1. Immunosuppressants
   2. Antihypertensives
   3. Steroids
   4. Antineoplastics
   5. Diuretics
   6. Cholesterol-lowering drugs

5. Which laboratory tests are used to screen patients for infection? Select all that apply.
   1. White blood cell differentiated count
   2. Liver function
   3. Electrolytes
   4. Blood cultures
   5. Platelet count

C. Age-Related Changes

1. What of the following are the reasons for a delayed healing process in older adults? Select all that apply.
   1. Decreased tissue elasticity
   2. Decreased lean muscle mass
   3. Decreased blood supply to tissues
   4. Decreased renal function
   5. Decreased neurons in the brain

D. Allergies and Allergens

Match each common allergic reaction in the numbered column with the most appropriate causative agent in the lettered column.

1. _____ Asthma
2. _____ Anaphylaxis
3. _____ Urticaria (hives)
4. _____ Atopic dermatitis (eczema)
5. _____ Allergic contact dermatitis

A. Food
B. Latex gloves, plants (poison ivy)
C. Pollens, dust
D. Soaps
E. Insect venom, antibiotics

E. Resistance

1. Which of the following are the reasons for the development of resistant bacterial strains? Select all that apply.
   1. Bacterial cells develop mutations
   2. Overuse of antibiotics
   3. Introduction of allergens
   4. Exposure to cigarette smoke
   5. Increased use of immunizations

2. Which nursing considerations are recommended by the Centers for Disease Control and Prevention to prevent antimicrobial resistance in long-term care patients? Select all that apply.
   1. Encourage patients to have annual influenza vaccine.
   2. Carefully monitor blood glucose.
   3. Prevent development of pressure ulcers.
   4. Promptly report diarrhea in patients on antibiotics; cause may be *C. difficile*.
   5. Carefully collect specimens for culture to prevent contamination.

F. Standard Precautions

For each disease or condition in the numbered column, indicate all of the appropriate types of precautions in the lettered column. Answers may be used more than once.

1. _____ Mumps
2. _____ Scabies
3. _____ Pneumonia
4. _____ Impetigo
5. _____ Rubeola (measles)
6. _____ Wound infections
7. _____ Varicella (chickenpox)
8. _____ Rubella
9. _____ Tuberculosis
10. _____ Diphtheria (pharyngeal)

A. Airborne precautions
B. Droplet precautions
C. Contact precautions

11. Contact with which substances requires the use of Standard Precautions when the nurse is performing procedures? Select all that apply.
    1. Patient's blood
    2. Sweat and perspiration
    3. Mucous membranes
    4. Intact skin
    5. Body fluids

G. Hyperbaric Oxygen Therapy

1. Which are complications for which the nurse monitors the patient during hyperbaric oxygen therapy? Select all that apply.
    1. Ear pain
    2. Eye pain
    3. Seizures
    4. Bradycardia
    5. Chest pain
    6. Allergic reaction

H. Autoimmunity

Match the autoimmune disorders in the numbered column with the most appropriate targets in the lettered column.

1. _____ Diabetes mellitus type 1
2. _____ Addison's disease
3. _____ Multiple sclerosis
4. _____ Myasthenia gravis
5. _____ Rheumatic fever
6. _____ Ulcerative colitis
7. _____ Crohn's disease
8. _____ Rheumatoid arthritis
9. _____ Autoimmune thrombocytopenic purpura

A. Colon
B. Adrenal gland
C. Ileum
D. Joints
E. Brain and spinal cord
F. Pancreas
G. Neuromuscular junction
H. Heart
I. Platelets

I. Antigens

1. Which of the following are antigens? Select all that apply.
    1. Microorganisms
    2. White blood cells
    3. Environmental substances
    4. Platelets
    5. Dust

J. Immune System Organs

1. Which body organs are involved in immunity? Select all that apply.
   1. Bone marrow
   2. Heart
   3. Lungs
   4. Lymph nodes
   5. Spleen
   6. Thyroid gland

2. *Using Figure 5.1 in the book as a reference, label organs involved in immunity (A–G).*

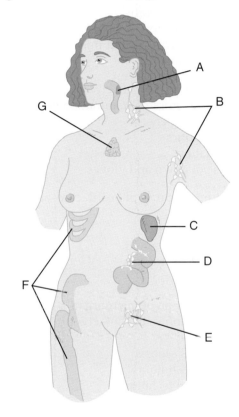

A. _____

B. _____

C. _____

D. _____

E. _____

F. _____

G. _____

K. Inflammatory Response

Indicate the stages of the inflammatory response following tissue injury outlined in Figure 5.2 in the book using the letters A–D. Answers may be used more than once.

1. _____ Release of chemical mediators

2. _____ Ingestion and destruction of foreign agents

3. _____ Repair and regeneration

4. _____ Normal tissue

5. _____ Movement of proteins, water, and white blood cells out of capillaries into injured tissues

6. _____ Exudate formation

7. _____ Intact cells

8. _____ Phagocytic lymphocytes enter area of injury

9. _____ Dilated blood vessels and increased capillary permeability

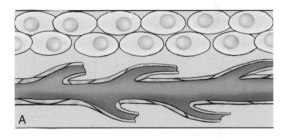

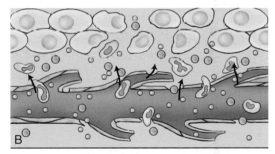

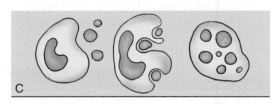

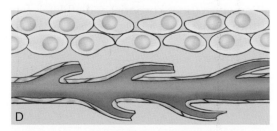

PART II: PUTTING IT ALL TOGETHER

L. Multiple Choice/Multiple Response
Choose the most appropriate answer or select all that apply.

1. Prostaglandins, histamine, and leukotrienes are examples of:
   1. hormonal factors.
   2. chemical mediators.
   3. erythrocytes.
   4. thrombocytes.

2. A hormone produced by the adrenal cortex that is antiinflammatory is:
   1. epinephrine.
   2. cortisol.
   3. aldosterone.
   4. thyroxine.

3. Cells that are produced to clean up inflammatory debris are called:
   1. fibroblasts.
   2. platelets.
   3. neutrophils.
   4. macrophages.

4. Which is a sign of local infection?
   1. Fever
   2. Chills
   3. Warm skin
   4. Pale skin

5. Many childhood illnesses such as measles and chickenpox and some forms of hepatitis are caused by:
   1. viruses.
   2. bacteria.
   3. protozoa.
   4. fungi.

6. It is seldom possible to kill viruses because:
   1. replication of the virus occurs within the host cell.
   2. the cell wall can be destroyed with drugs.
   3. the cell wall requires oxygen for functions.
   4. the host cell is separate from the virus.

7. Ringworm (tinea corporis) and athlete's foot (tinea pedis) are examples of disease caused by:
   1. bacteria.
   2. viruses.
   3. fungi.
   4. protozoa.

8. Which types of patients are most susceptible to health care–associated infections? Select all that apply.
   1. Patients with pneumonia
   2. Patients requiring insulin
   3. Patients with myocardial infarction
   4. Patients with AIDS
   5. Cancer patients receiving chemotherapy
   6. Patients with emphysema

9. The overgrowth of a second microorganism that can cause illness following antibiotic therapy for one microorganism is called:
   1. thrombophlebitis.
   2. superinfection.
   3. sexually transmitted infection.
   4. septicemia.

10. The most basic and effective method of preventing cross-contamination is:
    1. hand hygiene.
    2. antibiotics.
    3. isolation.
    4. use of gown and gloves.

11. The primary cause of health care–associated infections is:
    1. soiled hands.
    2. faulty equipment.
    3. airborne droplets.
    4. open wounds.

12. The elimination of microorganisms from any object that comes in contact with the patient is called:
    1. medical asepsis.
    2. clean technique.
    3. isolation technique.
    4. surgical asepsis.

13. How much fluid is required by patients with infection?
    1. 1 L/day
    2. 2 L/day
    3. 5 L/day
    4. 10 L/day

14. Teaching for patients undergoing hyperbaric oxygen therapy includes:
    1. do not take aspirin 1 week before.
    2. do not wear a watch.
    3. swallow first to prevent pressure buildup.
    4. wear everyday clothes.

15. An advantage of home health care for infected patients is that the patient is:
    1. exposed to fewer health care–associated infections.
    2. not capable of spreading infections to others.
    3. not exposed to poorly prepared food.
    4. vulnerable to poor hygiene.

16. Which type of precaution is used to prevent the transmission of methicillin-resistant *Staphylococcus aureus* (MRSA) infections?
    1. Airborne
    2. Droplet
    3. Respiratory
    4. Contact

17. People with generalized infections become dehydrated because of:
    1. poor skin turgor and dry mouth.
    2. dry mucous membranes and decreased metabolism.
    3. inflammation and pain.
    4. fever and anorexia.

18. A diet recommended for patients with infection is:
    1. low sodium.
    2. high fiber.
    3. high protein.
    4. low potassium.

19. A common side effect of broad-spectrum antibiotics is:
    1. superinfection.
    2. hemorrhage.
    3. hypotension.
    4. hypokalemia.

20. Food-borne illness is a common community-acquired infectious disease often caused by:
    1. pseudomonas.
    2. diphtheria.
    3. streptococcus.
    4. salmonella.

21. What percentage of the U.S. population suffers from allergies of some sort?
    1. Under 5%
    2. 20%–25%
    3. 40%–45%
    4. 50%–75%

22. Antigens that cause hypersensitivity reactions are called:
    1. antibodies.
    2. complement.
    3. allergens.
    4. interferon.

23. Allergy testing is performed by injecting small amounts of allergen:
    1. intradermally.
    2. intramuscularly.
    3. intravenously.
    4. interstitially.

24. In anaphylaxis, what is an effect of histamine?
    1. Bronchospasm
    2. Vasoconstriction
    3. Phagocytosis
    4. Decreased vascular permeability

25. Which drugs are used to treat anaphylaxis? Select all that apply.
    1. Atropine
    2. Diphenhydramine
    3. Corticosteroids
    4. Propranolol
    5. Aminophylline
    6. Epinephrine

26. A 36-year-old female patient has multiple sclerosis. Which tissues and organs are affected?
    1. Heart and kidney tissue
    2. White matter of brain and spinal cord
    3. Lung tissue and liver cells
    4. Spleen tissue and thymus gland

27. What are common portals of entry for flu and cold viruses? Select all that apply.
    1. Mouth
    2. Skin
    3. Nose
    4. Conjunctiva
    5. Lungs
    6. Outer ear canal

28. It is now necessary to give two or more drugs to tuberculosis patients because:
    1. it prolongs the effects of each drug.
    2. it potentiates the effect of each drug.
    3. strains of bacteria resistant to drugs have developed.
    4. more people are susceptible to tuberculosis.

29. A common protozoal infection that occurs as an opportunistic infection in persons who are HIV positive is:
    1. pneumocystic pneumonia.
    2. Rocky Mountain spotted fever.
    3. thrush.
    4. conjunctivitis.

30. Any items that have been touched or cross-contaminated by the host, such as bed linens or side rails, are:
    1. vectors.
    2. common vehicles.
    3. pathogens.
    4. fomites.

31. Which are effects of histamine on the body when it is released during anaphylaxis? Select all that apply.
    1. Shock from hypervolemia
    2. Decreased vascular permeability
    3. Edema
    4. Bronchospasm
    5. Vasoconstriction

PART III: CHALLENGE YOURSELF!

M. Getting Ready for NCLEX
Choose the most appropriate answer or select all that apply.

1. The nurse is taking care of a patient with influenza who is on droplet precautions. Which are true statements about droplet precautions?
    1. Wear gloves when entering the patient's room.
    2. The patient must wear a surgical mask when leaving the room.
    3. The door to the room must be closed.
    4. Staff and visitors must wear a surgical mask if they are within 3 feet of the patient.

2. The nurse is reviewing common reportable diseases in a staff development program. Which are common reportable diseases? Select all that apply.
    1. Syphilis
    2. Crohn's disease
    3. Hypertension
    4. Gonorrhea
    5. Diabetes mellitus
    6. Hepatitis

3. The nurse is caring for patients with the following illnesses. Which illnesses require the use of airborne precautions? Select all that apply.
    1. Pneumonia
    2. Measles
    3. Tuberculosis
    4. Pertussis
    5. Meningitis
    6. Varicella

4. The nurse is caring for patients with the following conditions. Which of the following require contact precautions? Select all that apply.
    1. Tuberculosis
    2. Influenza
    3. Impetigo
    4. Wound infection
    5. Viral conjunctivitis

5. What general health practices can help slow the development of MDROs in patients? Select all that apply.
    1. Encourage vaccinations for communicable diseases.
    2. Reserve antibiotics for serious infections.
    3. Wear gown and gloves at all times when working with patients who have MDROs.
    4. Remove gown and gloves immediately after leaving the patient's room.
    5. Place the patient in a private room.

6. The nurse is taking care of a patient with fecal incontinence who is placed on contact precautions. Which of the following procedures should the nurse follow with this patient? Select all that apply.
    1. Wear a gown when taking care of the patient.
    2. Place the patient in a private room.
    3. Remove the gown after leaving the patient's room.
    4. Place surgical mask on the patient before the patient leaves the room.
    5. Put gloves on after entering the patient's room.

7. The priority nursing responsibility when taking care of a patient with immunodeficiency is to:
    1. avoid rectal thermometers.
    2. encourage adequate nutritional intake.
    3. prevent infection.
    4. encourage the patient to turn, cough, and breathe deeply.

8. The nurse is taking care of a patient who has a temperature of 98.8°F, pulse 70, and respirations 18. The WBC is 3000/mm^3. Which food will be eliminated from the patient's diet?
   1. Fresh produce
   2. Aged cheeses
   3. Whole milk
   4. Peanut butter

9. The infection control nurse is teaching a class on infection control precautions to prevent the transmission of MDROs in health care settings. Which statement should the nurse incorporate when caring for a patient with an MDRO infection?
   1. Implement contact precautions for all patients known to be infected with MDROs in acute care settings.
   2. Wear a mask routinely to prevent transmission of MDROs from the patient to the nurse.
   3. Keep the door to the patient's room closed.
   4. The patient should wear a mask when visitors are present.

N. Next-Generation NCLEX® Examination-Style Questions

Read the following situations and answer the questions below.

1. A 32-year-old female client was prescribed Clindamycin for bacterial infection by her primary care physician (PCP). The nurse reviews the health history and vital signs.

   Health History:
   32-year-old female client prescribed Clindamycin for bacterial infection by her primary care physician (PCP) presents to the emergency department with complaints of five episodes of watery diarrhea. In the last 12 hours, loss of appetite, nausea, and abdominal pain and tenderness rated 6/10 on a numeric pain scale. Client states she has been taking the antibiotic for 7 days.

   Vital Signs:

Temperature	102.5°F (39.2°C)
Pulse	90 beats per minute
Respirations	20 breaths per minute
Blood Pressure	108/60 mmHg

   Which physician orders would the nurse anticipate being prescribed? Select all that apply.
   1. Regular diet
   2. Complete bedrest
   3. Colace (Docusate sodium) BID PO
   4. IV infusion normal saline at 125 mL/hour
   5. Stool specimen
   6. Droplet precautions
   7. Vancomycin 125 mg PO Q6H
   8. Continue clindamycin as ordered by PCP
   9. Zofran (Ondansetron) Q4H IV PRN
   10. Tylenol (acetaminophen) 325 mg PO Q6H PRN

2. An 80-year-old male client is admitted to the medical unit. The nurse reviews the physician's progress notes.

   Physician's Progress Notes:
   4/2/21 0800: 80-year-old male client admitted to the medical unit with a large draining wound on his sacrum. Wound care has been consulted. Wound cultures suggest methicillin-resistant *Staphylococcus aureus* (MRSA). *Collin Jacobs*, MD

   Drag the personal protective equipment from the choices below to fill in each blank in the following sentence.

1. The personal protective equipment required to care for this patient includes _____ and _____ .

   Personal Protective Equipment:
   1. Gown
   2. Surgical mask
   3. Gloves
   4. N95 mask
   5. Surgical cap
   6. Disposable shoe covers

Fluid, Electrolyte, and Acid-Base Balance

chapter

6

Go to http://evolve.elsevier.com/Linton/medsurg/ for additional activities and exercises.

NCLEX CATEGORIES

Health Promotion and Maintenance

Physiological Integrity: Basic Care and Comfort, Pharmacological Therapies, Reduction of Risk Potential, Physiological Adaptation

PART I: MASTERING THE BASICS

A. Body Water
Select the correct word to complete each sentence.

1. With increasing age, body water (increases/ decreases).

2. Fat cells contain (more/less) water than other cells.

3. Females have (higher/lower) body water percentages than males.

4. An obese person has a (higher/lower) percentage of body water than a thin person.

5. What are locations where skin turgor is best measured? Select all that apply.
   1. Wrist
   2. Sternum
   3. Inner aspects of thighs
   4. Cheeks
   5. Forehead
   6. Fingertips

6. What are common parts of the body against which skin is pressed to test for edema? Select all that apply.
   1. Ankle
   2. Tibia
   3. Fibula
   4. Femur
   5. Sternum
   6. Sacrum

B. Electrolytes

1. Which are electrolytes? Select all that apply.
   1. Bilirubin
   2. Urea
   3. Magnesium
   4. Phosphate
   5. Creatinine
   6. Sodium
   7. Potassium
   8. Protein
   9. Chloride
   10. Calcium

C. Fluid Balance

1. Which conditions have great potential for altering fluid balance? Select all that apply.
   1. Burns
   2. Multiple sclerosis
   3. Ulcerative colitis
   4. Dyspnea
   5. Vomiting
   6. Kidney disease
   7. Tachycardia
   8. Hypothermia
   9. Diarrhea
   10. Congestive heart failure

2. Which are related to fluid volume excess? Select all that apply.
   1. Stimulates thirst
   2. Retention of fluid
   3. Activity intolerance
   4. Increased ADH production
   5. Inhibits antidiuretic hormone (ADH)

D. Regulation of Body Fluid Volume and Changes in Vital Signs

Match the condition in the numbered column with the most appropriate effect in the lettered column.

1. _____ Hypokalemia
2. _____ Increased plasma osmolality
3. _____ Hyponatremia

A. Orthostatic hypotension
B. Increased thirst
C. Decreased muscle tone

E. Fluid and Electrolyte Changes

Choose the most appropriate answer or select all that apply.

1. Which vital sign changes (focused assessment findings) are related to a patient with fluid volume deficit due to dehydration? Select all that apply.
   1. Bounding pulse
   2. Increased blood pressure
   3. Fall in systolic blood pressure > 20 mm Hg from lying to standing
   4. Fever
   5. Increased respiratory rate
   6. Subnormal body temperature

2. What respiratory changes occur with metabolic alkalosis? Select all that apply.
   1. Deep, rapid respirations
   2. Slow, shallow respirations
   3. Dyspnea
   4. Intermittent apnea
   5. Tachypnea

F. Blood Gas Values

Refer to Table 6.7. Add arrows (↑, ↓) or normal in the table below.

Arterial Blood Gas Values with Uncompensated Respiratory and Metabolic Acidosis and Alkalosis				
Condition	**Cause**	**pH**	**HCO₃**	**PaCO₂**
Respiratory acidosis	Hypoventilation			
Respiratory alkalosis	Hyperventilation			
Metabolic acidosis	Diabetic ketoacidosis Lactic acidosis Diarrhea Renal insufficiency			
Metabolic alkalosis	Vomiting HCO₃ retention Volume depletion K + depletion			

PART II: PUTTING IT ALL TOGETHER

G. Multiple Choice/Multiple Response

Choose the most appropriate answer or select all that apply.

1. The major electrolytes in extracellular fluid are:
   1. sodium and chloride.
   2. potassium and phosphate.
   3. calcium and bicarbonate.
   4. magnesium and phosphate.

2. Which are anions? Select all that apply.
   1. Sodium
   2. Potassium
   3. Chloride
   4. Bicarbonate
   5. Phosphate

3. The concentration of electrolytes in a solution or body fluid compartment is measured in:
   1. milligrams (mg).
   2. grams (g).
   3. milliliters (mL).
   4. milliequivalents (mEq).

4. In what type of environment does water loss via the skin and lungs increase?
    1. Hot, moist environment
    2. Hot, dry environment
    3. Cool, dry environment
    4. Cool, moist environment

5. Because the retention of sodium causes water retention, aldosterone acts as a regulator of:
    1. acid balance.
    2. base balance.
    3. blood pH.
    4. blood volume.

6. One way the body tries to compensate for fluid volume deficits is to:
    1. increase heart rate.
    2. increase urine output.
    3. increase blood pressure.
    4. decrease production of ADH.

7. ADH is decreased in response to:
    1. deficient fluid volume.
    2. excess fluid volume.
    3. decreased urination.
    4. concentrated urine.

8. The body tries to compensate for excess fluid volume by:
    1. increasing the filtration and excretion of sodium and water.
    2. stimulating the production of ADH.
    3. inhibiting the production of epinephrine.
    4. stimulating thirst.

9. Which electrolytes cause a majority of health problems when there is an electrolyte imbalance? Select all that apply.
    1. Potassium
    2. Chloride
    3. Magnesium
    4. Bicarbonate
    5. Sodium

10. When the body goes without fluid intake, which hormone increases water reabsorption?
    1. Thyroxine
    2. Epinephrine
    3. ADH
    4. Aldosterone

11. Which disturbances result from low levels of serum potassium? Select all that apply.
    1. Metabolic function
    2. Neuromuscular function
    3. Cardiac function
    4. Bone structure
    5. Acid-base balance

12. Which drugs cause hypokalemia? Select all that apply.
    1. Narcotics
    2. Anticholinergics
    3. Potassium-wasting diuretics
    4. Calcium channel blockers
    5. Corticosteroids

13. If more calcium is needed in the bones, it is taken from the blood, as well as being reabsorbed through the:
    1. lungs.
    2. kidneys.
    3. heart.
    4. liver.

14. One liter of fluid retention equals a weight gain of:
    1. 1 pound.
    2. 2.2 pounds.
    3. 5.4 pounds.
    4. 10 pounds.

15. Puffy eyelids and fuller cheeks suggest:
    1. excess fluid volume.
    2. deficient fluid volume.
    3. potassium excess.
    4. potassium deficit.

16. If a depression remains in the tissue after pressure is applied with a fingertip, the edema is described as:
    1. excessive.
    2. pitting.
    3. depressed.
    4. minimal.

17. A deep and persistent pit that is approximately 1 inch deep is described as:
    1. 1+.
    2. 2+.
    3. 3+.
    4. 4+.

18. If the veins take longer than 3–5 seconds to fill when placed in a dependent position, the patient may have:
    1. hypokalemia.
    2. hyperkalemia.
    3. hypovolemia.
    4. hypervolemia.

19. Weakness and muscle cramps are symptoms of:
    1. hyponatremia.
    2. hypokalemia.
    3. fluid volume deficit.
    4. respiratory acidosis.

20. The normal range for urine pH is:
    1. 2.0–7.0.
    2. 4.0–12.0.
    3. 4.6–6.8.
    4. 7.8–12.0.

21. A urine specimen that is not tested within 4 hours of collection may become:
    1. alkaline.
    2. acidic.
    3. more concentrated.
    4. less concentrated.

22. Which is the best measure of fluid balance?
    1. pH
    2. Urine potassium
    3. Creatinine clearance
    4. Specific gravity

23. In most instances, normal urine specific gravity is between:
    1. 1.016 and 1.022.
    2. 2.001 and 4.035.
    3. 4.001 and 6.035.
    4. 5.0 and 7.0.

24. A 24-hour urine specimen is required to determine:
    1. creatinine clearance.
    2. pH.
    3. specific gravity.
    4. osmolality.

25. Blood urea nitrogen (BUN) provides a measure of:
    1. blood volume.
    2. renal function.
    3. cardiac function.
    4. liver function.

26. Which is a symptom of hyponatremia?
    1. Palpitations
    2. Hypertension
    3. Confusion
    4. Insomnia

27. What amount of fluid per day is needed by the average person for adequate hydration?
    1. 3 liters for women and men daily
    2. 2 liters for women/2.2 liters for men daily
    3. 2.2 liters for women/3.0 liters for men daily
    4. 64 fluid ounces daily

28. To prevent hyponatremia in patients with feeding tubes, what should be used for irrigation?
    1. Sterile water
    2. Normal glucose
    3. Normal saline
    4. Sterile dextrose

29. The heart rate of patients on digitalis should be closely watched because hypokalemia can contribute to:
    1. congestive heart failure.
    2. pericarditis.
    3. digitalis toxicity.
    4. diuresis.

30. To prevent gastrointestinal irritation, oral potassium supplements should be given with:
    1. meals.
    2. a full glass of water or fruit juice.
    3. a full glass of milk.
    4. a teaspoon of applesauce.

31. When the respiratory system fails to eliminate the appropriate amount of carbon dioxide to maintain the normal acid-base balance, what occurs?
    1. Respiratory alkalosis
    2. Respiratory acidosis
    3. Metabolic acidosis
    4. Metabolic alkalosis

32. The most common cause of respiratory alkalosis is:
    1. hypoventilation.
    2. hyperventilation.
    3. drowning.
    4. obesity.

33. Patients may develop high levels of magnesium in their blood for which reason?
    1. Decreased gastrointestinal absorption
    2. Increased urinary loss
    3. Excessive use of magnesium-containing medications
    4. Excessive use of alcohol

34. Which patient should be encouraged to breathe slowly into a paper bag?
    1. Patient who is hyperventilating
    2. Patient with emphysema
    3. Patient with respiratory acidosis
    4. Patient with hypokalemia

35. When the body retains too many hydrogen ions or loses too many bicarbonate ions, what occurs?
    1. Respiratory acidosis
    2. Respiratory alkalosis
    3. Metabolic acidosis
    4. Metabolic alkalosis

36. Potassium is a critical factor for the transmission of nerve impulses because it is necessary for:
    1. muscular activity.
    2. acid-base balance.
    3. fluid balance.
    4. membrane excitability.

37. In addition to its role in regulating fluid balance, sodium is also necessary for:
    1. nerve impulse conduction.
    2. bone structure.
    3. protein structure.
    4. breakdown of glycogen.

38. The most common cause of hypocalcemia is related to problems with which hormone?
    1. ADH
    2. Aldosterone
    3. Thyroxine
    4. Parathyroid hormone (PTH)

39. What is the normal total daily intake of fluids?
    1. 1000 mL
    2. 1200 mL
    3. 1500 mL
    4. 2500 mL

40. What is the best position for the patient who is experiencing dyspnea?
    1. Keep the bed flat.
    2. Elevate the head of the bed 30 degrees.
    3. Elevate the head of the bed 60 degrees.
    4. Elevate the head of the bed 90 degrees.

41. A bounding pulse occurs in patients with:
    1. dehydration.
    2. hypovolemia.
    3. circulatory overload.
    4. hyperthermia.

42. What is the patient at risk for when the total intake is substantially less than the total output?
    1. Excess fluid volume
    2. Deficient fluid volume
    3. Hypoventilation
    4. Hyperventilation

43. What is the normal hourly adult urine output?
    1. 30–40 mL/hour
    2. 40–80 mL/hour
    3. 50–60 mL/hour
    4. 100 mL/hour

44. A rapid weight gain of 8% is considered to be:
    1. minimal.
    2. mild.
    3. moderate.
    4. severe.

45. If the patient has a rapid weight loss of 2 Kilograms, what is the equivalent loss of fluid?
    1. 1 liter
    2. 2 liters
    3. 4 liters
    4. 6 liters

PART III: CHALLENGE YOURSELF!

H. Getting Ready for NCLEX
Choose the most appropriate answer or select all that apply.

1. The nurse is taking care of a patient with a fluid and electrolyte imbalance. The nurse notices a fall in systolic pressure of more than 20 mm Hg when the patient changes from the lying to standing position. Which does this indicate in the patient?
    1. Excess fluid volume
    2. Deficient fluid volume
    3. Sodium deficit
    4. Sodium excess

2. The nurse has attended an in-service program on fluid imbalances and learned about conditions associated with hypovolemia. Which factors are related to causes of hypovolemia? Select all that apply.
    1. Decreased oral fluid intake
    2. Vomiting
    3. Decreased ADH production
    4. High fever
    5. Diarrhea
    6. Excessive sweating

3. An older patient in an assisted-living facility is showing signs of dehydration. Which are indicators of dehydration? Select all that apply.
    1. Hypotension
    2. Decreased pulse
    3. Decreased respirations
    4. Increased temperature
    5. Weight loss
    6. Decreased hematocrit (Hct) and hemoglobin (Hgb)

4. An older patient is being treated for dehydration and has received excessive fluid replacement. The nurse should observe the patient for which sign of excess fluid volume?
    1. Decreased pulse
    2. Decreased blood pressure
    3. Dyspnea
    4. Decreased respirations

5. A patient with cardiac failure is retaining fluid. Which indicators of excess fluid volume are likely to be present in this patient? Select all that apply.
    1. Increased blood pressure
    2. Bounding pulse
    3. Decreased respirations
    4. Weight loss
    5. Irritability

6. What is the treatment for a patient with excess fluid volume?
    1. Increase sodium intake
    2. Increase water intake
    3. Give diuretics
    4. Give antiemetics

7. Which are nursing interventions for the patient with excess fluid volume? Select all that app.
    1. Offer ice chips.
    2. Offer clear liquids.
    3. Use small fluid containers.
    4. Turn every 2 hours.
    5. Inspect skin for breakdown.
    6. Check temperature.

8. Which aspects of the health and physical exam are important in determining the fluid and electrolyte status of a patient? Select all that apply.
    1. History of Gout
    2. _____Vomiting
    3. Use of diuretics
    4. Use of salicylates
    5. Dyspnea
    6. Skin turgor

9. A patient with heart failure has just been placed on a low-sodium diet. Which foods should the patient avoid? Select all that apply.
    1. Natural cheese
    2. Sausage
    3. Cooked oatmeal
    4. Fresh chicken
    5. Pizza
    6. Frozen peas

10. A patient who has been taking a diuretic for 1 week has hypokalemia. Which foods should be on a recommended diet for this patient? Select all that apply.
    1. Lima beans
    2. Mangoes
    3. Artichokes
    4. Bananas
    5. Ginger ale
    6. Fresh apples

11. A patient with a chronic lung disease is showing signs of an acid-base imbalance. Which are manifestations of acid-base imbalance? Select all that apply.
    1. Dyspnea
    2. Confusion
    3. Vomiting
    4. Muscle weakness
    5. Numbness
    6. Decreased skin turgor

12. Which factor places an older person at high risk for fluid and electrolyte imbalance?
    1. Decreased renal response
    2. Decreased lean muscle mass
    3. Increased sense of thirst
    4. Increased total body water

13. The nurse is observing a patient in a long-term care facility. Which focused assessment finding is the *least* reliable indicator of fluid status in an 80-year-old patient?
    1. Pitting peripheral edema
    2. Poor tissue turgor
    3. Intake and output
    4. Mucous membrane moisture

14. When the blood is more concentrated in a patient with deficient fluid volume, which blood study result is expected?
    1. Decreased BUN
    2. Increased creatinine
    3. Increased hematocrit
    4. Decreased hemoglobin

15. When breathing problems occur in a patient with excess fluid volume, the nurse instructs the patient to:
    1. lie flat in bed.
    2. have head of bed elevated 30 degrees.
    3. ambulate frequently.
    4. be in the side-lying position.

16. The patient with heart failure has excess fluid volume with pitting edema. What is the priority nursing intervention for this patient?
    1. Turn the patient every 2 hours.
    2. Have the patient cough and deep-breathe every 2 hours.
    3. Ambulate the patient every 2 hours.
    4. Check the blood pressure every 2 hours.

17. The nurse is taking care of a patient with hypokalemia. Which are nursing interventions for this patient? Select all that apply.
    1. Monitor serum potassium levels.
    2. Monitor arterial blood gas results.
    3. Record intake and output.
    4. Monitor heart rate and rhythms.
    5. Encourage green, leafy vegetables in the diet.
    6. Encourage oranges and bananas in the diet.

18. The nurse plans to prevent a serious fluid and electrolyte imbalance in the patient with renal failure. What is the best way to decrease the incidence of serious fluid and electrolyte imbalances?
    1. Monitor blood pressure carefully.
    2. Monitor temperature carefully.
    3. Monitor rate and rhythm of the pulse carefully.
    4. Monitor records of fluid intake and output carefully.

The Patient With Cancer

chapter

7

Go to http://evolve.elsevier.com/Linton/medsurg/ for additional activities and exercises.

NCLEX CATEGORIES

Safe and Effective Care Environment:
Coordinated Care, Safety and Infection Control

Health Maintenance

Psychosocial Integrity

Physiological Integrity: Basic Care and Comfort, Pharmacological Therapies, Reduction of Risk Potential, Physiological Adaptation

PART I: MASTERING THE BASICS

A. Key Terms
Match the definition in the numbered column with the most appropriate term in the lettered column.

1. _____   Tending to progress in virulence; has the characteristics of becoming increasingly undifferentiated, invading surrounding tissues, and colonizing distant sites

2. _____   Cancer-causing agent

3. _____   The use of radiation in the treatment of cancer and other diseases

4. _____   Process by which cancer spreads to distant sites

5. _____   Agents that work by affecting biologic processes

6. _____   Chemical agents specifically used to treat cancer

7. _____   Tumor; cells that reproduce abnormally and in an uncontrolled manner

8. _____   Use of chemicals to treat illness

9. _____   Relatively harmless, nonmalignant tumors that do not spread

A. Radiotherapy
B. Benign
C. Chemotherapy
D. Metastasis
E. Neoplasm
F. Malignant
G. Antineoplastic
H. Carcinogen
I. Biotherapy

B. Radiation Therapy
Choose the most appropriate answer or select all that apply.

1. Which normal cells are most sensitive to radiation? Select all that apply.
   1. Nail beds
   2. Digestive and urinary tract linings
   3. Respiratory tract lining
   4. Skin
   5. Lymph tissue
   6. Ovaries
   7. Kidneys
   8. Lungs
   9. Testes
   10. Hair follicle
   11. Bone marrow

2. Due to damage to the most sensitive cells during radiation therapy, which are the related side effects of therapy? Select all that apply.
   1. Bone marrow suppression
   2. Alopecia
   3. Anorexia
   4. Heart failure
   5. Liver failure
   6. Nausea and vomiting

3. Regardless of the site treated with radiation therapy, which two common side effects occur? Select all that apply.
   1. Dry mouth
   2. Skin changes
   3. Diarrhea
   4. Fatigue
   5. Esophagitis

C. Warning Signs of Cancer

1. Which are warning signs of cancer? Select all that apply.
   1. Nausea and vomiting
   2. Nagging cough and hoarseness
   3. Change in bowel or bladder habits
   4. Heart palpitations and tachycardia
   5. Sores that do not heal
   6. Dyspnea and trouble breathing
   7. Change in warts or moles

D. Stages of Tumors

Match the definition in the numbered column with the most appropriate stage in the lettered column.

1. _____ There is limited spread of the cancer in the local area, usually to nearby lymph nodes.

2. _____ The malignant cells are confined to the tissue of origin; there is no invasion of other tissues.

3. _____ The cancer has metastasized to distant parts of the body.

4. _____ The tumor is larger or has spread from the site of origin into nearby tissues, or both; regional lymph nodes are likely to be involved.

A. Stage I
B. Stage II
C. Stage III
D. Stage IV

E. Health Maintenance: Nutrition Considerations

Match the nutrition conditions in the numbered column with the associated types of cancer caused in the lettered column.

1. _____ High-fat diets
2. _____ Obesity

3. _____ High alcohol intake
4. _____ Diets high in salt-cured, smoked, and nitrate-cured foods

A. Esophageal and stomach cancers
B. Cancers of the colon, breast, prostate, gallbladder, ovary, and uterus
C. Cancers of the breast, colon, and prostate
D. Cancers of the oral cavity, larynx, pharynx, esophagus, liver, colon, rectum, and breast

5. Which are included in the recommended diet for health maintenance and prevention of cancer? Select all that apply.
   1. Low fat
   2. Decreased fiber
   3. Limited smoked and nitrate-preserved foods
   4. Two servings of fruits and vegetables daily
   5. Decreased calories

PART II: PUTTING IT ALL TOGETHER

F. Multiple Choice/Multiple Response

Choose the most appropriate answer or select all that apply.

1. What is the second most common cause of death in the United States?
   1. Heart disease
   2. Cancer
   3. Accident
   4. Stroke

2. What is the effect on cells and tissue when DNA of a normal cell is exposed to a carcinogen and irreversible changes occur in the DNA?
   1. The cell appears abnormal but continues to function normally.
   2. The cell is in a latent period before increased growth forms tumors.
   3. A tumor develops.
   4. Transformed cells relocate to remote sites.

3. A patient whose primary tumor has grown and spread to regional lymph nodes but not to distant sites is staged:
   1. $T_1N_2M_1$.
   2. $T_2N_1M_0$.
   3. $T_0N_3M_1$.
   4. $T_4N_0M_0$.

4. A patient has cancer that has been staged $T_1N_0M_0$. The nurse would interpret this information as:
   1. minimal size and extension of tumor.
   2. no sign of tumor.
   3. malignancy in epithelial tissue but not in basement membrane.
   4. progressively increasing size and extension.

5. A treatment likely to be curative when tumors are confined in one area is:
   1. radiotherapy.
   2. chemotherapy.
   3. immunotherapy.
   4. surgery.

6. Radiation has immediate and delayed effects on cells; the immediate effect is:
   1. cell death.
   2. alteration of DNA, which impairs cell's ability to reproduce.
   3. interruption of the clotting cascade.
   4. cell starvation.

7. Which side effect occurs in patients undergoing radiotherapy and also in patients taking antineoplastic drugs?
   1. Phlebitis at infusion site
   2. Erythema and peeling of skin
   3. Alopecia
   4. Cardiomyopathy

8. The highest rate of death from all cancers occur among:
   1. Caucasians.
   2. Latinos.
   3. Native Americans.
   4. African Americans.

9. What is the most dangerous side effect of antineoplastic drugs?
   1. Alopecia
   2. Nausea and vomiting
   3. Electrolyte imbalance
   4. Bone marrow suppression

10. A drug that boosts the body's natural defenses to combat malignant cells is:
    1. vincristine.
    2. interferon.
    3. doxorubicin (Adriamycin).
    4. paclitaxel (Taxol).

11. Invasive procedures are minimized in patients with:
    1. leukopenia.
    2. thrombocytopenia.
    3. anemia.
    4. agranulocytosis.

12. Compromised host precautions may be needed for patients with:
    1. leukopenia.
    2. thrombocytopenia.
    3. anemia.
    4. weight loss.

13. Which tumor is malignant?
    1. Fibroma
    2. Lipoma
    3. Melanoma
    4. Myoma

14. Which diagnostic procedure is used to detect cancers of the central nervous system, spinal column, neck bones, and joints?
    1. Magnetic resonance imaging (MRI)
    2. Computed tomography (CT)
    3. Positron emission tomography (PET)
    4. Contrast radiographs

15. Which are major systemic side effects of antineoplastic drugs? Select all that apply.
    1. Dry mouth
    2. Bone marrow suppression
    3. Urinary retention
    4. Sedation
    5. Nausea and vomiting
    6. Constipation
    7. Dizziness
    8. Alopecia
    9. Electrolyte imbalance

16. Match the side effect in the numbered column with the most appropriate drug in the lettered column.
    1. _____ May cause hypertension if eating foods rich in tyramine
    2. _____ Neurotoxicity resulting in numbness and tingling of extremities
    3. _____ Toxic effects on the heart that may lead to heart failure
    4. _____ Fluid retention

    A. Vincristine (Oncovin)
    B. Doxorubicin (Adriamycin)
    C. Procarbazine (Matulane)
    D. Dexamethasone (Decadron)

17. The nurse observes that a female patient with breast cancer is experiencing alopecia as a side effect of her chemotherapy. Which is a correct response of the nurse to the patient?
    1. "Increase protein in your diet to encourage new hair growth."
    2. "Increase fluid intake so new hair growth will not be dry."
    3. "Examine your scalp for bleeding, which may be a temporary response to chemotherapy."
    4. "Your new hair may be a different color and texture."

18. A patient with cancer is complaining of nausea and vomiting associated with chemotherapy. Which food and beverages should the nurse recommend for this patient? Select all that apply.
    1. Clear broth
    2. Coffee
    3. White rice
    4. Crackers or pretzels
    5. Yogurt
    6. Cooked broccoli

19. A patient is receiving radiation treatment to her head and neck. Which is a special problem for this patient, putting her at risk for infections of the gums and teeth?
    1. Dry mouth (xerostomia)
    2. Nausea and vomiting
    3. Bone marrow suppression
    4. Anorexia

20. A patient receiving Adriamycin for treatment of cancer is experiencing signs of cardiomyopathy. Which finding should the nurse report to the health care provider?
    1. Dehydration
    2. Dyspnea
    3. Alopecia
    4. Urinary retention

21. A cancer patient has had the lower abdomen irradiated. Which is a priority nursing activity for this patient?
    1. Monitor the patient for edema.
    2. Increase fluid intake and have patient empty bladder often.
    3. Encourage patient to eat foods high in iron.
    4. Observe patient for palpitations, pallor, and excessive fatigue.

22. Which patient should be placed in a private room?
    1. Patient with internal radiation
    2. Patient with external radiation
    3. Patient with chemotherapy
    4. Patient requiring standard precautions

PART III: CHALLENGE YOURSELF!

G. Getting Ready for NCLEX
Choose the most appropriate answer or select all that apply.

1. A patient experiences erythema and peeling of skin while receiving radiation therapy. Which are appropriate nursing interventions for this patient? Select all that apply.
    1. Increase fluid intake.
    2. Use lotions.
    3. Watch for excessive bruising and bleeding.
    4. Report fever.
    5. Keep skin moist.
    6. Wear cotton clothing.

2. The outcome criterion of a patient's completing essential activities without exhaustion is related to patients with:
    1. alopecia.
    2. loss of a body part.
    3. anemia.
    4. denial.

3. The priority care for patients experiencing neurotoxicity from antineoplastic drugs is to:
   1. monitor for edema.
   2. protect the patient from infection.
   3. protect extremities from injury.
   4. assess skin turgor.

4. What is appropriate teaching for the patient who is having external radiation therapy?
   1. "The treatment may be painful for the first 5 minutes, but the pain will subside."
   2. "You will be radioactive as long as the machine is turned on."
   3. "Skin markings made by the radiologist are used to mark areas that will not be irradiated."
   4. "Skin over the area being treated may become inflamed."

5. Which are characteristics of malignant tumors? Select all that apply.
   1. Usually slow growth rate
   2. Invade surrounding tissue
   3. Cells closely resemble those of tissue of origin
   4. Recurrence common after removal
   5. Frequent metastasis
   6. Little tissue destruction

6. The nurse is assisting with a staff education program on common oncologic emergencies. Which are common oncologic emergencies? Select all that apply.
   1. Superior vena cava syndrome
   2. Pulmonary edema
   3. Hypertension
   4. Hypercalcemia
   5. Syndrome of inappropriate antidiuretic hormone (SIADH)
   6. Spinal cord compression
   7. Disseminated intravascular coagulation

7. A patient receiving chemotherapy has a white blood cell count of 2000/mm^3. The nurse anticipates that the patient will be placed on:
   1. airborne precautions.
   2. contact precautions.
   3. neutropenic precautions.
   4. droplet precautions.

8. A patient has received a radiation implant. Which teaching points should the nurse emphasize with this patient? Select all that apply.
   1. "You will be placed in a private room."
   2. "Do not wash off the skin markings made by the radiation therapist."
   3. "Visitors and staff are restricted in the amount of time they can spend in your room."
   4. "Your skin over the irradiated area may become irritated."
   5. "Staff and visitors will maintain some distance from you while they are in your room."

H. Next-Generation NCLEX® Examination-Style Questions

Read the following situations and answer the questions below. For more information, refer to Nursing Care Plan, The Patient with Cancer, in your textbook.

A 63-year-old man recently diagnosed with lung cancer is being treated with radiotherapy and chemotherapy. The nurse reviews the health history, previous shift's nurse's notes, and vital signs.

> **Health History:**
> 63-year-old man recently diagnosed with lung cancer being treated with radiotherapy and chemotherapy. Client is married, the father of three grown children, and is an insurance salesman. He smoked one pack of cigarettes a day for 30 years, having quit smoking 10 years ago. He continues to work part time.
>
> **Nurse's Notes:**
> 6/2/21 0730: Client states he is fatigued and weak since starting his therapy. Client has severe nausea and has vomited 200 cc of green emesis in the last 2 hours. He complains of a dry mouth and is having some dysphagia. Client reports that the skin over the area being irradiated is tender. The client states that his pain is a 8/10 on a 0 to 10 pain intensity scale. *K. Harris, RN*
>
> **Vital Signs:**
>
> | Temperature | 98.8 degrees F (37.1 C) |
> |---|---|
> | Pulse | 88 beats per minute |
> | Respirations | 20 breaths per minute |
> | Blood pressure | 180/88 mmHg |

1. Highlight the assessment findings that require immediate follow-up by the nurse.

A 25-year-old client diagnosed with lung cancer has been admitted to the oncology unit. The nurse reviews the health history and vital signs.

> **Health History:**
> 25-year-old client diagnosed with lung cancer has been admitted to the oncology unit. Client has been undergoing radiation therapy for 3 months. He complains of fatigue, weakness, and occasional shortness of breath. He states that he has been having bleeding from his gums when he brushes his teeth and notes a large bruise to his right leg from bumping into his nightstand. He denies pain at this time.
>
> **Vital Signs:**
>
> | Temperature | 99 degrees F (37.2 C) |
> |---|---|
> | Pulse | 76 beats per minute |
> | Respirations | 16 breaths per minute |
> | Blood Pressure | 92/68 mmHg |

2. Based on the client's assessment findings, which of the following potential nursing interventions would be appropriate for the care of the client at this time? Select all that apply.
   1. Initiate contact precautions
   2. Use a soft toothbrush.
   3. Schedule activities to prevent overtiring.
   4. Protect from injury
   5. Encourage the patient to report increase in fever
   6. Administer antihypertensives
   7. Apply ice to the right leg
   8. Advise the patient to eat small, frequent feedings

Pain

chapter 8

Go to http://evolve.elsevier.com/Linton/medsurg/ for additional activities and exercises.

NCLEX CATEGORIES

Safe and Effective Care Environment:
Coordinated Care, Safety and Infection Control

Psychosocial Integrity

Physiological Integrity: Pharmacological Therapies, Reduction of Risk Potential, Physiological Adaptation

PART I: MASTERING THE BASICS

A. Key Terms

Match the definition in the numbered column with the most appropriate term in the lettered column.

1. _____ Pain receptor

2. _____ Unpleasant sensory and emotional experience associated with actual or potential tissue damage, existing whenever the person says it does

3. _____ Drug that acts on the nervous system to relieve or reduce the suffering or intensity of pain

4. _____ A physiologic result of repeated doses of an opioid where the same dose is no longer effective in achieving the same analgesic effect; higher doses needed to achieve pain relief

5. _____ Behavioral pattern of compulsive drug use characterized by craving for an opioid and obtaining and using the drug for effects other than pain relief

6. _____ Physiologic adaptation of the body to an opioid so that a person exhibits withdrawal symptoms when the opioid is stopped abruptly after repeated administration

7. _____ Amount of pain a person is willing to endure before taking action to relieve pain

8. _____ Pain that persists or recurs for more than 3–6 months

9. _____ Point at which a stimulus causes the sensation of pain

10. _____ Pain that is temporary, and its cause is known and treatable; it also serves as a warning of tissue damage and subsides when healing takes place

A. Pain
B. Addiction
C. Acute pain
D. Pain tolerance
E. Nociceptor
F. Physical dependence
G. Tolerance
H. Chronic pain
I. Pain threshold
J. Analgesic

B. Gate Control Theory

1. Which are factors that close the gate, according to the gate control theory? Select all that apply.
   1. Distraction
   2. Massage
   3. Position change
   4. Fear of pain
   5. Guided imagery
   6. Heat application

C. Addiction

1. Which of the following describe addiction? Select all that apply.
    1. Physiologic changes that occur from repeated doses of opioids
    2. Compulsive obtaining and use of drug for psychic effects
    3. Withdrawal symptoms may occur if the opioid is stopped abruptly (e.g., irritability, chills, sweating, nausea)
    4. Psychological dependence characterized by continued craving for opioid for other than pain relief
    5. The need for higher doses to achieve pain relief

PART II: PUTTING IT ALL TOGETHER

D. Multiple Choice/Multiple Response

Choose the most appropriate answer or select all that apply.

1. One difference between acute and chronic pain is that a patient with acute pain:
    1. often becomes depressed.
    2. shows little facial expression.
    3. feels isolated.
    4. has a fast heart rate.

2. Which are physical factors that influence the response to pain? Select all that apply.
    1. Age
    2. Type of surgery
    3. Culture
    4. Pain tolerance
    5. Pain threshold
    6. Anxiety

3. When the pain threshold is lowered, the person experiences pain:
    1. less easily.
    2. more easily.
    3. as excruciating.
    4. as mild.

4. Which age group tends to report their pain as much less severe than it really is?
    1. Older adults
    2. Middle adults
    3. Young adults
    4. Adolescents

5. Surgery in which area is reported to be the most painful for patients?
    1. Skull region
    2. Thoracic region
    3. Upper abdominal region
    4. Lower abdominal region

6. An autonomic nervous system response to pain includes:
    1. urinary frequency.
    2. constricted pupils.
    3. increased heart rate.
    4. diarrhea.

7. Postoperative pain and pain in childbirth are examples of:
    1. chronic pain.
    2. permanent pain.
    3. acute pain.
    4. nonmalignant pain.

8. An example of acute pain with recurrent episodes is associated with:
    1. low back pain.
    2. migraine headaches.
    3. rheumatoid arthritis.
    4. cancer pain.

9. What is chronic non-cancer pain that interferes with sleep and function?
    1. Acute persistent pain
    2. Acute metastatic pain
    3. Persistent pain
    4. Metastatic pain

10. When possible, the information about pain should obtained from the:
    1. nurse.
    2. patient.
    3. doctor.
    4. patient's family.

11. Which are examples of cutaneous stimulation methods for pain control? Select all that apply.
    1. Guided imagery
    2. Application of heat
    3. Application of cold
    4. Listening to music
    5. Transcutaneous electrical nerve stimulation (TENS)
    6. Massage

12. The longest time a cold application can be used without tissue injury would be:
    1. 3 minutes.
    2. 15 minutes.
    3. 30 minutes.
    4. 60 minutes.

13. Fentanyl (Duragesic) transdermal patches are used to treat chronic pain by delivering:
    1. NSAIDs.
    2. salicylates.
    3. opioids.
    4. steroids.

14. Relaxation is most effective for:
    1. delusional pain.
    2. mild to moderate pain.
    3. moderate to severe pain.
    4. severe pain.

15. When pain is unpredictable, analgesics are more effective when given:
    1. once a day.
    2. twice a day.
    3. around the clock.
    4. PRN.

16. The initial treatment choice for mild pain is:
    1. opioid analgesics.
    2. nonopioid analgesics.
    3. narcotics.
    4. anesthetics.

17. Aspirin, acetaminophen, and NSAIDs are examples of:
    1. opioid analgesics.
    2. nonopioid analgesics.
    3. narcotics.
    4. anesthetics.

18. Ketorolac tromethamine (Toradol) is generally used for the short-term management of:
    1. cancer pain.
    2. heart failure.
    3. urinary tract infection.
    4. postoperative pain.

19. Drugs such as nonopioids that do not improve analgesia beyond a certain dosage are said to have a(n):
    1. peak effect.
    2. duration effect.
    3. ceiling effect.
    4. onset effect.

20. Nonopioids tend to block pain transmission:
    1. at the central nervous system.
    2. during cell wall synthesis.
    3. at the myocardium.
    4. at the peripheral nervous system.

21. Nalbuphine, butorphanol, and pentazocine (Talwin) are examples of:
    1. nonopioid analgesics.
    2. anticholinergics.
    3. opioid agonist-antagonists.
    4. opioid agonists.

22. What must happen **first** when a patient receiving morphine IM for pain will now be given equianalgesic dose PO?
    1. Reduce level of analgesia as much as patient can tolerate.
    2. Evaluate pain intensity to determine if patient is able to switch.
    3. Ensure dose is calculated to ensure approximately same level of analgesia.
    4. Ensure patient's family is capable of administering correctly.

23. If the patient is nauseated or has difficulty swallowing, which route is useful for administering opioids?
    1. Oral
    2. Rectal
    3. Topical
    4. Intradermal

24. To evaluate the patient for constipation, the nurse monitors for:
    1. black, tarry stools and anorexia.
    2. decreased blood pressure, itching, and respiratory distress.
    3. abdominal distention, cramping, and abdominal pain.
    4. intake and output, nausea, and vomiting.

25. Which nonpharmacologic pain intervention increases the pain threshold and reduces muscle spasm?
    1. Jaw relaxation
    2. Simple imagery
    3. Music
    4. TENS

26. When a prescription for pain medication states 10–20 mg IM q 4–6 hours PRN for pain, what will the nurse do when a 10-mg dose has been given and it is not effective?
    1. Adjust the next dose up as prescribed until pain is relieved with minimal or no side effects.
    2. Give an additional 10 mg as soon as possible.
    3. Wait 6 hours and give 20 mg the next time.
    4. Determine if the patient has developed pain tolerance.

PART III: CHALLENGE YOURSELF!

E. Getting Ready for NCLEX
Choose the most appropriate answer or select all that apply.

1. A patient asks the nurse about his pain that is "lasting for such a long time." Which are characteristics of chronic pain? Select all that apply.
   1. Lasts 3–6 months
   2. Responds to analgesics
   3. Pain is a sign of tissue injury
   4. Normal heart rate and blood pressure
   5. Oral route is preferred route for pain medication
   6. Minimal facial expression

2. A patient is experiencing acute pain. Which are examples of conditions that cause acute pain? Select all that apply.
   1. Low back pain
   2. Rheumatoid arthritis
   3. Neuralgia (herpes zoster)
   4. Sickle cell crisis
   5. Phantom limb pain
   6. Migraine headaches

3. The nurse has attended an in-service education program at the hospital on adjuvant analgesics and medications for the treatment of pain. She plans to share this information with her coworkers. Which are examples of pain medications? Select all that apply.
   1. Antidepressants
   2. Muscle relaxants
   3. Anticonvulsants
   4. Antipsychotics
   5. Diuretics

4. The nurse is monitoring a patient for parasympathetic responses to pain. Which are parasympathetic responses to pain? Select all that apply.
   1. Constipation
   2. Increased blood pressure
   3. Dilated pupils
   4. Urinary retention
   5. Perspiration

5. The nurse is caring for an older adult with cognitive impairment. What are common pain behaviors in cognitively impaired older adults that should be documented? Select all that apply.
   1. Grimacing
   2. Crying
   3. Increased wandering
   4. Increased appetite
   5. Noisy breathing

6. A 46-year-old patient has received nitrous oxide during surgery and says he does not have pain postoperatively. Which factor best explains his response to pain?
   1. Pain threshold
   2. Religious beliefs
   3. Age
   4. Anesthetic

7. A stoic 75-year-old Asian woman who has been experiencing back pain states that she does not want to bother the nurse. Which factors best explain her response to pain? Select all that apply.
   1. Age
   2. Fear
   3. Anxiety
   4. Culture
   5. Pain tolerance

8. Following assessment of a patient's pain, list in the proper sequence the steps in pain management. Use 1 as the first step and 6 as the last step.
   A. _____   Determine the status of the pain.
   B. _____   Describe the pain (location, quality, intensity, aggravating factors).
   C. _____   Identify coping methods.
   D. _____   Accept the patient's report of pain.
   E. _____   Examine the site.
   F. _____   Record assessment, interventions, and evaluation.

9. The application of cold is contraindicated in patients with:
   1. hip fracture.
   2. muscle sprain.
   3. allergic reaction.
   4. peripheral vascular disease.

10. The nurse is giving preoperative medication, Phenergan and Demerol, to a surgical patient. Which effect of opioids is not potentiated by the use of promethazine (Phenergan)?
    1. Sedation
    2. Respiratory depression
    3. Hypotension
    4. Analgesia

11. A patient is complaining of neuropathic pain. A drug classification that is effective in treating neuropathic pain is:
    1. muscle relaxants.
    2. benzodiazepines.
    3. antidepressants.
    4. corticosteroids.

12. A patient who has had back surgery complains of muscle spasms. Which drug may be most effective in relieving his pain?
    1. Muscle relaxant
    2. Opioid
    3. NSAID
    4. Aspirin

13. When observing sedation in a patient, which stage would the nurse consider to be an emergency?
    1. Sleeping, but arouses when called
    2. Drowsy, but easily aroused
    3. Frequently drowsy to drifting off to sleep during conversations
    4. Minimal response to physical stimulation

14. The nurse is taking care of one patient with acute pain and one patient with chronic pain. The nurse knows that a behavioral sign of acute pain is:
    1. tired-looking.
    2. minimal facial expression.
    3. attention on things other than pain.
    4. restless.

F. Next-Generation NCLEX® Examination-Style Questions

Read the following situations and answer the questions below.

1. The nurse is caring for a 42-year-old male client admitted to the medical-surgical unit from the emergency department with multiple fractures in the right arm. The nurse reviews the nurse's notes.

   > Nurse's Notes:
   > 2000: Client reports pain to right arm 7/10 on numeric pain scale. Client states, "It hurts the most when I move." Capillary refill less than 3 seconds, denies numbness or tingling to right arm. *Sally Peterson, RN*
   > 2015: Applied cold compress to right arm and administered 10 mg of morphine IM as ordered. *Sally Peterson, RN*
   > 2100: Client rates pain to right arm 2/10 on numeric pain scale. Client states, "It feels like the pain is slowly going away." *Sally Peterson, RN*

   Which evidence indicates that the pain was relieved? Select all that apply.
   1. Morphine 10 mg IM was given.
   2. Client stated that the pain was slowly going away.
   3. Pain intensity rated by the client decreased from 7 to 2.
   4. A cold compress was applied to the right arm.
   5. Client stated that it hurt the most with movement.
   6. Capillary refill is less than 3 seconds.

2. A 30-year-old client was admitted to the Emergency Department following a motor vehicle accident. The client had a crush injury to his left leg and contusions to the bilateral upper extremities. The nurse reviews the flow sheet data nurse's notes.

> Nurse's Notes:
> 0800: Client alert and oriented × 3, and able to move both arms and his right leg. He is unable to move his left leg and has diminished pulses to the left lower extremity. Client rates pain 10/10 on a 0–10 pain intensity scale.
>
> | Vital signs Flowsheet: | 0800 |
> | --- | --- |
> | Temperature | 98.6°F (37°C) |
> | Pulse | 102 beats/minute |
> | Respirations | 24 breaths/minute |
> | Blood Pressure | 140/78 mmHg |

Complete the following sentence by choosing from the lists of options.

The assessment findings that require immediate follow-up include

_____1 (Select), _____ 2 (Select),

and _____ 3 (Select).

> Options for 1:
> Alert and oriented × 3
> 10/10 left leg pain
> Respirations = 24 breaths/min

> Options for 2:
> Unable to move left leg
> BP = 140/78 mmHg
> Pulse = 102 beats per minute

> Options for 3:
> Diminished pulses to left lower extremity
> Contusions to bilateral upper extremities
> Temperature 98.6°F (37°C)

Shock

chapter

9

Go to http://evolve.elsevier.com/Linton/medsurg/ for additional activities and exercises.

NCLEX CATEGORIES

Safe and Effective Care Environment:
Coordinated Care, Safety and Infection Control

Psychosocial Integrity

Physiological Integrity: Pharmacological Therapies, Reduction of Risk Potential, Physiological Adaptation

PART I: MASTERING THE BASICS

A. Key Terms

Match the definition in the numbered column with the correct term in the lettered column.

1. _____ Systemic inflammatory response to an infection and is one of the leading causes of morbidity and mortality worldwide

2. _____ Generalized inflammatory condition that follows serious physiologic threat; characterized by damage to vascular endothelium and hypermetabolic state

3. _____ Deficiency of blood flow

4. _____ Life-threatening organ dysfunction caused by a dysregulated host response to infection

5. _____ Syndrome characterized by inadequate tissue perfusion resulting in impaired cellular metabolism

A. Ischemia
B. Multiple organ dysfunction syndrome (MODS)
C. Sepsis
D. Shock
E. SIRS

B. Types of Shock

1. Which descriptions are related to hypovolemic shock? Select all that apply.
   1. Caused by rapid blood loss, dehydration, hemorrhage, severe diarrhea or vomiting, and excessive perspiration
   2. Complicated by increased capillary permeability
   3. Occurs with physical impairment of blood flow
   4. Associated with pulmonary embolism and tension pneumothorax
   5. Occurs when the circulating blood volume is inadequate to maintain the supply of oxygen and nutrients to tissue

2. Which descriptions relate to distributive shock? Select all that apply.
   1. Fluid pools in dependent areas of the body
   2. Related to excessive blood or fluid loss, inadequate fluid intake, or a shift of plasma from blood into body tissues
   3. Occurs when heart fails as a pump
   4. Problem is with excessive dilation of blood vessels
   5. Related to burns, peritonitis, and intestinal obstruction
   6. Associated with congestive heart failure (CHF), acute myocardial infarction (MI), and heart rhythm disturbances

3. Which are three types of distributive shock? Select three that apply.
   1. Hypovolemic
   2. Cardiogenic
   3. Anaphylactic
   4. Septic
   5. Obstructive
   6. Neurogenic

4. Match the description of causes of ineffective tissue perfusion in the numbered column with the correct terms in the lettered column. Ineffective tissue perfusion related to:
   1. _____ myocardial contractility
   2. _____ impaired circulatory blood flow
   3. _____ blood volume loss
   4. _____ widespread vasodilation

   A. Hypovolemic
   B. Obstructive
   C. Cardiogenic
   D. Distributive

C. Drug Therapy

1. Which medications are commonly used in the treatment of cardiogenic shock? Select all that apply.
   1. Inotropics
   2. Vasopressors
   3. Corticosteroids
   4. Histamine-1 blockers
   5. Antimicrobials
   6. Antidysrhythmics

PART II: PUTTING IT ALL TOGETHER

D. Multiple Choice/Multiple Response

Choose the most appropriate answer or select all that apply.

1. Which are compensatory mechanisms in shock related to the sympathetic nervous system response? Select all that apply.
   1. Decreased heart rate
   2. Peripheral vasodilation
   3. Decreased blood flow to the kidneys
   4. Renin-angiotensin-aldosterone system activation
   5. Increased rate and depth of respirations
   6. Increased water excretion

2. Following an automobile accident, a 35-year-old man experienced severe hemorrhage. This type of shock is classified as:
   1. hypovolemic.
   2. cardiogenic.
   3. obstructive.
   4. distributive.

3. A woman experiences burns over 80% of her body. The nurse suspects she has:
   1. hypovolemic shock.
   2. cardiogenic shock.
   3. obstructive shock.
   4. distributive shock.

4. A person has a severe allergic reaction that results in bronchoconstriction and increased capillary permeability. This type of shock is:
   1. anaphylactic.
   2. cardiogenic.
   3. hypovolemic.
   4. septic.

5. Which type of shock occurs suddenly following exposure to a substance for which the patient had already developed antibodies?
   1. Neurogenic
   2. Septic
   3. Anaphylactic
   4. Cardiogenic

6. The body of a patient with neurogenic shock is unable to compensate with vasoconstriction because:
   1. the vasomotor center is incapacitated.
   2. chemicals released as a result of tissue ischemia depress the myocardium.
   3. bronchoconstriction and airway obstruction occur.
   4. systemic inflammatory response syndrome occurs.

7. One of the effects of shock on the neuroendocrine system is:
   1. release of catecholamines.
   2. decreased antidiuretic hormone (ADH).
   3. increased cerebral blood flow.
   4. decreased aldosterone.

8. One of the effects of shock on the respiratory system is:
   1. metabolic alkalosis.
   2. tissue hypoxia.
   3. depressed immune system.
   4. bronchodilation.

9. Assessment findings in the compensatory stage are likely to include:
   1. drowsiness.
   2. slightly increased blood pressure.
   3. increased blood glucose.
   4. increased bowel sounds.

10. Which assessment data would the nurse expect to find in a patient in the end-organ dysfunction stage of shock?
    1. Increased pulse pressure
    2. Weak, thready pulse
    3. Warm, flushed skin
    4. Increased blood pressure

11. The purpose of giving blood and fluids to improve cardiac output in a patient with cardiogenic shock is to:
    1. promote delivery of oxygen to cells.
    2. correct acid-base imbalances.
    3. improve fluid and electrolyte imbalances.
    4. decrease the incidence of infection.

12. Which type of shock does *not* have replacement of fluid as a priority?
    1. Distributive
    2. Neurogenic
    3. Hypovolemic
    4. Cardiogenic

13. Vasopressin is given to patients with septic shock because it is a:
    1. vasoconstrictor.
    2. vasodilator.
    3. bronchodilator.
    4. positive inotrope.

14. For which type of shock are antimicrobials prescribed?
    1. Hypovolemic
    2. Cardiogenic
    3. Distributive
    4. Septic

15. Why is atropine prescribed for neurogenic shock?
    1. Raise heart rate
    2. Raise blood pressure
    3. Treat pain
    4. Dilate blood vessels

16. For which type of shock are inotropic and antidysrhythmic agents prescribed?
    1. Neurogenic
    2. Distributive
    3. Cardiogenic
    4. Anaphylactic

17. Hypermetabolism in shock causes which type of malnutrition?
    1. Increased carbohydrate
    2. Decreased protein
    3. Decreased glucose
    4. Increased nitrogen

18. Which assessment finding would the nurse expect to see in a patient with septic shock that would not be present in a patient with hypovolemic shock?
    1. Cool skin
    2. Fever
    3. Low blood pressure
    4. Dizziness

19. List in order the three stages of shock, starting with the earliest stage as 1 and the latest stage as 3.
    A. _____ Shock
    B. _____ Pre-shock
    C. _____ End-organ dysfunction

PART III: CHALLENGE YOURSELF!

E. Getting Ready for NCLEX
Choose the most appropriate answer.

1. List in order of priority the steps to be taken in the first-aid treatment of a patient in shock.
    A. _____ Control external bleeding with direct pressure or pressure dressing.
    B. _____ Keep the patient in a flat position with legs elevated (unless further injury could be caused by raising legs).
    C. _____ Summon medical assistance.
    D. _____ Protect the patient from cold but do not overheat.
    E. _____ Establish/maintain patent airway.

2. The nurse is taking care of a 24-year-old patient following a spinal cord injury. The nurse notices that the patient has developed hypotension and bradycardia. This type of shock is:
   1. hypovolemic.
   2. septic.
   3. anaphylactic.
   4. neurogenic.

3. A patient who has had recent abdominal surgery has a blood pressure (BP) of 90/60 mm Hg and a pulse of 120. What is the priority treatment goal for this patient?
   1. Correct acid-base imbalances.
   2. Manage cardiac dysrhythmias.
   3. Administer antishock drugs.
   4. Improve blood flow and oxygen supply to vital organs.

4. A patient has just come to the hospital system clinic with hypovolemic shock. Which position is best to maintain blood flow to vital organs for this patient?
   1. Supine with head lowered
   2. Fowler's
   3. Supine with legs elevated 45°
   4. Left side-lying

5. The nurse is monitoring a patient in shock who has just arrived at a community clinic. The nurse knows that improving blood flow and oxygen supply to the vital organs is necessary for this patient. Why is this a priority in shock treatment?
   1. Brain cells begin to die after 4 minutes without oxygen.
   2. Cells resort to anaerobic metabolism, producing lactic acid immediately.
   3. Acidosis has a depressant effect on myocardial cells.
   4. If compensatory mechanisms are effective, the blood pressure will remain normal.

6. A patient in shock has a pulse of 120 bpm, BP of 80/40 mm Hg, and respirations of 28. These signs represent:
   1. fluid volume deficit.
   2. inadequate circulation.
   3. impaired tissue perfusion.
   4. electrolyte imbalance.

7. A patient in shock is also experiencing pain and agitation. Why is prompt treatment of the pain and agitation essential for this patient?
   1. Restores fluid volume
   2. Reduces unnecessary oxygen consumption
   3. Improves bronchodilation
   4. Decreases signs of infection

8. The nurse is taking care of a patient who has been in an accident and is experiencing rapid blood loss. Which sign should the nurse expect to see?
   1. Increased heart rate
   2. Peripheral vasoconstriction
   3. Increased water excretion
   4. Dilation of renal arteries

9. The nurse is taking care of a patient with congestive heart failure, resulting in inadequate cardiac output. Which problem is a priority for the nurse to address with this patient?
   1. Fluid volume deficit
   2. Potential injury
   3. Potential infection
   4. Inadequate peripheral circulation

10. A patient is being treated for hypovolemic shock. What is the reason the nurse emphasizes handling the patient gently and coordinating care to allow time for the patient to rest?
    1. Decrease fluid volume deficit
    2. Decrease fluid overload
    3. Maintain adequate body heat
    4. Reduce oxygen requirement

F. Next-Generation NCLEX® Examination-Style Questions

Read the following situations and answer the questions below.

1. The nurse is caring for a 42-year-old female client admitted to the emergency department following a motor vehicle accident. The nurse reviews the nurse's notes and vital signs.

> Nurse's Notes:
> 0800: A 42-year-old female client is admitted to the emergency department following a motor vehicle accident. First responders report an estimated blood loss of 500 cc at the scene of the accident. Client presents with an open femur fracture to the right lower extremity with active bleeding at the site, severe lacerations to the bilateral upper extremities, and ecchymosis to the chest, abdomen, and head. Alert and oriented ×2.
>
> Vital signs:
>
> | Temperature | 98.6° F (37°C) |
> | --- | --- |
> | Respirations | 26 BPM |
> | Pulse | 140 BPM |
> | SPO2 | 88% |
> | Blood Pressure | 70/52 mmHg |

Which physician orders would the nurse anticipate being prescribed? Select all that apply.
1. Soft diet
2. Strict intake and output
3. Head CT scan
4. IV infusion NS at 50 mL/hour
5. CT scan of the abdomen
6. Apply O₂ via nasal canula
7. Administration of packed red blood cells
8. Apply cooling blanket
9. Echocardiogram

2. A 80-year-old male client is brought to the Emergency Department admitted with septic shock. The oncoming nurse reviews the nurse's notes.

> Nurse's Notes:
> 0600: Pt alert and oriented to person, place, and time. Client states he was diagnosed with a UTI by his PCP 4 days ago but he did not complete antibiotics. IV inserted. BP 90/60. ER provider at bedside.
> 0700: Change of shift report received. Assumed care of client. Client resting in bed. Disoriented to place. BP 70/40. 1000 ML normal saline bolus administered as ordered. Client complains of pain to right lower extremity. Pedal pulses diminished in right foot.
> 0800: BP 72/40. Provider notified. Orders received to obtain CBC, lactic acid, doppler to right lower extremity, and administer 1000 ML normal saline bolus.

Select 1 condition and 1 client assessment finding to fill in each blank in the following sentence.

The client is at risk for developing _____, due to _____.

> Condition:
> Constipation
> Sensory deprivation
> Inadequate tissue perfusion
> Ascites

> Client Assessment Finding:
> Microvascular thrombosis
> Immobility
> Isolation
> Infection

The Older Adult Patient

Go to http://evolve.elsevier.com/Linton/medsurg/ for additional activities and exercises.

NCLEX CATEGORIES

Safe and Effective Care Environment:
Coordinated Care

Health Promotion and Maintenance

Psychosocial Integrity

Physiological Integrity: Pharmacological Therapies, Reduction of Risk Potential, Physiological Adaptation

PART I: MASTERING THE BASICS

A. Age-Related Changes

1. Which age-related changes decrease in older people? Select all that apply.
   1. Tolerance for extremes in temperature
   2. Conduction speed of CNS impulses
   3. Pulmonary gas exchange
   4. Force of pulse
   5. Intellectual capability
   6. Total body water

2. Which age-related changes increase in older people? Select all that apply.
   1. Loss of neurons (brain cells)
   2. Functional ability of brain cells
   3. Conduction speed associated with synaptic transmission
   4. Vital capacity
   5. Long-term memory
   6. Calcification of coronary arteries

3. Which system shows only a slight decline with age?
   1. Renal system
   2. Central nervous system
   3. Respiratory system
   4. Cardiovascular system

4. With increasing age, a person's reduced tolerance for physical work may be due to the decreased:
   1. number of neurons in the brain.
   2. capacity of heart cells to utilize oxygen.
   3. size of the heart.
   4. resistance to blood flow in many organs.

5. Which change occurs in aging kidneys?
   1. Decreased filtration rate
   2. Increased extracellular fluid
   3. Increased cell mass
   4. Decreased residual urine

6. What are the six key assessment areas of the SPICES assessment tool that can be used for routine focused assessments of the older adult?

   S _____

   _____

   P _____

   _____

   I _____

   _____

   C _____

   _____

   E _____

   _____

   S _____

   _____

PART II: PUTTING IT ALL TOGETHER

B. Multiple Choice/Multiple Response
Choose the most appropriate answer or select all that apply.

1. Which is a frequent concern of older adults?
    1. Long-term memory loss
    2. Creativity loss
    3. Short-term memory loss
    4. Judgment loss

2. Which result in decreased vital capacity in older people? Select all that apply.
    1. Vertebrae more prone to fracture
    2. Calcification of costal cartilage
    3. Deterioration of vascular tone
    4. Weakening of esophageal muscle contractions
    5. Kyphosis

3. Which is a frequent respiratory complaint of older adults?
    1. Orthostatic hypotension
    2. Inability to breathe
    3. Increased respirations
    4. Exertional dyspnea

4. Why is respiratory care of increased importance to older adults?
    1. They are reluctant to get flu and pneumonia vaccinations.
    2. Decreased activity due to aging lowers oxygenation.
    3. Increased demands on the aging body increase risks of infection.
    4. Chronic pulmonary disease is the third leading cause of death in older adults.

5. Which is an age-related change that occurs due to loss of oils in the skin?
    1. Infection
    2. Itching
    3. Wrinkles
    4. Brown spots

6. What is the leading cause of disability in old age?
    1. Urinary tract infection
    2. Macular degeneration
    3. Pressure ulcers
    4. Arthritis

7. What is the name for the curvature of the thoracic spine that causes a bent-over appearance in some older adults?
    1. Kyphosis
    2. Arthritis
    3. Scoliosis
    4. Lordosis

8. Which is a cause of presbycusis in older people?
    1. Changes in the lens
    2. Ototoxicity from medications
    3. Hardening of the outer ear canal
    4. Atrophic changes in the cochlea

9. What percentage of adults older than age 69 are hearing-impaired?
    1. 10%
    2. 25%
    3. 50%
    4. 75%

10. What is the leading cause of new age-related blindness in older people?
    1. Glaucoma
    2. Cataracts
    3. Corneal abrasion
    4. Macular degeneration

11. Which is a normal age-related change?
    1. Increased absorption of calcium and zinc
    2. Increased acidity of saliva
    3. Increased peristalsis
    4. Decreased gastric emptying

12. A developmental challenge in old age is to:
    1. develop close relationships with other people; to learn and experience love.
    2. find a vocation or hobby where the individual can help others or in some way contribute to society.
    3. establish trusting relationships with other people.
    4. review life and gain a feeling of accomplishment or fulfillment.

13. For the nurse to provide effective gerontological care, the crucial basis for deciding care needs is:
    1. medical diagnosis.
    2. functional assessment.
    3. activities of daily living.
    4. community resources.

14. Which age-related changes affect the inactivation of drugs in the body? Select all that apply.
    1. Decreased liver size
    2. Reduced blood flow through the liver
    3. Decreased body water
    4. Reduced liver enzyme activity
    5. Decreased renal function

15. Which is a cause of progressive slowing of responses and reflexes in older adults?
    1. Decreased impulse conduction speed
    2. Loss of neurons in the brain
    3. Inadequate tissue oxygenation
    4. Atherosclerosis and decreased cellular respiration

16. Which are ways an older person can use adaptive strategies and modifying behavior to deal with age-related neurologic changes? Select all that apply.
    1. Avoid temperature extremes.
    2. Exercise moderately.
    3. Begin walking, climbing stairs, and bicycling exercises.
    4. Approach tasks at a slower pace.
    5. Attend to one task at a time.

17. Which factor contributes to constipation in an older person?
    1. Lack of dietary fiber
    2. Decreased hydrochloric acid
    3. Slower gastric emptying of fluids
    4. Abdominal bloating

18. Which nursing intervention is recommended for the care of an older person who is experiencing decreased loss of muscle strength?
    1. Increased calcium in diet
    2. Weight-bearing exercises
    3. Limited walking and bicycling activities
    4. Use of a cane when walking

PART III: CHALLENGE YOURSELF!

C. Getting Ready for NCLEX
Choose the most appropriate answer or select all that apply.

1. The nurse is taking care of an older female patient who was admitted to the hospital 1 day ago with pneumonia. This illness has impaired her ability to compensate. The nurse should monitor this patient, recognizing that she is at risk for:
   1. disorientation.
   2. hypotension.
   3. loss of brain neurons.
   4. sedation.

2. A 74-year-old man with cirrhosis is admitted to the hospital and he has started taking a diuretic. Which age-related change may result in decreased drug clearance in this patient?
   1. Increased body fat
   2. Decreased body water
   3. Decreased hepatic blood flow
   4. Decreased serum albumin

3. An 80-year-old woman is being seen by the nurse at a medical clinic. Due to a decreased number and sensitivity of sensory receptors and neurons in this patient, the nurse provides nursing care so that this patient can:
   1. avoid temperature extremes and accomplish tasks at a slower pace.
   2. do deep-breathing exercises and positioning to facilitate lung expansion.
   3. use mnemonics and rehearsal memory training to improve memory performance.
   4. use assistive devices for walking and preventing falls.

4. The nurse is taking care of a 70-year-old patient whose blood pressure is 150/90 mm Hg. What is an age-related cause of this blood pressure?
   1. Decreased neurons and conduction speed at synapses
   2. Arteries dilate, lengthen, and become more rigid
   3. Chronic hypoxic state of the brain
   4. Decreased heart rate and stroke volume

5. The nurse is taking care of a 75-year-old patient whose resting cardiac output has fallen 40%. Which is an explanation for this finding?
   1. Decreases in filtration and plasma flow rate
   2. Increased valvular rigidity
   3. Incomplete closure of the aortic and pulmonic valves
   4. Decreased heart rate and stroke volume

6. The nurse is taking care of an 82-year-old man with atherosclerosis and chronic hypoxia. Which is a behavior that the nurse should expect to observe in this patient?
   1. Difficulty remembering planned events for the day
   2. Slow responses
   3. Decrease in creativity
   4. Inability to learn new material

7. The nurse has attended a program on respiratory nursing care for older patients. The program focused on factors that make older persons more susceptible and less likely to recover from respiratory infections. What information learned is beneficial for this nurse to teach coworkers about these factors in the older adult? Select all that apply.
   1. Less effective cough reflex
   2. Less efficient ciliary action
   3. Thinning of capillary walls
   4. Increased number of capillaries surrounding the alveoli
   5. Thickening of coronary arteries

8. The nurse is taking care of an 85-year-old man who is taking streptomycin for a bacterial infection. An adverse reaction that may occur in this patient is:
   1. confusion.
   2. nephrotoxicity.
   3. hemorrhage.
   4. hypotension.

9. The nurse is explaining to a 78-year-old patient with decreased renal function that medication toxicity must be monitored due to:
   1. increased storage of fat-soluble drugs.
   2. decreased drug metabolism.
   3. increased concentration of drug in tissues.
   4. decreased drug elimination.

10. The nurse is observing a 90-year-old patient for drug interactions among over-the-counter medications and prescription medications. The patient is taking sodium bicarbonate. Which classification of prescription medications may result in a drug interaction with large amounts of sodium bicarbonate?
    1. Anticoagulants
    2. Diuretics
    3. Sedatives
    4. Cholesterol-lowering medications

11. The nurse is collecting data about an 82-year-old patient. Which are indicators that this patient is moving toward ego integrity? Select all that apply.
    1. Recognizes and accepts changes in physical and mental capabilities
    2. Develops new meaningful intimate relationships
    3. Learns about home and time management
    4. Revises life goals
    5. Adapts to new lifestyles

Falls

chapter

11

Go to http://evolve.elsevier.com/Linton/medsurg/ for additional activities and exercises.

NCLEX CATEGORIES

Safe and Effective Care Environment: Safety and Infection Control

Physiological Integrity: Basic Care and Comfort, Pharmacological Therapies, Physiological Adaptation

PART I: MASTERING THE BASICS

A. Key Terms

Match the definition in the numbered column with the most appropriate term in the lettered column.

1. _____ Anything that restricts movement
2. _____ Unplanned descent to the floor with or without injury
3. _____ Factors related to the internal functioning of an individual, such as the aging process or physical illness that can cause falls
4. _____ Psychotropic medication given to subdue agitated or confused patients
5. _____ Law enacted in 1987 to protect patients from unnecessary restraints in nursing homes
6. _____ Factors in the environment that can cause falls

A. Chemical restraints
B. Extrinsic factors
C. Fall
D. Omnibus Reconciliation Act (OBRA)
E. Physical restraint
F. Intrinsic factors

B. Risk Factors

1. Which of the following are factors associated with people at greatest risk for injury from falls? Select all that apply.
   1. Peripheral neuropathy
   2. Pneumonia
   3. Kidney disease
   4. Confusion
   5. Hypertension
   6. Osteoporosis
   7. Benzodiazepine use
   8. Antibiotic therapy
   9. Sensory impairment
   10. Gait disorders
   11. Short-term memory loss
   12. Balance disorders

2. Which of the following are intrinsic risk factors for falling? Select all that apply.
   1. Impaired hearing
   2. Balance and gait problems
   3. Environmental factors
   4. Loose rugs
   5. Foot disorders
   6. Postural hypotension
   7. Glare from shiny floors

C. Restraints

1. Which are damaging psychological effects of restraints on older patients? Select all that apply.
   1. Decreased dependency
   2. Anger
   3. Increased confusion
   4. Decreased disorientation
   5. Withdrawal
   6. Aggressive behavior
   7. Loss of self-image
   8. Fear
   9. Security

D. Nursing Interventions

Match each risk factor in the numbered column with the most appropriate intervention in the lettered column.

1. _____ Musculoskeletal disorders
2. _____ Impaired adaptation to the dark
3. _____ Balance disorders
4. _____ Stroke
5. _____ Reduced visual acuity
6. _____ Postural hypotension
7. _____ Impacted cerumen (earwax)
8. _____ Peripheral neuropathy
9. _____ Impaired color perception
10. _____ Foot disorders
11. _____ Presbycusis

A. Maintain adequate lighting; reduce glare from shiny floors and allow time for eyes to adjust to light levels (e.g., from a dark room to outside); use nightlight in bedroom and bathroom.
B. Trim toenails; use appropriate footwear.
C. Speak slowly; use low voice; decrease background noise; encourage use of hearing aid.
D. Remove earwax.
E. Use bright colors as markers, especially orange, yellow, and red.
F. Be sure that patient wears glasses, if appropriate; keep glasses clean; encourage regular eye examinations.
G. Use correctly sized footwear with firm soles.
H. Encourage balance, gait training, and muscle-strengthening exercises.
I. Encourage dorsiflexion exercises; use pressure-graded stockings; elevate head of bed; teach individual to get up from chair or bed slowly to avoid tipping head backward.
J. Encourage balance exercises.
K. Place call bell in visual field and within reach of arm that has use; anticipate needs for toileting, dressing, eating, and bathing; assist with transfer; provide passive range-of-motion exercises to improve functional ability.

12. Which are interventions to prevent falls for a patient with impaired dark adaptation? Select all that apply.
    1. Be sure the patient wears glasses, if appropriate.
    2. Maintain adequate lighting.
    3. Reduce glare from shiny floors.
    4. Allow time to adjust to light levels (as patient moves from a dark room to outside).
    5. Keep glasses clean.
    6. Encourage regular eye examinations.
    7. Use a nightlight in the bathroom.

E. Documentation

1. Which factors are important to document at the time when a fall occurs? Select all that apply.
    1. What the patient was doing
    2. Vital signs of the patient at the time of the fall
    3. Mental status of the patient
    4. Nutritional status of the patient
    5. Environmental factors

F. Prevention

1. Which are basic strategies for reducing all types of falls? Select all that apply.
    1. Decrease physical activities.
    2. Increase exercise.
    3. Modify the environment.
    4. Reduce visual impairment.
    5. Increase use of over-the-counter (OTC) medication.

2. Which are environment-oriented fall prevention techniques used in long-term care facilities? Select all that apply.
    1. Assist patient to void every 4 hours.
    2. Keep rooms and hallways free from clutter.
    3. Place TV controls within reach.
    4. Clean up spills, including urine.
    5. Encourage exercise to strengthen muscles and prevent weakness.

3. Which of the following are fall prevention guidelines for the home? Select all that apply.
    1. Watch for pets underfoot and scattered pet food.
    2. Check for even, nonglare lighting in every room.
    3. Use 60-watt light bulbs to provide proper lighting in rooms.
    4. Make sure there is a telephone in the room next to the bedroom.
    5. Be sure to use bifocals to assist with walking.

PART II: PUTTING IT ALL TOGETHER

G. Multiple Choice
Choose the most appropriate answer.

1. What is the estimated ratio of community-dwelling older adults who fall in a given year?
   1. 1 in 3
   2. 1 in 10
   3. 1 in 20
   4. 1 in 100

2. At what age is the risk of injury after a fall the greatest?
   1. 40
   2. 65
   3. 75
   4. 85

3. Which percentage of deaths due to falls does the U.S. Public Health Service state are preventable?
   1. One-fifth
   2. One-third
   3. One-half
   4. Two-thirds

4. Older patients are more likely than younger patients to be physically restrained because of their greater likelihood of:
   1. mental decline and weight loss.
   2. chronic illness and physical decline.
   3. heart disease and insomnia.
   4. falling and confusion.

5. Physical restraints should be removed and released for 10 minutes every:
   1. hour.
   2. 2 hours.
   3. 4 hours.
   4. 8 hours.

6. Psychoactive drugs should never be used for the purpose of:
   1. relief of headaches.
   2. insomnia.
   3. discipline.
   4. hallucinations.

7. Why are older adults at particular risk for injury from their accidents?
   1. They are more confused.
   2. They are more disoriented.
   3. They are likely to have poorer clinical outcomes.
   4. They are not as coordinated.

PART III: CHALLENGE YOURSELF!

H. Getting Ready for NCLEX
Choose the most appropriate answer or select all that apply.

1. Which of the following are major problems from using physical restraints? Select all that apply.
   1. Skin breakdown
   2. Impaired circulation
   3. Dizziness and vertigo
   4. Accidental strangulation
   5. Reduced visual acuity

2. The first step in preventing falls and injury is to determine:
   1. which medications the patient is taking.
   2. the hazards in the environmental setting.
   3. who is at greatest risk.
   4. whether the patient has alcohol or drug problems.

3. Which of the following interventions are recommended to reduce the risk of falls? Select all that apply.
   1. Calcium and vitamin D for susceptible patients
   2. Exercises to improve balance
   3. Frequent ambulation
   4. Muscle strengthening exercises
   5. High-protein diet

4. Which of the following nursing interventions are recommended for a patient with impaired hearing who is at risk for falls? Select all that apply.
   1. Maintain adequate lighting.
   2. Encourage balance and gait training.
   3. Speak slowly.
   4. Use a loud voice.
   5. Decrease background noises.
   6. Provide passive range-of-motion exercise.

I. Nursing Care Plan

Refer to Nursing Care Plan, Patient with a History of Falling, in the book, to answer questions 1-3.

A 75-year-old woman resides in a long-term care facility because of chronic health problems, including hypertension, emphysema, and mild dementia. She has a history of several falls at home, including one that resulted in a wrist fracture that led to the admission to the long-term care facility. This patient is at risk for falls related to (1) weakness, dizziness, and poor balance; (2) environmental hazards; and (3) postural hypotension.

1. Which factor in her health history puts this patient most at risk for a fracture from a fall?
   1. Emphysema
   2. Dementia
   3. High blood pressure
   4. History of several falls at home

2. What is the priority intervention for this patient to prevent her from falling?
   1. Discuss possible environmental hazards and measures to reduce risks with the patient.
   2. Keep bed at lowest level.
   3. Orient patient frequently to person, place, and time.
   4. Remove restraints at least every 2 hours for 10 minutes for range-of-motion exercises.

3. Which are interventions associated with this patient's risk for falls related to postural hypotension? Select all that apply.
   1. Provide call button and respond quickly.
   2. Keep bed at lowest level.
   3. Suggest elastic stockings to improve venous return.
   4. Teach patient to change positions slowly.
   5. Encourage adequate fluids to prevent dehydration.

J. Next-Generation NCLEX® Examination-Style Questions

Read the following situations and answer the questions below.

1. The nurse reviews the health history and vital signs of a 70-year-old male client residing in a long-term care (LTC) facility.

Health History:
70-year-old male client has a history of several falls, hypotension, COPD, dizziness, poor balance, and Alzheimer's. He ambulates with one person assist and a walker, but attempts to wander frequently. Weight 165 lbs (74.8 kg).

Vital Signs:

Blood Pressure	88/52 mm Hg standing
Pulse	80 beats/minute
Respirations	18 breaths/minute
Temperature	99°F (37.2°C)

Complete the following sentence by choosing from the list of options below.

Factors that contribute to his risk for falls include _____ 1, _____ 2, and _____ 3.

Options for 1	Options for 2	Options for 3
COPD	Respirations = 18 BPM	Dizziness
Blood pressure 88/52 mm Hg standing	History of falls	Male gender
Pulse 80	Temperature 99° F (37.2°C)	Weight 165 lbs (74.8 kg)

2. The nurse beginning her 2300–0700 shift reviews the previous shift's nurse's notes and vital signs of a 75-year-old female client admitted to the surgical unit following a right total hip replacement. The client has been receiving oxycodone 10 mg Q4H PRN for pain.

Using the nurse's notes and vital signs, highlight the assessment findings that require immediate follow-up by the nurse.

Nurse's Notes:

5/23/21 2230: Client reports pain to right hip rated 7/10 on numeric scale. Administered 10 mg oxycodone po as ordered.

5/23/21 2250: Client fell while ambulating to bathroom. Client complains of dizziness and is alert and oriented ×2. She appears drowsy. Provider notified. Report given to S. Johns, RN.

Vital Signs:

Blood Pressure	90/58 mm Hg sitting
Pulse	72 beats/minute
Respirations	16 breaths/minute
Temperature	98.6°F (37°C)

Immobility

chapter
12

Go to http://evolve.elsevier.com/Linton/medsurg/ for additional activities and exercises.

NCLEX CATEGORIES

Safe and Effective Care Environment: Safety and Infection Control

Health Promotion and Maintenance

Physiological Integrity: Basic Care and Comfort, Reduction of Risk Potential, Physiological Adaptation

A. Erythema
B. Pressure injury
C. Isometric exercise
D. Immobility
E. Range-of-motion exercise
F. Active exercise
G. Contracture
H. Shearing forces
I. Passive exercise

PART I: MASTERING THE BASICS

A. Key Terms
Match the definition in the numbered column with the most appropriate term in the lettered column.

1. _____ The inability to move; imposed restriction on entire body

2. _____ Exercise in which each joint is moved in various directions to the farthest possible extreme

3. _____ Exercise of the patient which is carried out by the therapist or nurse without the assistance of the patient

4. _____ Muscle contraction without movement used to maintain muscle tone

5. _____ Exercise carried out by the patient

6. _____ Redness of the skin; usually a sign that capillaries have become congested because of impaired blood flow

7. _____ Limited range of motion due to joint, muscle, or soft tissue limitations

8. _____ Two contacting parts sliding on each other

9. _____ An open wound caused by pressure on a bony prominence; also called a *bed sore* or *decubitus ulcer*

B. Pressure Injuries

1. Which of the following are elements of a pressure injury prevention protocol? Select all that apply.
   1. Reposition patient on bedrest at least every 4 hours.
   2. Utilize trapeze bars to enhance patient mobility.
   3. Teach wheelchair patients to shift their weight every 15 minutes if able.
   4. Position patients so that they are resting on pressure points of the skin.
   5. When the patient is in bed, keep the head raised as much as possible to reduce shearing force.
   6. Do not massage or use rubber rings to elevate heels or sacral areas.

2. Which characteristics are related to stage I pressure injuries? Select all that apply.
   1. Irregular, ill-defined area of pressure reflecting the shape of the object creating the pressure
   2. Some skin loss in the epidermis and/or dermis
   3. Nonblanchable erythema
   4. Ulcer is surrounded by a broad, indistinct, painful, reddened area that is hot or warmer than normal
   5. Little destruction of tissue; condition is reversible
   6. Pain and tenderness may be present, with swelling and hardening of the skin and associated heat

3. Which characteristics are related to stage III pressure injuries? Select all that apply.
   1. A shallow ulcer develops and appears blistered, cracked, or abraded
   2. Crater-like sore with a distinct outer margin
   3. Wound may be infected and is usually open and draining
   4. Ulcer is usually infected and may appear black with exudation, foul odor, and purulent drainage
   5. Full-thickness skin loss involving damage or necrosis of the dermis and subcutaneous tissues
   6. Full-thickness skin loss with extensive destruction of the deeper underlying muscle and possible bone tissue

C. Consequences of Immobility

Match the consequences of immobility in the numbered column with the body system in the lettered column. Answers may be used more than once.

1. _____ Increased risk of atelectasis and infection
2. _____ Decreased glomerular filtration rate
3. _____ Decreased tactile stimulation
4. _____ Thickening of joint capsule
5. _____ Pressure injuries
6. _____ Constipation
7. _____ Increased storage of fat
8. _____ Increased peripheral resistance
9. _____ Decreased glucose tolerance
10. _____ Loss of smoothness of cartilage surface

A. Integumentary
B. Gastrointestinal
C. Musculoskeletal
D. Pulmonary
E. Urinary
F. Metabolic
G. Sensory
H. Cardiovascular

D. Pressure Injury Locations

Refer to the figure below, Possible Locations of Pressure Injuries (Figure 12.1). Label the bony prominences (A–Z).

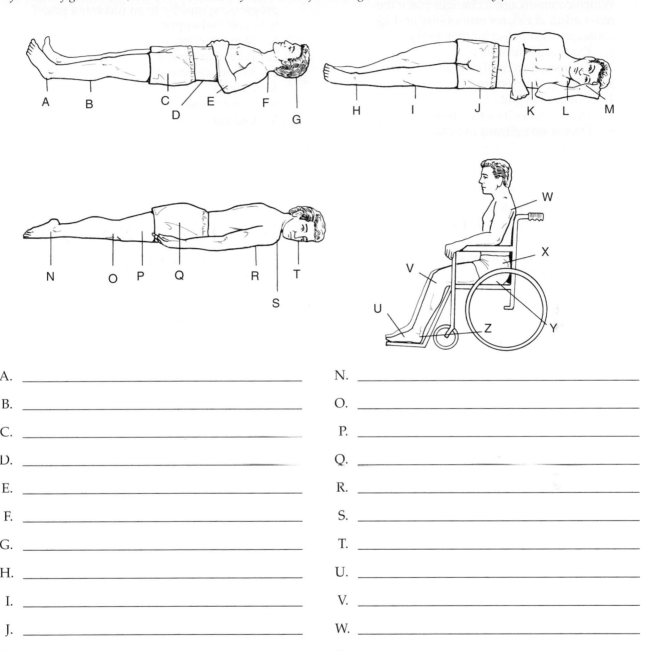

A. _____	N. _____
B. _____	O. _____
C. _____	P. _____
D. _____	Q. _____
E. _____	R. _____
F. _____	S. _____
G. _____	T. _____
H. _____	U. _____
I. _____	V. _____
J. _____	W. _____
K. _____	X. _____
L. _____	Y. _____
M. _____	Z. _____

E. Aging and Immobility

1. Which common aging changes place the older adult at risk for immobility and its consequences? Select all that apply.
   1. Decreased flexibility
   2. Decreased strength
   3. Changes in posture
   4. Changes in gait
   5. Decreased kidney function
   6. Decreased neurons in brain
   7. Likelihood of having one or more chronic illnesses

2. Which common medical illnesses place the older person at risk for immobility and its consequences? Select all that apply.
   1. Arthritis
   2. Cardiovascular disease
   3. Diabetes mellitus
   4. Stroke
   5. Anemia
   6. Thyroid disorders
   7. Parkinson disease
   8. Foot disorders

PART II: PUTTING IT ALL TOGETHER

F. Multiple Choice/Multiple Response

Choose the most appropriate answer or select all that apply.

1. What is the result of little or no motion of the joints?
   1. Contractures
   2. Tendonitis
   3. Bursitis
   4. Skin breakdown

2. What is the most frequent site of skin breakdown?
   1. Ischial tuberosities
   2. Sacrum
   3. Heels
   4. Trochanter

3. The best preventive measure for pressure injuries is:
   1. a high-protein diet.
   2. deep-breathing.
   3. frequent position changes.
   4. moderate exercise.

4. Which characteristics of patients with circulatory disease result in erythema progressing rapidly to an ulcerated stage? Select all that apply.
   1. Skin infection
   2. Poor skin turgor
   3. Malnourishment
   4. Obesity
   5. Lacerations
   6. Old age

5. Which conditions result from pressure injuries? Select all that apply.
   1. Falls
   2. Longer hospital stays
   3. Confusion
   4. Likelihood of long-term care facility placement
   5. Increased need for oxygen therapy
   6. Increased mortality

6. Which are contraindicated in the care of patients with pressure injuries? Select all that apply.
   1. Sheepskin
   2. Massage
   3. Egg-crate mattress
   4. Trapeze bars
   5. Rubber ring
   6. Heat lamp
   7. Use of moisturizers

7. What is the recommended treatment for stage I and stage II pressure injuries?
   1. Use antibiotic creams and ointments.
   2. Apply heat to the area around the pressure injury.
   3. Clean with alcohol and antiseptics.
   4. Clean with water or normal saline.

8. A 60-year-old patient with pneumonia has thick secretions pooled in the lower respiratory structures. These secretions interfere with the:
   1. exchange of white blood cells and red blood cells in the capillaries.
   2. circulation of blood to the extremities.
   3. detoxification process in the liver.
   4. exchange of oxygen and carbon dioxide in the lungs.

9. Which is the most common problem associated with immobility in relation to food and fluid intake?
   1. Hypoproteinemia
   2. Hypokalemia
   3. Anorexia
   4. Nausea

10. For patients with pressure injuries, the diet should be high in:
    1. potassium.
    2. fiber.
    3. protein.
    4. vitamins.

11. Which are the causes of constipation in patients with pressure injuries? Select all that apply.
    1. Anorexia
    2. Nausea
    3. Inactivity
    4. Decreased fluid intake
    5. Lack of fiber in diet

12. What is the most effective way to prevent urinary incontinence associated with immobility?
    1. High-protein diet
    2. Coughing and deep-breathing program
    3. Restriction of fluid intake
    4. Schedule for toileting

13. Which are therapeutic reasons for immobility? Select all that apply.
    1. Reduce the workload of the heart in a cardiac condition
    2. Prevent atelectasis and hypostatic pneumonia
    3. Treat urinary incontinence
    4. Promote healing and repair
    5. Prevent further injury of a body part
    6. Obtain relief from joint contractures

14. Which side effects of drugs may contribute to factors causing immobility? Select all that apply.
    1. Dizziness
    2. Hypertension
    3. Hypotension
    4. Hyperglycemia
    5. Tachycardia

PART III: CHALLENGE YOURSELF!

G. Getting Ready for NCLEX

Choose the most appropriate answer or select all that apply.

1. A patient is slumped down while sitting in bed. Which actions does the nurse take to prevent shearing? Select all that apply.
   1. Use moisturizers to prevent friction.
   2. Avoid friction when moving the patient to prevent damage to the uppermost layers of the skin.
   3. Reposition the patient in bed at least every 2 hours.
   4. Position the patient so that he is not resting on pressure points of the skin.
   5. Gently cleanse the skin when soiled.
   6. Keep the head of the bed lowered as much as possible to prevent the patient from sliding down in the bed.

2. The nurse is taking care of three patients who are newly admitted to an assisted-living facility. As the nurse collects data to assist in planning their care, the nurse focuses on prevention of pressure injuries. What is the first step in the prevention of pressure injuries?
   1. Reposition the patient in bed at least every 2 hours.
   2. Keep bed linens dry, smooth, and free of wrinkles.
   3. Use a special mattress or bed designed to reduce pressure.
   4. Identify patients at risk for developing pressure injuries.

3. A 74-year-old male patient is in a rehabilitation center following hospitalization for hip surgery. Which are ways to assist this immobile patient to gain independence? Select all that apply.
   1. Use of slip-on shoes
   2. Pressure-reducing pad for wheelchair
   3. Loose pullover shirts
   4. Velcro closures
   5. Increased fluid intake

4. A 65-year-old patient with heart failure is on bedrest and refuses to take deep breaths. Which is most likely to occur to the respiratory status of this patient?
   1. An accumulation of carbon dioxide that collects in the alveoli
   2. An accumulation of thick secretions that pool in the lower respiratory structures
   3. Decreased circulation to the lungs
   4. Decreased oxygen entering the lungs

5. The Norton scale is used by the nurse to identify patients at risk of developing pressure injuries. Which categories are included in the Norton scale? Select all that apply.
   1. Physical condition
   2. Mental condition
   3. Activity level
   4. Medications
   5. Mobility
   6. Incontinence

6. To prevent the side effects of immobility, the nurse has been changing the position of the patient at least every 2 hours. What should the nurse do if redness persists after 2 hours?
   1. Continue turning the patient every 2 hours.
   2. Maintain joints in their functional positions.
   3. Increase the fluid intake for this patient.
   4. Shorten the interval between repositioning.

H. Next-Generation Nclex® Examination-Style Questions

The nurse reviews the health history of an 84-year-old woman who has resided in an intermediate care facility for 2 years.

Health History:
84 year old female admitted to the intermediate care facility because she had been living at home alone and was unable to shop and cook for herself after falling and breaking her wrist. She had previously been active in the community, but in the residential home she has remained confined to her room and is not interested in interacting with other people. Client prefers to stay in bed or in a chair most of the time. She has fallen many times, usually on her way to the dining room to eat. Interdisciplinary team identified the following problems associated with her immobility: (1) continued falling, (2) incontinence, and (3) isolation and perhaps depression.

1. For each body system listed below, select one potential nursing intervention that would be appropriate for the care of the client at this time.

   Musculoskeletal _____ 1 (Select)

   Renal _____ 2 (Select)

   Sensory _____ 3 (Select)

Options for 1	Options for 2	Options for 3
• Use a wheelchair for mobility	• Develop a regular schedule of toileting	• Encourage client to stay in room to prevent overstimulation
• Assist with progressive ambulation	• Decrease fluid intake	• Increase social interaction with residents
• Encourage bedrest to prevent falls	• Urinary catheter	• Transfer client to a psychiatric facility

An 80-year-old female client admitted to the surgical unit post right total hip replacement has a history of impaired balance and weakness in the right lower extremity. The nurse reviews the clients health history and physical assessment.

Health History:
An 80-year-old female client admitted to the surgical unit post right total hip replacement has a history of impaired balance and weakness in the right lower extremity. She reports falling 2 days prior to surgery. She lives alone and is active in the community. She has been instructed to use a walker when ambulating and to call for assistance. She has been irritable and insists on caring for herself. On several occasions she has been unable to delay urination until she could get help.

Physical Assessment:
Alert and oriented ×3. Blood pressure 110/68 mm Hg, pulse 88 bpm; respirations 18 breaths per minute, temperature 97°F orally. Urine is dark with a strong odor. Erythema noted to sacrum. Pain to right hip 7/10 on numeric pain scale.

Drag or write the three assessment findings from the choices below to fill in each blank in the following sentence.

2. The assessment findings that require immediate follow-up include _____

    (1)_____, _____(2)_____ , and _____(3)_____.

Assessment Findings:
- Blood pressure 110/68 mm Hg
- Pulse 88 bpm
- Respirations 18 breaths/minute
- Urine is dark with a strong odor
- Erythema noted to sacrum
- Pain to right hip 7/10 on numeric pain scale
- Alert and oriented times 3
- Fall 2 days ago

Delirium and Dementia

Go to http://evolve.elsevier.com/Linton/medsurg/ for additional activities and exercises.

NCLEX CATEGORIES

Safe and Effective Care Environment:
Coordinated Care, Safety and Infection Control

Health Promotion and Maintenance

Psychosocial Integrity

Physiological Integrity: Pharmacological Therapies, Reduction of Risk Potential, Physiological Adaptation

PART I: MASTERING THE BASICS

A. Delirium and Dementia

1. Which descriptions are related to delirium? Select all that apply.
    1. Short-term confusional state
    2. Often irreversible confusion
    3. Acute confusional state
    4. Chronic confusion
    5. Often reversible confusion
    6. Characterized by disturbances in attention, thinking, and perception

2. Which descriptions are related to dementia? Select all that apply.
    1. Characterized by impaired intellectual function
    2. Caused by some underlying illness
    3. Develops over a short period of time
    4. Clearly defined hallucinations may be present
    5. Flat or indifferent affect
    6. Intermittent fear, perplexity, or bewilderment

3. Match the descriptions in the numbered column with the proper terms in the lettered column. Answers may be used more than once.
    1. _____ Speech may be slurred and disjointed with endless repetitions
    2. _____ Engaging in conversation may be difficult
    3. _____ Generally considered irreversible
    4. _____ Significant cognitive decline from a previous level of performance in one or more areas of cognitive domain
    5. _____ Difficulty paying attention; easily distracted
    A. Delirium
    B. Dementia (major neurocognitive disorder, major NCD)

PART II: PUTTING IT ALL TOGETHER

B. Multiple Choice/Multiple Response
Choose the most appropriate answer or select all that apply.

1. The use of physical restraints should be avoided with patients with delirium because restraints tend to:
    1. increase anxiety.
    2. disturb thought processes.
    3. increase impaired thinking.
    4. disturb sleep patterns.

2. When a patient with dementia resists activities such as bathing or dressing, the nurse should:
   1. orient the patient to reality.
   2. avoid confrontations.
   3. state clearly what needs to be done.
   4. offer a variety of choices to encourage decision-making.

3. Patients with dementia should be offered:
   1. three full meals a day.
   2. low-fiber foods.
   3. a diet low in salt.
   4. finger foods high in protein and carbohydrates.

4. When the nurse is taking care of patients with dementia, it is helpful to remember that they usually:
   1. benefit from reality orientation.
   2. forget things quickly.
   3. become agitated by extraneous stimuli.
   4. are able to learn new things.

5. Which approach may agitate patients with dementia?
   1. A nonconfrontational manner
   2. Use of calm, gentle mannerisms
   3. Reality orientation
   4. Use of simple, direct communication

6. When caring for a patient with delirium, the nurse should:
   1. provide frequent, routine toileting.
   2. provide frequent orientation to surroundings.
   3. cut the food into small portions.
   4. break tasks down into individual steps to be done one at a time.

7. Which medications may cause delirium? Select all that apply.
   1. Sedatives
   2. Opioids
   3. Antianxiety agents
   4. Antithyroids
   5. Antidepressants
   6. Steroids

8. Which are general medical illnesses or conditions that may result in dementia? Select all that apply.
   1. Alzheimer disease
   2. Postoperative status
   3. Trauma
   4. HIV infection
   5. Parkinson disease

9. Which are underlying medical illnesses or conditions that may cause delirium? Select all that apply.
   1. Dehydration
   2. Overmedication
   3. Alzheimer disease
   4. Parkinson disease
   5. Infection
   6. Fluid and electrolyte imbalance

10. Which are medications that most often cause confusion in older adults? Select all that apply.
    1. Anticholinergic drugs
    2. H_2-receptor blockers
    3. Laxatives
    4. Antacids
    5. Nonsteroidal antiinflammatory drugs (NSAIDs)

11. What do the majority of people fear most about aging?
    1. Increased loneliness
    2. Impaired cognition
    3. Impaired mobility
    4. Loss of independence

PART III: CHALLENGE YOURSELF!

C. Getting Ready for NCLEX
Choose the most appropriate answer or select all that apply.

1. The nurse in a long-term care facility is assisting with the admission of a patient with confusion. What is the first step in collecting data about a confused person?
   1. Observe the behavior of the patient.
   2. List any known acute or chronic illnesses.
   3. List all medications the patient is taking.
   4. Collect data about the nutritional status of the patient.

2. When the nurse is caring for a delirious patient who is experiencing hallucinations, the best response of the nurse would be:
   1. "What is it that you are seeing on the wall?"
   2. "You are sick in the hospital, and what you are seeing is part of the illness."
   3. "The time is 2:00 PM and the day of the week is Monday."
   4. "Tell me what you are seeing."

3. A female patient with dementia starts to become very restless and agitated. Which is an effective nursing intervention for this patient?
   1. Discuss the cause of her discomfort with her.
   2. Speak calmly and reassure her constantly.
   3. Orient her to time and place.
   4. Divert her attention and gently guide her to a new activity.

4. A patient with dementia tells the nurse that he is afraid of bathtubs. The nurse's best response is to:
   1. reassure the patient that there is nothing to be afraid of.
   2. explain the reason for taking a bath in the bathtub.
   3. offer a variety of choices to the patient about taking a bath.
   4. arrange another way to give personal care.

5. Which concepts should be used as a basis for providing care for patients with dementia? Select all that apply.
   1. Patients usually forget things relatively quickly.
   2. Orient the patients to time and person with clocks and calendars.
   3. Patients are usually unable to learn new things.
   4. Break down tasks into individual steps to be done one at a time.
   5. Provide frequent orientation to the surroundings.

6. A patient with delirium is having trouble falling asleep. Which is the most appropriate nursing intervention to help this patient fall asleep?
   1. A walk followed by a shower
   2. Pain medication and watching a movie
   3. A backrub, a glass of warm milk, and soothing conversation
   4. A sedative and reality orientation

D. Next-Generation NCLEX® Examination-Style Questions

Read the following situation and answer question 1. For more information, refer to Nursing Care Plan, The Patient with Delirium, in your textbook.

The nurse is caring for an 81-year-old male client admitted for hip replacement surgery 2 days ago. The nurse reviews the Health History.

Health History:
81-year-old man admitted for hip replacement surgery 2 days ago. Prior to admission client lived alone and cared for himself. Client previously active, alert, and independent. However, since his surgery, he has been combative with the nurses. Client may be suffering from delirium related to the anesthesia from surgery, should resolve within a few days.

---

1. Based on the client information provided, what would be the nurse's priority nursing intervention?
   1. State clearly what needs to be done.
   2. Speak calmly and reassure the patient constantly.
   3. Provide reality orientation frequently.
   4. Provide safety and reduce anxiety.
   5. Administer an antianxiety medication.
   6. Call security for assistance.
   7. Allow the client to ventilate his feelings

Read the following situation and answer question 2.

2. The nurse is caring for an 80-year-old male client who is admitted to a long-term care facility because he has been unsafe living alone at home. The nurse reviews the Physician's Progress Notes in the medical record.

Physician's Progress Notes:
9/13/21 0700: 80-year-old man is admitted to a long-term care facility because he has been unsafe living alone at home. Client occasionally has gait disturbances that cause him to lose balance when ambulating. Recently, he has begun wandering unassisted at night. He has become increasingly irritable and agitated when approached by staff members. He is disoriented to time, place, and person. Recently diagnosed him Alzheimer disease. *Henry James, MD*

Highlight the problems that place the client at risk for injury.

Incontinence

Go to http://evolve.elsevier.com/Linton/medsurg/ for additional activities and exercises.

NCLEX CATEGORIES

Safe and Effective Care Environment:
Coordinated Care, Safety and Infection Control

Physiological Integrity: Basic Care and Comfort,
Physiological Adaptation

PART I: MASTERING THE BASICS

A. Key Terms
Match the definition or description in the numbered column with the most appropriate term in the lettered column.

1. _____ Term used to describe the passage of urine

2. _____ The most common cause of incontinence in older adults involving overactive detrusor muscle

3. _____ Bladder dysfunction caused by neurologic dysfunction associated with a spinal cord injury, pelvic radiation, or surgery

4. _____ Associated with nerve damage that causes the muscles of the pelvic floor to become weak

5. _____ Procedure used to empty the bladder by using the open hand to gently press on the abdomen over the bladder to promote urine passage

6. _____ Usually related to anal sphincter dysfunction caused by anal surgery, trauma during childbirth, Crohn disease affecting the anus, diabetic neuropathy, and laxatives

A. Anorectal incontinence
B. Overactive bladder
C. Credé technique
D. Bowel (fecal) incontinence
E. Micturition
F. Neurogenic bladder

B. Physiology of Urination

1. Which factors are required for normal controlled voiding? Select all that apply.
   1. Patent urethra
   2. Healthy detrusor muscle
   3. Mental alertness
   4. Constricted bladder sphincter
   5. Nerve impulse transmission

C. Types of Urinary Incontinence
Choose the most appropriate answer.

1. Which type of urinary incontinence typically has a sudden or more recent onset and is associated with treatable factors?
   1. Established
   2. Persistent
   3. Transient
   4. Stress urinary incontinence

2. Which type of urinary incontinence is determined after reversible causes of incontinence have been addressed?
   1. Established (persistent)
   2. Prompted
   3. Transient
   4. Acute

3. List the treatable factors of transient urinary incontinence that can remembered by the acronym DRIP.

D _____

R _____

I _____

P _____

Match the definition or description in the numbered column with the most appropriate term in the lettered column.

4. _____ The term used when a person is incontinent because of an inability to get to the toilet due to physical or cognitive impairments, the inability to manage the mechanics of toileting, or environmental barriers

5. _____ The involuntary loss of urine associated with an overdistended bladder

6. _____ The involuntary loss of urine associated with a strong, sudden urge to void; most often results from an overactive detrusor (bladder)

7. _____ The involuntary loss of small amounts of urine during physical activity that increases abdominal pressure

8. _____ The co-occurrence of stress and urge incontinence

A. Stress urinary incontinence
B. Urge urinary incontinence
C. Overflow urinary incontinence
D. Mixed urinary incontinence
E. Functional urinary incontinence

D. Common Therapeutic Measures for Urinary Incontinence

Match the definition or description in the numbered column with the most appropriate term in the lettered column.

1. _____ Intended to help the patient recognize incontinence and to ask caregivers for help with toileting

2. _____ Timed voiding based on voiding diary kept for 3–5 days to determine voiding pattern

3. _____ Includes anticholinergics and smooth muscle relaxants

4. _____ Uses patient education, scheduled voiding, and positive reinforcement

5. _____ Internal, external, and self-catheterization

6. _____ A device that is applied to the penis to compress the urethra and prevent the passage of urine

7. _____ Products designed to absorb urine faster and wick it away from the skin, with a fabric-type layer that stays dry to minimize moisture on the skin and maceration

8. _____ Uses electronic or mechanical sensors to give feedback about physiologic activity

9. _____ Commonly called *Kegel exercises*

10. _____ Performed to remove obstructions, treat severe bladder overactivity, implant an artificial sphincter, reposition the sphincter unit, improve perineal support, and inject substances that increase urethral compression (suburethral bulking agents)

11. _____ A device similar to a diaphragm that is inserted into the vagina that lifts and holds the pelvic organs in place; may be used to treat stress incontinence

12. _____ Retained in the vagina to strengthen muscles of pelvic floor

13. _____ Used to gain control of the bladder to prevent leakage by interrupting bladder urge

A. Pelvic muscle exercises
B. Bladder training
C. Penile compression device
D. Habit training
E. Pessary
F. Drug therapy
G. Biofeedback
H. Incontinence garments and pads
I. Prompted voiding
J. Urine collection devices
K. Vaginal cones
L. Urge suppression
M. Surgical treatment

14. Which factors contribute to overflow incontinence? Select all that apply.
    1. Urethral obstruction
    2. Spinal cord injury
    3. Underactive bladder muscle
    4. Impaired nerve impulse transmission
    5. Postanesthesia
    6. Dementia

PART II: PUTTING IT ALL TOGETHER

E. Multiple Choice/Multiple Response

Choose the most appropriate answer or select all that apply.

1. Drugs that may cause urinary retention include:
    1. chlorothiazides and loop diuretics.
    2. antihypertensives and insulin.
    3. anticholinergic and antihistamine medications.
    4. antibiotics and antiviral drugs.

2. The amount of urine remaining in the bladder after voiding is called the:
    1. urodynamic series.
    2. clean catch.
    3. voiding duration.
    4. postvoid residual volume.

3. How much urine normally remains in the bladder after voiding?
    1. 50 mL or less
    2. 100 mL or less
    3. 200 mL or less
    4. 250 mL or less

4. The patient has overflow incontinence. What serious reaction may occur in this patient if the bladder becomes overdistended?
    1. Stress incontinence
    2. Orthostatic hypotension
    3. Autonomic dysreflexia
    4. Tachycardia

5. When a person has a normal bladder but voids inappropriately because of an inability to get to the toilet, this is called:
    1. urge incontinence.
    2. functional incontinence.
    3. overflow incontinence.
    4. stress incontinence.

6. Stimuli that may encourage voiding include:
    1. decreasing the fluid intake to less than 2000 mL/day.
    2. drinking caffeine and cola drinks.
    3. tapping the suprapubic area and stroking the inner thigh.
    4. pouring warm water over the perineum and drinking water while on the toilet.

7. What is the most common cause of incontinence in older adults?
    1. Bladder overactivity (urge incontinence)
    2. Obstruction of urine flow
    3. Relaxation of pelvic floor muscles
    4. Confusion and immobility

8. The treatment for fecal neurogenic incontinence is to:
    1. cleanse the colon, usually with enemas and suppositories.
    2. treat the underlying medical condition.
    3. schedule toileting based on the patient's usual time of defecation.
    4. teach pelvic muscle exercises and biofeedback.

9. What is the initial treatment for a patient with anorectal bowel incontinence?
    1. Cleansing the colon
    2. Identify and treat the cause
    3. Pelvic muscle exercises with or without biofeedback
    4. Scheduled toileting

10. The cause of overflow bowel incontinence is:
    1. nerve damage that causes weak pelvic muscles.
    2. colon or rectal disease.
    3. loss of anal reflexes in patients with dementia.
    4. constipation in which the rectum is constantly distended.

11. A patient with bowel overflow incontinence may need laxatives to:
    1. immediately relieve constipation.
    2. stimulate peristalsis.
    3. improve the loss of anal sphincter tone.
    4. reverse the loss of the anal reflex.

12. What is a common reason for urethral obstruction in males?
    1. Vasoconstriction
    2. Hypertension
    3. Kidney obstruction
    4. Prostate enlargement

13. Which diagnostic procedure is used to determine whether the patient is emptying the bladder completely?
    1. Postvoid residual volume
    2. Imaging procedures
    3. Cystometry
    4. Urodynamic testing

14. Which methods of treatment are used for urge urinary incontinence? Select all that apply.
    1. Anticholinergics
    2. Muscarinic receptor antagonist (antispasmodics)
    3. Beta agonists
    4. Catheterization
    5. Behavior modification

15. Which patients usually require intermittent catheterization only once or twice before normal bladder function returns? Select all that apply.
    1. Postoperative patient
    2. Spinal cord–injured patient
    3. Alzheimer patient
    4. Postpartum patient
    5. Patient with urinary tract infection

16. Which activities may lead to stress incontinence? Select all that apply.
    1. Coughing
    2. Laughing
    3. Lifting
    4. Nervous system disorder
    5. Urethral obstruction
    6. Sneezing

17. Which are contributing factors to stress incontinence? Select all that apply.
    1. Postpartum pelvic floor muscle relaxation
    2. Spinal cord injury
    3. Postanesthesia
    4. Obesity
    5. Aging

18. Which are methods of treatment for a person with stress incontinence? Select all that apply.
    1. Scheduled voiding
    2. Pelvic muscle exercises
    3. Bladder training
    4. Avoid fluids with caffeine
    5. Use of contigen (collagens)

19. Which are three general goals of treatment for the incontinent person? Select all that apply.
    1. Restoration or improvement of control for treatable incontinence.
    2. Management of irreversible incontinence.
    3. Recognition of incontinence as a normal age-related change.
    4. Prevention of complications.
    5. Pelvic muscle rehabilitation.
    6. Use of drug therapy.

20. Drug therapy is most effective in the treatment of:
    1. neurogenic incontinence.
    2. functional incontinence.
    3. stress incontinence.
    4. urge incontinence.

21. What does nursing care of the patient with incontinence address? Select all that apply.
    1. Measures to correct the specific type of incontinence
    2. Maintain skin integrity
    3. Improve situational low self-esteem
    4. Decreased fluid intake
    5. Improve knowledge of management

22. What does data collection relative to urinary incontinence include? Select all that apply.
    1. Physical findings
    2. Urine volume
    3. Scheduling surgical intervention
    4. Recording the voiding pattern
    5. Associated signs and symptoms
    6. Obtaining prescriptions for patient to begin drug therapy
    7. Medications patient is using
    8. Medical history

23. Assessment of bowel incontinence includes: (Select all that apply.)
    1. Performing an abdominal assessment
    2. Recording the usual bowel pattern
    3. Improve situational low self-esteem
    4. Characteristics of stool
    5. Related symptoms
    6. Training for pelvic floor exercises and biofeedback
    7. Activities
    8. Diet and fluid intake
    9. Medication being taken
    10. Use of aids to help elimination
    11. Encourage good grooming

PART III: CHALLENGE YOURSELF!

F. Getting Ready for NCLEX
Choose the most appropriate answer or select all that apply.

1. The nurse is taking care of a patient with bowel overflow incontinence. What is the first step in medical management of bowel overflow incontinence?
    1. Treat the underlying medical condition.
    2. Teach pelvic muscle exercises and biofeedback.
    3. Cleanse the colon, often with enemas and suppositories.
    4. Schedule toileting based on the patient's usual time of defecation.

2. A patient has bowel incontinence. What does the nurse provide for the patient to prevent constipation? Select all that apply.
    1. Protein
    2. Fiber
    3. Carbohydrates
    4. Potassium
    5. Fluids

3. A patient is scheduled for a cystoscopy and asks the nurse what this test is. The nurse answers that cystoscopy:
    1. evaluates the neuromuscular function of the bladder.
    2. may be prescribed to create images of the urinary structures.
    3. uses a scope inserted through the urethra to visualize the urethra and bladder.
    4. detects involuntary passage of urine when abdominal pressure increases.

4. A patient with neurogenic bowel incontinence is not able to voluntarily delay defecation. Which intervention can correct this condition?
    1. Scheduled toileting
    2. Pelvic floor muscle exercises
    3. Administer laxatives
    4. Relieve constipation

5. Which foods thicken the stool in a patient with bowel incontinence?
    1. Fruit juices
    2. Raw vegetables
    3. Chocolate
    4. Bananas

6. A patient with bowel incontinence asks the nurse which foods he can eat to avoid odor and gas. Which foods may cause odor and gas? Select all that apply.
    1. Broccoli
    2. Dairy products
    3. Cabbage
    4. Garlic
    5. Oatmeal
    6. Rice

G. Next-Generation NCLEX® Examination-Style Questions
Read the following situation and answer questions 1–2. For more information, refer to Nursing Care Plan, The Patient with Stress Urinary Incontinence, in your textbook.

The nurse is caring for an 80-year-old resident in a long-term care facility complains of having trouble "holding my urine." The nurse reviews the Physician's Progress Notes in the medical record.

> 09/17/21 1120: 80-year-old resident complains of having trouble "holding my urine." She is unable to control urine if she strains, coughs, or laughs. She is the mother of five children, all born at home. She reports no other complaints except for arthritis in her hips and knees and hypertension. Fear of losing control of her urine has caused her to avoid leaving her room except for meals. She is wearing perineal pads to keep her dry.
> Physical examination: Height 5' 3". Weight 179 lbs. Heart and breath sounds normal.

1. Highlight the symptoms are indicative of stress incontinence in this patient?

2. Drag the three contributing factors from the choices below to fill in each blank in the following sentence.

   The factors that have contributed to her stress incontinence include _____ 1 _____, _____ 2 _____, and _____ 3 _____.

Contributing Factors:
Age
Height 5'3
Arthritis
Hypertension
Mother of five
Obesity

3. What are the most important nursing interventions to improve her urinary control? Select all that apply.
   1. Instruct her how to do Kegel perineal exercises.
   2. Inspect the perineal area and buttocks, reporting signs of irritation.
   3. Advise to empty her bladder every 2 hours while awake.
   4. Decrease fluid intake.
   5. Discourage coffee, tea, and alcohol.

4. Which are the most important ways to reduce the risk for urinary tract infection in this patient? Select all that apply.
   1. Encourage her to empty her bladder as scheduled.
   2. Use strict aseptic technique during catheterization.
   3. Encourage an intake of 1500–3000 mL of fluid per day as tolerated.
   4. Decrease fluid intake to decrease incontinence.
   5. Pour warm water over the perineum and run water in the sink.
   6. Emphasize the importance of trying to delay voiding until the scheduled time.

Read the following situation and answer question below.

The nurse is caring for a 70-year-old man admitted to the surgical unit post left total knee replacement. The nurse reviews the Health History and vital signs.

Health History:
Urge incontinence
Enlarged prostate
Parkinson's disease.
Client has been taking Levodopa to manage his Parkinson's. He usually drinks three cups of coffee per day and smokes a pack of cigarettes every day.

BP	142/82 mm Hg
Pulse	88 BPM
Respirations	18 BPM
Temperature	99.7 F

3. Choose the most likely options for the information missing from the statements below by selecting from the list of options provided.

   His urge incontinence is most likely the result of _____ 1 _____, _____ 2 _____, _____ 3 _____, _____ and _____ 4 _____.

Options:
Hypertension
Medication effects
Coffee intake
Cigarette smoking
Enlarged prostate
Parkinson's disease
Infection

Nutrition

Go to http://evolve.elsevier.com/Linton/medsurg/ for additional activities and exercises.

NCLEX CATEGORIES

Psychosocial Integrity

Physiological Integrity: Basic Care and Comfort, Reduction of Risk Potential

PART I: MASTERING THE BASICS

A. Key Terms
Match the definition in the numbered column with the most appropriate term in the lettered column.

1. _____ Used to teach patients to identify, challenge, and correct negative thoughts about weight loss

2. _____ Focuses on the settings or chain of events that precede eating, the kinds of foods consumed, and the consequences of eating

3. _____ A condition caused by the lack of adequate glucose that causes an excessive breakdown of tissue protein, loss of sodium and other cations, and involuntary dehydration

4. _____ Feeling of fullness after eating

5. _____ Defined as having a BMI of 30 or higher

6. _____ A protein that contains all nine essential amino acids in sufficient quantity and ratio to meet the body's needs

A. Cognitive restructuring
B. Ketosis
C. Obesity
D. Satiety
E. Stimulus control
F. Complete protein

B. Nutritional Requirements of Healthy Adults

1. Which of the following are macronutrients? Select all that apply.
   1. Minerals
   2. Vitamins
   3. Hormones
   4. Carbohydrates
   5. Fats
   6. Proteins

2. Which are sources of protein in a healthy diet? Select all that apply.
   1. Fish
   2. Poultry
   3. Dry beans
   4. Eggs
   5. Rice
   6. Meat
   7. Nuts
   8. Soy products

List the number of kilocalories per gram provided by fats, carbohydrates, and protein.

3. Fats: _____

4. Carbohydrates: _____

5. Protein: _____

6. The four types of DRIs are:

   1. _____

   2. _____

   3. _____

   4. _____

C. MyPlate Guidelines

See Figure 15.1 in the book.

United States Department of Agriculture

10 tips
Nutrition
Education Series

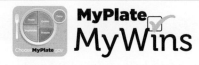
MyPlate
MyWins
Choose MyPlate

Based on the
Dietary Guidelines for Americans

Use MyPlate to build your healthy eating style and maintain it for a lifetime. Choose foods and beverages from each MyPlate food group. Make sure your choices are limited in sodium, saturated fat, and added sugars. Start with small changes to make healthier choices you can enjoy.

1 Find your healthy eating style
Creating a healthy style means regularly eating a variety of foods to get the nutrients and calories you need. MyPlate's tips help you create your own healthy eating solutions—"MyWins."

2 Make half your plate fruits and vegetables
Eating colorful fruits and vegetables is important because they provide vitamins and minerals and most are low in calories.

3 Focus on whole fruits
Choose whole fruits—fresh, frozen, dried, or canned in 100% juice. Enjoy fruit with meals, as snacks, or as a dessert.
Fruits

4 Vary your veggies
Try adding fresh, frozen, or canned vegetables to salads, sides, and main dishes. Choose a variety of colorful vegetables prepared in healthful ways: steamed, sauteed, roasted, or raw.
Vegetables

5 Make half your grains whole grains
Look for whole grains listed first or second on the ingredients list—try oatmeal, popcorn, whole-grain bread, and brown rice. Limit grain-based desserts and snacks, such as cakes, cookies, and pastries.
Grains

6 Move to low-fat or fat-free milk or yogurt
Choose low-fat or fat-free milk, yogurt, and soy beverages (soymilk) to cut back on saturated fat. Replace sour cream, cream, and regular cheese with low-fat yogurt, milk, and cheese.
Dairy

7 Vary your protein routine
Mix up your protein foods to include seafood, beans and peas, unsalted nuts and seeds, soy products, eggs, and lean meats and poultry. Try main dishes made with beans or seafood like tuna salad or bean chili.
Protein

8 Drink and eat beverages and food with less sodium, saturated fat, and added sugars
Use the Nutrition Facts label and ingredients list to limit items high in sodium, saturated fat, and added sugars. Choose vegetable oils instead of butter, and oil-based sauces and dips instead of ones with butter, cream, or cheese.
Limit

9 Drink water instead of sugary drinks
Water is calorie-free. Non-diet soda, energy or sports drinks, and other sugar-sweetened drinks contain a lot of calories from added sugars and have few nutrients.

10 Everything you eat and drink matters
The right mix of foods can help you be healthier now and into the future. Turn small changes into your "MyPlate, MyWins."

Center for Nutrition Policy and Promotion
USDA is an equal opportunity provider, employer, and lender.

Go to **ChooseMyPlate**.gov
for more information.

DG TipSheet No. 1
June 2011
Revised October 2016

1. What are the five food groups included in the USDA MyPlate guidelines?

   _____

   _____

   _____

   _____

   _____

Refer to the food checklist in Figure 15.2 in your book to answer questions 2–4.

United States Department of Agriculture

 MyPlate Daily Checklist
Find your Healthy Eating Style

Everything you eat and drink matters. Find your healthy eating style that reflects your preferences, culture, traditions, and budget—and maintain it for a lifetime! The right mix can help you be healthier now and into the future. The key is choosing a variety of foods and beverages from each food group—*and making sure that each choice is limited in saturated fat, sodium, and added sugars.* Start with small changes—**"MyWins"**—to make healthier choices you can enjoy.

Food Group Amounts for 1,800 Calories a Day

Fruits	Vegetables	Grains	Protein	Dairy
1 1/2 cups	**2 1/2 cups**	**6 ounces**	**5 ounces**	**3 cups**
Focus on whole fruits	Vary your veggies	Make half your grains whole grains	Vary your protein routine	Move to low-fat or fat-free milk or yogurt
Focus on whole fruits that are fresh, frozen, canned, or dried.	Choose a variety of colorful fresh, frozen, and canned vegetables—make sure to include dark green, red, and orange choices.	Find whole-grain foods by reading the Nutrition Facts label and ingredients list.	Mix up your protein foods to include seafood, beans and peas, unsalted nuts and seeds, soy products, eggs, and lean meats and poultry.	Choose fat-free milk, yogurt, and soy beverages (soy milk) to cut back on your saturated fat.

Limit Drink and eat less sodium, saturated fat, and added sugars. Limit:
- Sodium to **2,300 milligrams** a day.
- Saturated fat to **20 grams** a day.
- Added sugars to **45 grams** a day.

Be active your way: Children 6 to 17 years old should move **60 minutes** every day. Adults should be physically active at least **2 1/2 hours** per week.
Use SuperTracker to create a personal plan based on your age, sex, height, weight, and physical activity level.
SuperTracker.usda.gov

MyPlate Daily Checklist

Write down the foods you ate today and track your daily MyPlate, MyWins!

Food group targets for a 1,800 calorie* pattern are:

		Write your food choices for each food group	Did you reach your target?
Fruits	**1 1/2 cups** 1 cup of fruits counts as • 1 cup raw or cooked fruit; or • 1/2 cup dried fruit; or • 1 cup 100% fruit juice.	_____	Y N
Vegetables	**2 1/2 cups** 1 cup vegetables counts as • 1 cup raw or cooked vegetables; or • 2 cups leafy salad greens; or • 1 cup 100% vegetable juice.	_____	Y N
Grains	**6 ounce equivalents** 1 ounce of grains counts as • 1 slice bread; or • 1 ounce ready-to-eat cereal; or • 1/2 cup cooked rice, pasta, or cereal.	_____	Y N
Protein	**5 ounce equivalents** 1 ounce of protein counts as • 1 ounce lean meat, poultry, or seafood; or • 1 egg; or • 1 Tbsp peanut butter; or • 1/4 cup cooked beans or peas; or • 1/2 ounce nuts or seeds.	_____	Y N
Dairy	**3 cups** 1 cup of dairy counts as • 1 cup milk; or • 1 cup yogurt; or • 1 cup fortified soy beverage; or • 1 1/2 ounces natural cheese or 2 ounces processed cheese.	_____	Y N

Limit Limit:
- Sodium to **2,300 milligrams** a day.
- Saturated fat to **20 grams** a day.
- Added sugars to **45 grams** a day.

Y N

Activity Be active your way:
Adults:
- Be physically active at least **2 1/2 hours** per week.

Children 6 to 17 years old:
- Move at least **60 minutes** every day.

Y N

* This 1,800 calorie pattern is only an estimate of your needs. Monitor your body weight and adjust your calories if needed.

MyWins Track your MyPlate, MyWins
_____

Center for Nutrition Policy and Promotion
January 2016
USDA is an equal opportunity provider and employer.

2. In the daily food plan consisting of 1800 calories, what are the recommended amounts of foods in the following categories?

   a. Vegetables: _____

   b. Protein foods: _____

3. How much physical activity is recommended for adults?

   _____

   _____

4. What are limits on the following items in the My Daily Food Plan?

   a. Sugar: _____

   b. Saturated fat: _____

   c. Sodium: _____

D. Nutrition Labels

Refer to the figure below (Figure 15.3 in your book) to answer questions 1–6.

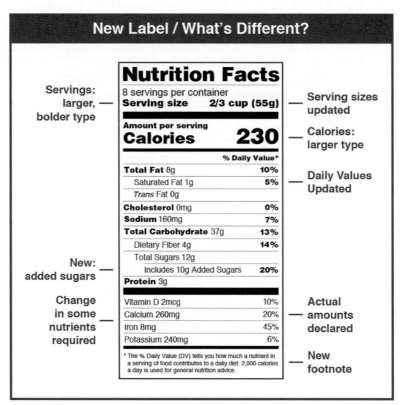

Example of a nutrition label. Courtesy of the U.S. Food and Drug administration.

1. How many calories per serving are provided? _____

2. How many servings are in this container? _____

3. What is the size of one serving? _____

4. What percentage daily value of vitamin A is provided in one serving? _____

5. How many calories are provided in one container? _____

6. a. What is the recommended daily fiber amount for a person on a 2000-calorie diet?

      _____

   b. How much many grams of dietary fiber are in each serving? _____

E. Vegetarian and Vegan Diets
Match the definition in the numbered column with the most appropriate term in the lettered column.

1. _____ A diet that includes milk, cheese, and other dairy products but excludes meat, fish, poultry, and eggs

2. _____ A person who consumes no foods of animal origin

3. _____ A diet that includes dairy products and eggs but excludes meat, fish, and poultry

A. Vegan
B. Lactovegetarian
C. Lacto-ovo-vegetarian

F. Management of Obesity

1. What is the ideal BMI?
   1. 20–25
   2. 30 and above
   3. 14
   4. 120 lbs.

2. What are strategies for modifying one's lifestyle? Select all that apply.
   1. Goal setting
   2. Stimulus control
   3. Cognitive restructuring
   4. Increasing intake of complete proteins
   5. Lowering cholesterol
   6. Problem solving
   7. Relapse prevention

3. Indicate what a balanced, calorie-restricted diet generally consists of.
   1. _____
   2. _____
   3. _____
   4. _____
   5. _____

4. Vitamins and minerals are needed when daily intakes of calories are below what level?

   Male _____ Female _____

G. Underweight
Choose the most appropriate answer or select all that apply.

1. What does a person who is in the state of starvation produce less of, therefore creating a negative balance?
   1. Nitrogen
   2. Glucose
   3. Glycogen
   4. Hormones

2. An underweight person is what percentage below the normal standard?
   1. 15%–20%
   2. 30%
   3. 10%
   4. 50%

3. What are some factors that may cause a patient to be underweight? Select all that apply.
   1. Insufficient food intake to meet activity needs
   2. Excessive activity
   3. Poor absorption and use of food consumed
   4. Consuming only vegetables
   5. Wasting disease
   6. Psychological or emotional stress

H. Nutritional Delivery Methods for Feeding Problems
*Match the definition in the numbered column with the most appropriate term in the lettered column. **Answers may be used more than once.***

1. _____ Feedings that deliver nutrients directly into the stomach or small intestine for patients who cannot take oral feedings

2. _____ Complications of this type of feeding can include nasal irritation, sinusitis, pharyngeal or vocal cord paralysis, nausea or vomiting, diarrhea, GI bleeding, aspiration pneumonia, electrolyte imbalances, hyperglycemia, and nutrition deficiencies

3. _____ Changing from one type of feeding to another; must be done gradually to prevent nutritional recovery syndrome with hypophosphatemia and possible hypokalemia

4. _____   Used for a short period of time
              because it does not supply all
              nutritional requirements

A. Peripheral parenteral
B. Transitional
C. Enteral

PART II: PUTTING IT ALL TOGETHER

I. Multiple Choice/Multiple Response

Choose the most appropriate answer or select all that apply.

1. What is the recommended daily fiber intake for adult women and men?
   1. 30–33 g for women and 60–63 g for men
   2. 10–14 g for women and 15–20 g for men
   3. 25–28 g for women and 31–34 g for men
   4. 10–20 g for women and 15–25 g for men

2. What is the recommended percentage of saturated fats in the diet ?
   1. 25%
   2. 14%
   3. 100%
   4. Less than 10%

3. What is the recommended daily reference intake of protein for adult?
   1. 115 g for men and 100 g for women
   2. 56 g for men and 46 g for women
   3. 75 g for men and 70 g for women
   4. 35 g for men and 20 g for women

4. Which diseases are associated with obesity? Select all that apply.
   1. Coronary artery disease
   2. Hyperkalemia
   3. Lipid disorder
   4. Type 2 diabetes mellitus
   5. Stroke
   6. Anemia

5. The areas covered during a nutritional assessment include: (Select all that apply.)
   1. Dietary history
   2. Electrocardiogram
   3. Laboratory data (if available)
   4. Anthropometric data
   5. Physical examination data

6. Which measurements are used to determine body composition?
   1. Height divided by weight
   2. Skinfold thickness and hydrostatic weighing
   3. Serum albumin lab
   4. Nitrogen balance

7. What information can be determined during a nutritional assessment when using the common 24-hour recall and food frequency tools?
   1. BMI
   2. Risk for type 2 diabetes mellitus
   3. Dietary deficits and excesses
   4. Goals for weekly weight loss

8. In addition to the diseases associated with obesity, it is also considered a risk factor for which medical conditions? Select all that apply.
   1. Some kinds of cancer
   2. Scurvy
   3. Joint disease
   4. Pellagra
   5. Gallstones
   6. Respiratory problems

9. Which conditions interfere with the taking in of liquids, and therefore may require enteral feeding? Select all that apply.
   1. Oral surgery
   2. Hyperglycemia
   3. Dysphagia
   4. Alkalosis
   5. Unconsciousness
   6. Anorexia
   7. Esophageal obstruction

10. List the feeding methods for enteral nutrition.

    1. _____

    2. _____

    3. _____

    4. _____

    5. _____

11. What are the major types of parenteral feedings? Select the correct two answers.
    1. Transitional feeding
    2. Nasogastric tube
    3. TPN or CPN
    4. PPN

12. What is a complication of enteral tube feedings when viscous formulas and crushed medications are inadequately flushed?
    1. Dumping syndrome
    2. Diarrhea
    3. GI bleeding
    4. Tube blockage

13. When moving from enteral to oral feedings, the patient may experience:
    1. breathing difficulties.
    2. bleeding at the TPN site.
    3. heart palpitations.
    4. poor appetite.

14. What is the condition that occurs when hypertonic fluid enters the jejunum; water is drawn into the lumen of the intestine to dilute the fluid, causing a drop in circulating blood volume?
    1. Dumping syndrome
    2. Tube blockage
    3. Hyponatremia
    4. Aspiration pneumonia

15. Dehydration is the most common fluid and electrolyte disturbance in older adults. How much daily water intake is recommended?
    1. 6–8 glasses/day
    2. 30–35 mL/kg of ideal body weight
    3. One glass of water with each meal
    4. 15–20 mL/kg of ideal body weight

16. The diet for older adults should include:
    1. low-fat foods.
    2. low-sodium foods.
    3. all of the food groups.
    4. high-protein foods.

17. For what deficiency are older adults with chronic diseases at increased risk?
    1. Protein deficiency
    2. Vitamin deficiency
    3. Mineral deficiency
    4. Carbohydrate deficiency

18. Which nutrient must be eaten daily, as it cannot be stored in the body?
    1. Carbohydrates
    2. Protein
    3. Lipids
    4. Minerals

19. What nutrition-related metabolic change occurs in older adults?
    1. BMR decreases.
    2. Lean body mass increases.
    3. Plasma glucose levels decrease.
    4. Tolerance to glucose decreases.

20. What is measured by skin calipers?
    1. Cholesterol
    2. Body surface area (BSA)
    3. Muscle tissue
    4. Subcutaneous fat tissue

21. What are the signs and symptoms of protein deficiency? Select all that apply.
    1. Edema
    2. Dehydration
    3. Wasting
    4. Subcutaneous fat tissue
    5. Thickening and hardening of the skin
    6. Decreased enzyme development
    7. Diminished immune response
    8. Weakness
    9. Lack of energy

PART III: CHALLENGE YOURSELF!

J. Getting Ready for NCLEX
Choose the most appropriate answer or select all that apply.

1. Which are grain products? Select all that apply.
   1. Oatmeal
   2. White bread
   3. Lima beans
   4. Saltine crackers
   5. Spaghetti

2. A health care provider has suggested a soft/low-residue diet for a patient with colitis. Which of these foods would be appropriate for a low-residue diet? Select all that apply.
   1. Pastas
   2. Casseroles
   3. Moist, tender meats
   4. Salads
   5. Bran
   6. Canned/cooked fruits and vegetables
   7. Desserts, cakes, and cookies without nuts or coconut

3. A postmenopausal woman asks the nurse about calcium requirements to prevent osteoporosis. What amount of daily calcium intake is recommended?
   1. 250 mg/day
   2. 4000 IU
   3. 1000–1500 mg/day
   4. Weekly injections of 3000 mg

4. The laboratory data of a patient whose nutritional status is being assessed has a transferrin saturation of 15%. Which condition does this indicate?
   1. Anemia
   2. Iron overload
   3. Anorexia
   4. Obesity

5. The nurse is taking care of an older adult. One nutrient that older people need less of is:
   1. complex carbohydrate.
   2. sugar.
   3. protein.
   4. lipid.

6. The nurse is taking the history of an older adult who has anorexia. The nurse explains to the patient that this may be due to an age-related change of:
   1. decreased tolerance to glucose.
   2. change in appetite responses.
   3. periodontal disease.
   4. decreased salivary secretions.

7. The nurse is collecting data for the dietary history of a patient. Which are signs of malnutrition? Select all that apply.
   1. Shiny hair
   2. Smooth skin
   3. Pale face
   4. Red conjunctiva
   5. Swollen lips
   6. Bleeding gums

8. The nurse is taking care of a patient who has returned from surgery to the medical floor. He is on a clear liquid diet. Which of the following are included in a clear liquid diet? Select all that apply.
   1. Ice cream
   2. Custard
   3. Cream soup
   4. Fat-free broth
   5. Coffee
   6. Popsicles

9. The nurse is taking care of a patient who is on a mechanical soft diet. Which foods on the patient's tray should the nurse question?
   1. Cottage cheese
   2. Rice
   3. Bananas
   4. Cookies without nuts

10. The nurse is teaching a patient about foods allowed on a high-fiber diet. The patient has been on a low-residue diet for 5 days. Which of the following food is not allowed on a low-residue diet, but is allowed on a high-fiber diet?
    1. Pastas
    2. Canned cooked vegetables
    3. Fresh uncooked fruits
    4. Cream soups

Intravenous Therapy

chapter

16

Go to http://evolve.elsevier.com/Linton/medsurg/ for additional activities and exercises.

NCLEX CATEGORIES

Physiological Integrity: Pharmacological Therapies, Reduction of Risk Potential

PART I: MASTERING THE BASICS

A. Key Terms
Match the definition in the numbered column with the most appropriate term in the lettered column. Not all terms may be used.

1. _____ A liquid containing one or more dissolved substances

2. _____ A term used to describe a solution that has a higher concentration of electrolytes than normal body fluids

3. _____ A term used to describe a solution that has the same concentration of electrolytes as normal body fluids

4. _____ A term used to describe a solution that has a lower concentration of electrolytes than normal body fluids

5. _____ A measure of the concentration of electrolytes in a fluid

6. _____ Describes both a needle and a catheter

A. Hypotonic
B. Cannula
C. Solution
D. Hypertonic
E. Extravasation
F. Isotonic
G. Tonicity

Match the definition or description in the numbered column with the most appropriate term in the lettered column.

7. _____ Leakage of fluid from a blood vessel

8. _____ Piece of catheter breaks off in a vein

9. _____ Skin torn or irritated by tape or insertion of cannula

10. _____ Blood clot

11. _____ Obstruction caused by trapped embolus

12. _____ Collection of infused fluid in tissue surrounding the cannula

13. _____ Unattached blood clot or other substance in the circulatory system

14. _____ Inflammation of the vein

A. Thrombus
B. Embolism
C. Infiltration
D. Catheter embolus
E. Embolus
F. Trauma
G. Phlebitis
H. Extravasation

PART II: PUTTING IT ALL TOGETHER

B. Multiple Choice/Multiple Response
Choose the most appropriate answer or select all that apply.

1. Irrigation of an occluded IV cannula is not recommended because:
   1. the IV cannula may become infiltrated.
   2. clots may be forced into the bloodstream.
   3. the IV cannula may become dislodged.
   4. thrombophlebitis may occur.

2. An IV solution of 0.45% sodium chloride is given if the patient has experienced:
   1. excessive water loss.
   2. cerebral edema.
   3. excessive sodium loss.
   4. burns.

3. In which position should the nurse place a patient if air accidentally enters a central line?
   1. On the left side
   2. On the right side
   3. Semi-Fowler's
   4. Fowler's

4. Which statement is true about factors affecting the IV infusion rate?
   1. When the fluid container is raised, the fluid flows slower.
   2. As the fluid container empties, the rate slows down.
   3. Thick fluids flow faster than thin fluids.
   4. By straightening out the extremity, the fluid flows slower.

5. The nurse notices that the IV on the patient is running too fast. To slow the rate down, the nurse:
   1. vents the IV container.
   2. splints the arm with an arm board.
   3. turns the arm so that the IV site is free.
   4. uses the roller clamp to adjust flow rate.

6. Which are symptoms of an air embolus? Select all that apply.
   1. Pulmonary edema
   2. Frothy, pink sputum
   3. Shortness of breath
   4. Chest pain
   5. Hypertension
   6. Possible shock

7. Edema, coolness, and pain at the IV insertion site are indications of:
   1. thrombophlebitis.
   2. infection.
   3. air embolus.
   4. infiltration.

8. Which IV complication is characterized by redness, swelling, and warmth?
   1. Phlebitis
   2. Infiltration
   3. Hemorrhage
   4. Catheter embolus

9. A patient's IV has been running too fast over the past hour. Which are signs of fluid volume excess? Select all that apply.
   1. Confusion
   2. Bounding pulse
   3. Inflammation
   4. Redness
   5. Increased blood pressure
   6. Dyspnea

10. If signs of fluid volume excess occur, the nurse should:
    1. turn the patient to the right side.
    2. elevate the head of the bed.
    3. check the vital signs.
    4. use strict aseptic technique.

11. The patient with an air embolus is placed on the left side to trap air in the:
    1. left atrium so that it can be gradually absorbed.
    2. right ventricle so that it is not transferred to the lungs.
    3. left ventricle so that it is not transferred to the lungs.
    4. right atrium so that it can be gradually absorbed.

12. Which nursing intervention may prevent fluid volume excess during IV therapy?
    1. Encourage the patient to ambulate.
    2. Encourage the patient to cough.
    3. Time-tape the IV bag and monitor closely.
    4. Keep an accurate intake and output record.

13. What does a "drop factor of 15" mean?
    1. The infusion set will deliver 15 mL of fluid for every drop.
    2. The infusion set will deliver 1 mL of fluid for every 15 drops.
    3. The infusion set will deliver 1 mL of fluid in 15 minutes.
    4. The infusion set will deliver 15 mL of fluid in 1 minute.

14. How much air does it take to cause an air embolism in an adult?
    1. 5 mL
    2. 10 mL
    3. 15 mL
    4. 25 mL

15. An IV fluid container should not be used for more than:
    1. 12 hours.
    2. 24 hours.
    3. 48 hours.
    4. 72 hours.

16. When should central lines be used for IV therapy, rather than peripheral veins? Select all that apply.
    1. The client has healthy veins
    2. The client requires long-term therapy
    3. The client has poor peripheral veins
    4. The client needs irritating or vesicant drugs or fluids to be administered

17. Which descriptions indicate the best sites for IV insertion? Select all that apply.
    1. Use the least restrictive site.
    2. Use a small vein that is in good condition.
    3. Use a soft, straight vein.
    4. Use the nondominant arm.
    5. Begin with the most proximal vein and move distally as needed.

18. How many calories does a patient receive for each 1% of dextrose in a liter of fluid?
    1. 0 calories
    2. 34 calories
    3. 10 calories for each pound of patient's weight
    4. 117 calories

19. What devices are available for intravenous therapy? Select all that apply.
    1. Outside-needle catheters
    2. Subcutaneously implanted pumps
    3. Over-the-needle catheters
    4. Needles
    5. Subcutaneous infusion ports

20. What are the "six rights" that should be checked when administering intravenous fluids?

    1. _____
    2. _____
    3. _____
    4. _____
    5. _____
    6. _____

21. What influences the rate when an infusion flows by gravity? Select all that apply.
    1. The height of the fluid container
    2. Fluid volume in the container
    3. Fluid viscosity
    4. Cannula diameter
    5. Venting of the fluid container
    6. Type of port
    7. Position of extremity

22. What is the possible complication of irrigating to clear an obstructed cannula?
    1. Delay of the infusion
    2. Irritation of the site
    3. Air embolism
    4. Forcing a blood clot into the bloodstream

23. What precaution is necessary with central lines to avoid an air embolism, which can be fatal?
    1. Use correct cannula size.
    2. Make sure drug is compatible with infusion fluid.
    3. Prevent air entering the line.
    4. Determine the correct rate of infusion.

PART III: CHALLENGE YOURSELF!

C. Getting Ready for NCLEX
Choose the most appropriate answer or select all that apply.

1. The nurse is taking care of a patient with decreased cardiac output related to blood loss through a disrupted intravenous line. Which is the outcome criterion for this patient?
   1. Pulse and blood pressure within normal limits
   2. Patient activities completed without disruption of intravenous therapy
   3. Normal body temperature; no purulent drainage or redness at venipuncture site
   4. Fluid output equal to intake; no dyspnea or edema

2. The nurse is checking a patient with an IV in the left arm. Which signs of complications of IV therapy, if observed in this patient, should be documented and reported to the charge nurse? Select all that apply.
   1. Palpitations
   2. Cyanosis
   3. Blood return
   4. Edema
   5. Redness
   6. Swelling at the infusion site

3. The nurse is making rounds at 7:00 AM, and notes that the patient's IV has 900 mL and is running at 75 mL/hour as prescribed. When checking the IV on 10:00 AM rounds, the nurse notes that there is only 100 mL remaining. Which observation indicates to the nurse that the patient is experiencing a complication of the IV therapy?
   1. Flushing of the face
   2. Nausea and vomiting
   3. Bounding pulse
   4. Diarrhea

4. A patient complains of crushing chest pain and difficulty breathing and has a rapid, thready pulse. The nurse suspects that the patient is experiencing an air embolism. Which interventions are appropriate?
   1. Turn the patient onto his left side, raise the head of the bed, and notify the charge nurse or health care provider.
   2. Turn the patient onto his left side, lower the head of the bed, and notify the charge nurse or health care provider.
   3. Place the patient on his back, lower the head of the bed, and notify the charge nurse.
   4. Ambulate the patient for 15 minutes and notify the charge nurse.

5. The nurse checks a patient's IV site and finds that the vein is swollen and warm to touch . The IV is running well, but the site is red; the patient tells the nurse that the site is "sore when touched." These findings are indications of:
   1. infiltration.
   2. catheter embolus.
   3. air embolus.
   4. phlebitis.

6. The nurse checked the patient's IV 1 hour ago, and it was running at the correct rate of 50 mL/hour. Now the IV is running at 100 mL/hour. What may be the cause of this increased rate?
   1. The tubing has a kink in it.
   2. The clamp has slipped.
   3. The fluid container is too low.
   4. The filter is blocked.

7. Because older people often have less efficient cardiac function, the nurse should monitor an older person with an IV for:
   1. fluid volume excess.
   2. bleeding.
   3. infection.
   4. infiltration.

8. An older patient is receiving IV fluids to treat dehydration. When the patient complains of pain and a burning sensation at the IV site, assessment observations reveal that the IV site is pale, puffy, and cool. Which complication does the nurse suspect?
   1. Phlebitis
   2. Infiltration
   3. Fluid volume excess
   4. Embolism

9. The patient is an 80-year-old male with a history of high blood pressure. When the nurse comes in to give him a bath, she notices that his IV of D_5W, which was hung 1 hour before she came into his room, contains 500 mL. The prescription was for 1000 mL to run over 8 hours. The nurse should observe him for signs of:
   1. infection.
   2. shock.
   3. hemorrhage.
   4. heart failure.

10. While a patient is receiving an IV, his blood pressure is 145/90 mm Hg, the pulse is 110 bpm and bounding, and the patient reports difficulty breathing. After the nurse slows the infusion, what nursing intervention is appropriate?
    1. Monitor his vital signs hourly.
    2. Inspect the infusion site for swelling and bleeding.
    3. Elevate the head of his bed.
    4. Check connections to be sure they are secure.

11. A patient was admitted for nausea and vomiting that had lasted for the past 3 days. Intravenous fluids were begun at 150 mL/hour via a 21-gauge cannula. The IV was started at 1:00 PM. How much fluid should have been administered by 3:30 PM that same day? _____

12. The nurse has a prescription to discontinue a patient's IV after 24 hours. There were no complications of IV therapy. What must be recorded after discontinuing his IV? Select all that apply.
    1. Size of cannula
    2. Appearance of IV site
    3. Blood pressure
    4. Weight
    5. How the patient tolerated the procedure
    6. Respirations

13. The nurse is taking care of a patient with an IV. Which assignment is appropriate for the LPN to make to the unlicensed assistive personnel (UAP)?
    1. Ask the UAP to slow the infusion rate when it is flowing too fast.
    2. Ask the UAP to determine the best site.
    3. Ask the UAP to start the IV.
    4. Ask the UAP to protect the IV infusion while providing basic care.

14. The nurse is preparing to discontinue an IV in a patient. Place the following steps of this procedure in the proper order, with 1 being the first step and 5 being the last step.
    A. _____ Loosen or remove the tape and dressing.
    B. _____ Remove the cannula, keeping the hub parallel to the skin.
    C. _____ Gently press a dry gauze pad over the site.
    D. _____ Put on gloves.
    E. _____ Stop the flow of the fluid.

15. A patient is receiving intermittent infusions. How often should the nurse change the administration sets?
    1. 96 hours
    2. 24 hours
    3. 12 hours
    4. 8 hours

16. A patient is receiving continuous infusions that do not contain blood, blood products, or lipids. How often should the nurse change the administration sets?
    1. 96 hours
    2. 24 hours
    3. 12 hours
    4. 8 hours

Surgery

Go to http://evolve.elsevier.com/Linton/medsurg/ for additional activities and exercises.

NCLEX CATEGORIES

Safe and Effective Care Environment:
Coordinated Care

Physiological Integrity: Pharmacological
Therapies, Reduction of Risk Potential,
Physiological Adaptation

PART I: MASTERING THE BASICS

A. Types of Surgery

Match the descriptions of surgery types in the numbered column with surgery term in the lettered column. Some answers may be used more than once.

1. _____ Done to make an accurate diagnosis

2. _____ Refers to the removal of organs from a living donor or a deceased person for transplantation into another person.

3. _____ The blood in wound drainage decreases and the fluid becomes pinkish

4. _____ Done to remove a malignant tumor obstructing the intestines even though cancer is widespread in the body

5. _____ Often involves removal and study of tissue with biopsy of skin lesion or removal of a lump in the breast

6. _____ Performed to remove diseased tissue

7. _____ Restores function lost because of congenital defects.

8. _____ Surgery that restores function or structure to damaged or malfunctioning tissue

9. _____ Done to relieve symptoms or improve functions without correcting the basic problem

10. _____ When body organs protrude through an open wound

11. _____ Wound drainage is bright red postoperatively

12. _____ If peristalsis stops completely and the patient has abdominal distention

13. _____ The reopening of the surgical wound involving one or more layers of tissue

14. _____ Wound drainage becomes progressively lighter and thinner until it is straw colored and clear.

A. Ablative surgery
B. Palliative surgery
C. Diagnostic surgery
D. Restorative surgery
E. Constructive surgery
F. Dehiscence
G. Evisceration
H. Paralytic ileus
I. Procurement for transplant
J. Sanguineous
K. Serosanguineous
L. Serous

B. Surgical Complications

1. Which are reasons that older adults are often at greater risk for surgical complications? Select all that apply.
   1. Secretions are more copious.
   2. Impaired healing and recovery, if chronic illness is present.
   3. Takes longer to regain strength following periods of inactivity.
   4. Ciliary activity is less effective.
   5. Age-related changes in the heart and brain.

2. Which are reasons that smoking increases the risk of pulmonary complications? Select all that apply.
   1. Ineffective breathing patterns
   2. Risk for suffocation
   3. More tenacious secretions
   4. Less effective ciliary activity
   5. Impaired nutrition

3. How does smoking delay wound healing?
   1. Increases the potential for infection
   2. Produces more secretions that restrict blood flow to the wound
   3. Capillary constriction from the nicotine
   4. Coughing increases the risk of dehiscence
   5. Withdrawal from smoking causes anxiety and depression

4. Which are complications of wound healing? Select all that apply.
   1. Dehiscence
   2. Evisceration
   3. Infection
   4. Hypotension
   5. Bradycardia

5. Which are factors that may cause impaired peristalsis after surgery? Select all that apply.
   1. Hypertension
   2. Opioid analgesics
   3. Immobility
   4. Inability to cough
   5. Nausea

C. Preoperative Nursing Care

1. Which are diagnostic tests that are done preoperatively? Select all that apply.
   1. ECG
   2. Urine tests
   3. Culture and sensitivity tests
   4. Chest radiograph
   5. Thyroid function tests
   6. Blood studies

2. Which are components of a consent form for surgery? Select all that apply.
   1. Patient must be informed about the procedure to be done.
   2. Results of preoperative workup are explained.
   3. Alternative treatments are discussed.
   4. Discharge instructions are included.
   5. Risks involved are mentioned.
   6. Patient agrees to The procedure.

3. Which are safety nursing interventions following administration of the preoperative medication? Select all that apply.
   1. Instruct patient to remain in bed.
   2. Have the consent form signed.
   3. Raise the side rails of the bed.
   4. Have the patient void.
   5. Encourage passive exercises in bed.

D. Anesthesia

1. Which are the complications of local anesthesia? Select all that apply.
   1. Allergic responses
   2. Seizures
   3. Overdose
   4. Local tissue damage
   5. Respiratory depression
   6. Muscle relaxation

2. Which are the methods by which general anesthetic agents can be given? Select all that apply.
   1. Inhalation
   2. Intravenous infusion
   3. Oral administration
   4. Rectal administration
   5. Intramuscular injection

3. Which drugs have the potential to interact with general anesthetics? Select all that apply.
   1. Aspirin
   2. Herbal remedies
   3. Potassium-wasting diuretics
   4. Atropine
   5. CNS depressants

E. Safety Precautions

1. What safety precaution should be taken when patients are transferred to their own beds on the nursing unit?
   1. Lower the bed.
   2. Monitor intake and output.
   3. Take vital signs every 4 hours.
   4. Place the head of the bed in high Fowler's position.

F. Postoperative Care/Coughing

1. Which are the types of surgeries in which coughing is contraindicated? Select all that apply.
   1. Appendectomy
   2. Cataracts
   3. Brain surgery
   4. Mastectomy
   5. Hip replacement
   6. Hernias

G. Paralytic Ileus

1. Which of the following is a characteristic of paralytic ileus?
   1. Abdominal pain
   2. Presence of bowel sounds
   3. Increased temperature
   4. Increased blood pressure
   5. Abdominal distention

H. Drug Therapy/Preoperative Medications

1. Which are classifications of preoperative and operative drugs that depress respiratory function and cause pulmonary secretions to be drier and thicker during the postoperative phase? Select all that apply.
   1. Preoperative anticholinergics
   2. Opioid analgesics
   3. Corticosteroids
   4. General anesthetics
   5. Antihypertensives

I. Surgical Complications

1. What are causes of urinary retention following surgery? Select all that apply.
   1. Altered tissue perfusion
   2. Inadequate circulation
   3. Anxiety about voiding
   4. Trauma to the urinary tract
   5. Smooth muscle relaxation

2. List five things that most patients appreciate knowing about the operating room (OR).

   1. _____

   2. _____

   3. _____

   4. _____

   5. _____

PART II: PUTTING IT ALL TOGETHER

J. Multiple Choice/Multiple Response
Choose the most appropriate answer or select all that apply.

1. Why is there a risk of shock in the immediate postoperative period? Select all that apply.
   1. Loss of blood
   2. Ineffective breathing patterns
   3. Altered tissue perfusion
   4. Effect of anesthesia
   5. Electrolyte imbalance

2. Why may hypoxia occur in the immediate postoperative period? Select all that apply.
   1. Tongue falls back and blocks the airway.
   2. Secretions are more copious.
   3. Cough and swallowing reflexes are depressed by anesthesia.
   4. Ciliary activity is less effective.
   5. Laryngospasm or bronchospasm occur.

3. Which measures are taken to prevent the postoperative complication of shock? Select all that apply.
   1. Observe wound dressing.
   2. Report excessive drainage or bleeding.
   3. Ensure adequate fluids and nutrition.
   4. Assist to cough and deep breathe.
   5. Monitor intake and output.
   6. Note early changes in vital signs.
   7. Withhold oral fluids until nausea subsides.
   8. Splint incision during activity.

4. Which are criteria that determine when the patient can be moved from the recovery room to the nursing unit? Select all that apply.
   1. Patient is able to void.
   2. Gag reflex is present.
   3. Patient is able to ambulate.
   4. Vital signs are stable.
   5. Patient has minimal pain.
   6. Patient can be awakened easily.

5. What measures are used to prevent thrombophlebitis and related pulmonary emboli? Select all that apply.
   1. Early ambulation
   2. Leg exercises
   3. Coughing and deep breathing
   4. Monitoring vital signs
   5. Antiembolic stockings

6. Which are signs and symptoms that would alert the nurse to possible pulmonary emboli? Select all that apply.
    1. Hypotension
    2. Decreased respiratory rate
    3. Chest pain
    4. Dyspnea
    5. Bradycardia

7. Which is used for evaluating the outcomes of nursing goals related to risk for infection?
    1. Gag reflex present
    2. Intact wound margins
    3. Minimal swelling
    4. Patient statement of pain relief

8. Using Figure 17.9 from the book, label each method of wound closure in the figure below.

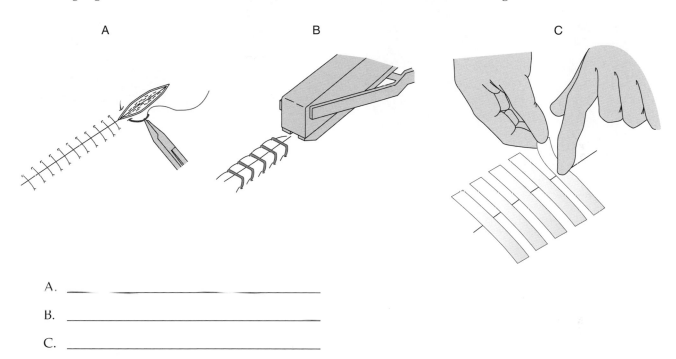

A   B   C

A. _____

B. _____

C. _____

9. Using Figure 17.8 from the book, label each complication of wound healing in the figure below.

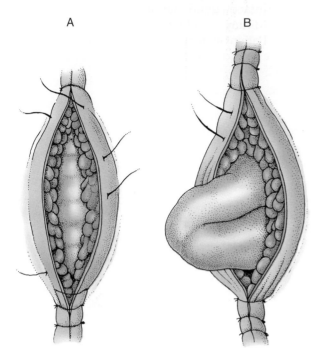

A   B

A. _____

B. _____

10. Which descriptions refer to dehiscence? Select all that apply.
    1. Most likely to occur between the 5th and 12th postoperative days
    2. Protrusion of body organs through the open wound
    3. Reopening of the surgical wound
    4. Likely to happen when there is excessive strain on the suture line
    5. Obesity is a risk factor

11. Using Figure 17.7 from the book, answer the questions that follow and specify by listing the letter. Some letters may be used more than once.

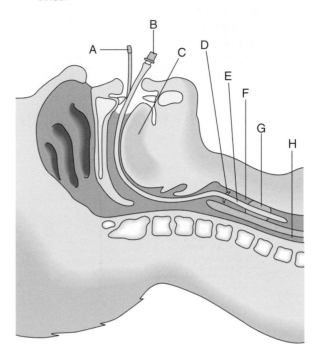

1. Which letter shows the endotracheal tube? _____
2. Which part of the figure shows the inflated cuff? _____
3. Through which tube is inhalation anesthetic administered? _____
4. What prevents aspiration of gastric contents while the patient is unconscious? _____
5. Which is the part that prevents leakage during mechanical ventilation? _____

12. Which postoperative problems are obese surgical patients more likely to have?
    1. Infection and increased temperature
    2. Excessive bleeding and hemorrhage
    3. Headache and bradycardia
    4. Respiratory and wound healing complications

13. Electrolyte imbalances may predispose the surgical patient to:
    1. cardiac arrhythmias.
    2. lung complications.
    3. liver malfunction.
    4. bone tissue loss.

14. If the patient is a minor, who signs the surgical consent form?
    1. Physician
    2. Registered nurse
    3. Parent or guardian
    4. Close relative

15. Which medications should be withheld before surgery? Select all that apply.
    1. Anticoagulants
    2. Aspirin
    3. Ginger and ginseng
    4. Antidepressants
    5. Digitalis

16. The use of local anesthetics that block the conduction of nerve impulses in a specific area is called:
    1. general anesthesia.
    2. sedative anesthesia.
    3. anticonvulsant anesthesia.
    4. regional anesthesia.

17. The injection of an anesthetic agent into and under the skin around the area of treatment is called:
    1. local infiltration.
    2. topical administration.
    3. nerve block technique.
    4. intravenous infusion.

18. One complication of spinal anesthesia is:
    1. tachycardia.
    2. hemorrhage.
    3. headache.
    4. shock.

19. Postspinal headache can be relieved by:
    1. elevating the head of the bed.
    2. lying flat.
    3. early ambulation.
    4. coughing and deep breathing.

20. A "blood patch" may help treat:
    1. hemorrhage.
    2. postspinal headache.
    3. shock.
    4. tachycardia.

21. Which adverse effects of anesthetic agents may be reduced by giving preanesthetic medications?
    1. Tachycardia
    2. Dry mouth
    3. Urinary retention
    4. Vomiting

22. Which are characteristics of malignant hyperthermia, a life-threatening complication of inhalation anesthesia? Select all that apply.
    1. Increased metabolic rate
    2. Hypertension
    3. Cyanosis
    4. Muscle rigidity
    5. Bradycardia

23. When peristalsis is slow and there is increased gas build up, what is the result?
    1. Abdominal cramping and distention
    2. Diarrhea and tachycardia
    3. Fever and infection
    4. Nausea and vomiting

24. "Gas pains" typically occur:
    1. during surgery.
    2. immediately after surgery.
    3. 6 hours after surgery.
    4. on second or third day after surgery.

25. An outcome criterion related to the absence of thrombophlebitis is:
    1. adequate oxygenation.
    2. normal arterial blood gases.
    3. no redness or swelling in the legs.
    4. normal wound healing.

26. What is used to monitor the oxygenation of blood?
    1. Sphygmomanometer
    2. Incentive spirometer
    3. Oximeter
    4. Stethoscope

27. When regional block anesthesia is used during surgery, the nurse must remember that after surgery:
    1. sensation in the area is impaired.
    2. circulation in the area is impaired.
    3. infection is likely to occur.
    4. fever may make the patient drowsy.

28. Once the immediate postoperative phase has passed, which risks lessen?
    1. Fever and infection
    2. Pneumonia and atelectasis
    3. Shock and hemorrhage
    4. Thrombophlebitis and decubitus ulcer

29. Clean sutured incisions heal by:
    1. first intention.
    2. second intention.
    3. third intention.
    4. fourth intention.

30. A soft tube that permits passive movement of fluids from the wound is called a(n):
    1. active drain.
    2. Hemovac.
    3. Penrose drain.
    4. Jackson-Pratt drain.

31. In the postoperative phase, place the colors of the wound drainage in order. Place 1 by the immediate postoperative phase, and 4 when the amount of blood in the drainage decreases.
    A. _____ Straw-colored
    B. _____ Clear
    C. _____ Bright red
    D. _____ Pink

32. Which sudden change in condition may precede wound dehiscence?
    1. Decrease in wound drainage
    2. Increase in wound drainage
    3. Increase in temperature
    4. Increase of purulent drainage

33. If evisceration occurs, the usual practice is to cover the wound with:
    1. dry sterile dressings.
    2. saline-soaked gauze with a dry dressing over it.
    3. antibiotic ointment and dry dressings.
    4. steroid ointment and dry dressings.

34. Signs and symptoms of wound infection usually do not develop until:
    1. the first hour after surgery.
    2. 12 hours after surgery.
    3. the first and second days after surgery.
    4. the third to fifth day after surgery.

35. A postoperative patient complains of pain, fever, swelling, and purulent drainage. These signs and symptoms are indications of:
    1. thrombophlebitis.
    2. evisceration.
    3. dehiscence.
    4. wound infection.

36. Pulmonary emboli usually originate from thrombi that develop in veins of the:
    1. chest.
    2. arms and shoulders.
    3. legs and pelvis.
    4. abdomen.

37. Emboli may be treated with:
    1. phenytoin (Dilantin) and anticonvulsants.
    2. morphine and analgesics.
    3. heparin and thrombolytic agents.
    4. furosemide (Lasix) and diuretics.

38. Catheterization is usually done postoperatively if the patient does not void in:
    1. 2 hours.
    2. 4 hours.
    3. 8 hours.
    4. 10 hours.

39. When a patient passes small amounts of urine frequently without feeling relief of fullness, this indicates:
    1. retention with overflow.
    2. stress incontinence.
    3. urge incontinence.
    4. kidney failure.

40. When a patient is unable to void postoperatively, what procedure may be necessary if all other interventions fail?
    1. An ultrasound to confirm the bladder is full
    2. Provide patient privacy while they attempt to void
    3. Catheterization
    4. Warm water poured over the perineum or hands

41. When do most patients pass flatus?
    1. 15 minutes after surgery
    2. 1 hour after surgery
    3. 48 hours after surgery
    4. 1 week after surgery

42. Which surgical drain works by creating negative pressure when the receptacle is compressed?
    1. Penrose
    2. Urinary
    3. Hemovac
    4. Passive

43. Which drug supplements the effects of local anesthetics?
    1. Propranolol (Inderal)
    2. Atropine
    3. Morphine
    4. Epinephrine

44. A patient states that his wound feels as if it is "pulling apart." This is an indication of:
    1. healing by first intention.
    2. dehiscence.
    3. evisceration.
    4. singultus.

45. Which postoperative drugs cause urinary retention?
    1. Antibiotics
    2. Thrombolytics
    3. Opioid analgesics
    4. Anticoagulants

46. The use of IV drugs to reduce pain intensity or awareness without loss of reflexes is called:
    1. regional anesthesia.
    2. conscious sedation.
    3. general anesthesia.
    4. balanced anesthesia.

47. Which is a commonly used IV drug for moderate sedation?
    1. Succinylcholine
    2. Isoflurane
    3. Nitrous oxide
    4. Benzodiazepine

48. Enflurane (Ethrane) and nitrous oxide are administered by:
    1. inhalation.
    2. IV infusion.
    3. intramuscular (IM) injection.
    4. rectal insertion.

49. If withdrawal from recreational drugs is anticipated after surgery, how can this complication be minimized?
    1. Delay the surgery.
    2. Admit patient to an inpatient rehab program.
    3. Intraoperative and postoperative drug therapy.
    4. Increased dose of the anesthetic agent.

50. Where can emboli formed in the legs possibly travel? Select all that apply.
    1. Kidneys
    2. Heart
    3. Lymph nodes
    4. Lungs
    5. Brain

PART III: CHALLENGE YOURSELF!

K. Getting Ready for NCLEX

Choose the most appropriate answer or select all that apply.

1. The surgical patient who is malnourished is at risk for:
   1. excessive bleeding and hemorrhage.
   2. drug toxicity and ineffective metabolism.
   3. cardiac complications and dyspnea.
   4. poor wound healing and infection.

2. The patient develops rupture of the suture line and states, "My incision is breaking open." Which action should the nurse take to prevent complications in this patient?
   1. Keep the patient in bed.
   2. Administer opioid analgesics as prescribed.
   3. Have the patient cough and deep breathe every 2 hours.
   4. Auscultate breath sounds.

3. After the first 24 hours following surgery, which finding should be reported to the health care provider if it is observed?
   1. Respirations of 20/minute
   2. Temperature of 98.8°F
   3. Blood pressure of 110/70 mm Hg
   4. Continued or excessive bleeding

4. Which finding in a postoperative patient should be reported to the health care provider?
   1. Redness that spreads to the surrounding area
   2. Redness at the wound suture site
   3. Low-grade fever
   4. Serosanguineous drainage

5. A week after surgery, the patient develops pain, fever, swelling, and purulent drainage around the wound site. Which action should the nurse take to prevent complications?
   1. Keep the patient in bed
   2. Early, frequent ambulation
   3. Monitor intake and output
   4. Good hand hygiene

6. What are four essential components for transferring the primary responsibility of care from one health care provider to another? Select all that apply.
   1. Assessment
   2. Recommendation
   3. Care plan
   4. Background
   5. Teaching plan
   6. Situation

7. Which are minimal information reports that must be communicated about a surgical procedure during a "hand-off"? Select all that apply.
   1. Any medication given
   2. Latest vital signs
   3. Laboratory tests prescribed
   4. Blood administered
   5. Any drains in place
   6. Discharge instructions

8. What are the causes of shock during the postoperative period? Select all that apply.
   1. Effect of anesthesia
   2. Loss of blood
   3. Dehydration without adequate replacement
   4. High blood volume
   5. Opioid administration before the anesthesia has worn off

9. The nurse has just received a change-of-shift report. Which patient should she check on first?
   1. A patient who is 2 days post-lobectomy
   2. A patient with an oral temperature of 101°F who has emphysema
   3. A patient who had an appendectomy 3 days ago
   4. A patient who had a hip replacement 1 week ago

10. A postoperative patient is receiving morphine for pain and is experiencing decreasing blood oxygenation levels in the recovery unit. Which factor in the patient's history increases the risk for postoperative airway obstruction?
    1. Diabetes mellitus
    2. Hypothyroidism
    3. Depression
    4. Obstructive sleep apnea

11. A patient with liver disease is scheduled for knee surgery. The patient faces a postoperative risk for:
    1. impaired blood clotting.
    2. infection.
    3. dizziness.
    4. nausea.

12. A patient with diabetes mellitus is scheduled for removal of a skin lesion. This patient is at risk postoperatively for:
    1. imbalanced fluid and electrolytes.
    2. infection.
    3. bleeding.
    4. decreased cardiac output.

13. The nurse has just attended a workshop on the Universal Protocol for Preventing Wrong Site, Wrong Procedure, and Wrong Person Surgery Principles. Which are requirements for the "time-out" procedure? Select all that apply.
    1. Do not start the procedure until all questions or concerns are resolved.
    2. The "time-out" must be done before an incision is made.
    3. Have the patient identify the site and procedure if possible.
    4. Mark the procedure site.
    5. Complete a surgical scrub before the "time-out."

14. When assessing an older patient preoperatively, what is especially important to remember about the skin? Select all that apply.
    1. It is fragile and may tear or bruise more easily when the patient is moved from stretcher to bed.
    2. Older patients' skin must not be palpated due increased risk of bruising.
    3. Any preoperative cuts, discoloration, or bruises must be documented to compare with any new injuries postoperatively.
    4. A decrease in turgor is a symptom of aging.

L. Next-Generation NCLEX® Examination-Style Questions

Read the following situation and answer the question below.

A 60-year-old woman required right total knee replacement due to a history of chronic osteoarthritis. The nurse reviews the health history, physical assessment, and vital signs.

Health History:
A 60-year-old woman admitted for right total knee replacement due to a history of chronic osteoarthritis. Client is a heavy smoker with a history of hypertension. Otherwise, she has been healthy and active. She is 2 days postop, but has only been out of bed once on the previous shift due to complaints of pain to her right knee.

Physical Assessment:
Client appear anxious when getting out of bed to ambulate with physical therapy. She complains of dyspnea and tightness in her chest. Client is alert and oriented times 3. Dressing on right hip is dry and intact. IV fluids infusing in the left hand.

Vital Signs:

Pulse	110 beats/minute
Respirations	24 breaths/minute
Temperature	99°F
Blood Pressure	172/70 mm Hg

---

1. Choose the most likely options for the information missing from the statements below by selecting from the lists of options provided.

   The nurse recognizes that _____1_____,

   _____1_____, and

   _____1_____ may indicate a pulmonary embolism. Nonpharmacologic nursing measures that could have decreased the risk of developing this complication include

   _____2_____, _____2_____,

   and _____2_____.

Options for 1	Options for 2
BP 172/70 mm Hg	Leg Exercises
Temperature 99°F	Early Ambulation
Dyspnea	Deep-breathing exercises
Chest Pain	Bedrest
Pulse 110 beats/minute	Antiembolic stockings

The nurse is caring for a client admitted to the surgical unit following abdominal surgery for a hernia repair. The client is postoperative day 1. The nurse reviews the physical assessment findings.

Physical Assessment:
Client is alert and oriented times 3. Hypoactive bowel sounds. Tolerating clear liquid diet. Abdominal distention. Last bowel movement 3 days ago. Complaints of gas pain 5/10. No flatus passed since surgery.

---

2. Which physician orders would the nurse anticipate being prescribed? Select all that apply.
   1. Advance to regular diet
   2. Complete bedrest
   3. Abdominal CT scan
   4. Stool specimen for ova and parasites
   5. Repeat complete metabolic profile (CMP)
   6. Assist patient to ambulate q2H
   7. Administer 10 mg bisacodyl suppository per rectum once daily
   8. Positioning client on the right side when in bed
   9. Apply heat to abdomen

The Patient With an Ostomy

Go to http://evolve.elsevier.com/Linton/medsurg/ for additional activities and exercises.

NCLEX CATEGORIES

Psychosocial Integrity

Physiological Integrity: Basic Care and Comfort, Reduction of Risk Potential, Physiological Adaptation, Coping Mechanism, Unexpected Body Changes

PART I: MASTERING THE BASICS

A. Key Terms
Match the definition in the numbered column with the most appropriate term in the lettered column.

1. _____ Site of opening on the skin
2. _____ Surgically created opening in the kidney to drain urine
3. _____ Surgically created opening into the urinary bladder
4. _____ Artificial opening into a body cavity
5. _____ Creates an internal reservoir in order to retain feces or urine
6. _____ Opening in the ureter; one or both ureters are brought out through opening in the abdomen or flank

7. _____ A urinary drainage system made from a portion of the small or large intestine
8. _____ Communication or connection between two organs or parts of organs
9. _____ Surgical opening in the ileum to drain fecal material from the small intestine
10. _____ Surgically created opening in the colon
11. _____ A "new" bladder constructed from a section of the bowel

A. Reanastomosis
B. Colostomy
C. Continent
D. Ileal or colonic conduit
E. Nephrostomy
F. Ostomy
G. Stoma
H. Ureterostomy
I. Vesicostomy
J. Ileostomy
K. Neobladder

B. Application of Ostomy Pouch

Match the steps in the numbered column below with the corresponding correct letters (A–F, showing stages of application) in the figure below (Figure 18.11 in the book).

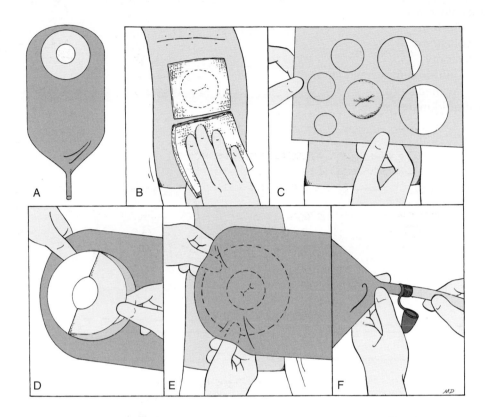

1. _____ Remove the backing from the adhesive of the new pouch.

2. _____ Connect the drain to the tubing or close the drain, if appropriate. Secure the tubing to the sheets or according to agency policy.

3. _____ Wash hands, put on gloves, and gather supplies.

4. _____ Use a stoma template to measure the size of the stoma and cut an opening the same size as the stoma into the skin barrier and adhesive.

5. _____ Remove the old pouch, clean the area around the stoma, and place a gauze square over the stoma to absorb the drainage.

6. _____ Place the opening in the new pouch over the stoma and gently press into place with the pouch drain pointed toward the floor.

7. Why is sizing the ostomy pouch so important during the first 6–8 weeks postoperatively?

   _____

   _____

   _____

   _____

8. If edema occurs after the first week postoperatively, this most likely indicates:
   1. improperly fitting collection device.
   2. infection.
   3. capillary hemorrhage.
   4. poor circulation.

C. Colostomy Types

Use the figure below (Figure 18.6 in the book). Label each type of colostomy (A–D) and indicate the type of drainage passed by each (E–G).

A. Descending colostomy
B. Ascending colostomy
C. Transverse colostomy
D. Sigmoid colostomy
E. Passes semiliquid to semiformed stool
F. Passes softly formed stool
G. Passes semiliquid material

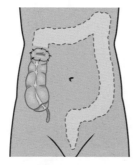

1. _____

    _____

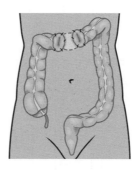

2. _____

    _____

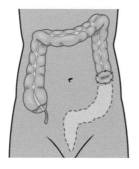

3. _____

    _____

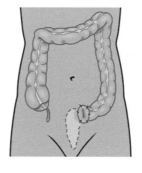

4. _____

    _____

5. What are the two main long-term complications of colostomies?

    1. _____

    2. _____

6. What type of medication can be inserted into a colostomy stoma to stimulate evacuation?
    1. Laxative liquid
    2. Hyperosmolar laxative
    3. Rectal suppository
    4. Nystatin

D. Types of Urinary Diversions

1. What are two serious consequences of urinary tract infections following ureterostomy? Select two that apply.
   1. Stenosis
   2. Hemorrhage
   3. Kidney damage
   4. Septicemia
   5. Prolapse

2. What is the treatment for yeast infections around the ureterostomy stoma?
   1. Antifungal powder
   2. Antibiotic ointment
   3. Steroid ointment
   4. Soap and water

3. If odor is a problem with ureterostomy, the pouch can be soaked for 20–30 minutes in:
   1. 50% alcohol.
   2. normal saline.
   3. vinegar and water.
   4. baking soda and water.

4. Name the most common types of urinary diversion.

   1. _____
   2. _____
   3. _____
   4. _____
   5. _____

5. Which types of urinary diversion require a collection pouch and meticulous skin care?
   1. IPAA
   2. Orthotopic neobladder
   3. Continent internal reservoirs
   4. Ureterostomies and ileal conduits

PART II: PUTTING IT ALL TOGETHER

E. Multiple Choice/Multiple Response
Choose the most appropriate answer or select all that apply.

1. A colostomy is performed by bringing a loop of the intestine through the wall of the:
   1. bladder.
   2. rectum.
   3. abdomen.
   4. stomach.

2. Which complication of colostomy involves the narrowing of the abdominal opening around the base of the stoma?
   1. Prolapse
   2. Stenosis
   3. Obstruction
   4. Evisceration

3. What is the result of the loss of bicarbonate in ileostomy drainage?
   1. Hypokalemia
   2. Hypercalcemia
   3. Metabolic acidosis
   4. Excess of fluid volume

4. The nurse notices that the patient's ileal conduit stoma has turned black. The nurse notifies the health care provider immediately because it may mean that:
   1. ureteral obstruction has occurred.
   2. circulation is impaired.
   3. wound infection is present.
   4. prolapse has occurred.

5. After bowel resection for the ileal conduit procedure, the nurse should expect:
   1. necrosis of the wound.
   2. temporary ileus.
   3. gray-black stoma.
   4. ureteral calculi.

6. The Kock pouch is made with a section of the:
   1. sigmoid colon.
   2. jejunum.
   3. ileum.
   4. ascending colon.

7. Which foods tend to produce thicker stools?
   1. Milk and cottage cheese
   2. Fresh fruits
   3. Green, leafy vegetables
   4. Pasta and boiled rice

8. Why is a nasogastric tube placed in a patient with bowel obstruction?
   1. Dilate the digestive tract
   2. Decompress the bowel
   3. Provide method of feeding
   4. Improve peristalsis

9. What is a complication of colostomy irrigation?
   1. Obstruction
   2. Diarrhea
   3. Infection
   4. Perforated bowel

10. A patient with an ileoanal reservoir is prescribed metronidazole (Flagyl) and steroids and asks the nurse why these drugs are prescribed. The nurse answers that they are given to treat:
    1. pain.
    2. bleeding.
    3. inflammation and infection.
    4. fluid volume deficit.

11. A patient with a colostomy is experiencing weakness when the colostomy is irrigated. Which manifestation requires the nurse to contact the health care provider?
    1. Prolapse
    2. Perforated bowel
    3. Diarrhea
    4. Red stoma

12. Which is a sign of bowel obstruction?
    1. Bloody stools
    2. Fever
    3. Abdominal distention
    4. Hypotension

13. Which is a major long-term complication caused by coughing in a patient with a colostomy?
    1. Prolapse
    2. Stenosis
    3. Obstruction
    4. Inflammation

14. Which is a complication of ureterostomy?
    1. Obstruction
    2. Perforation
    3. Hydronephrosis
    4. Prolapse

15. What are the different types of intestinal ostomies? Select all that apply.
    1. Colostomy
    2. Ileal pouch–anal anastomosis
    3. Ileostomy
    4. Urostomy
    5. Continent ileostomy

16. Which nurses with specialized training in ostomy management are an important resource for staff nurses and ostomy patients? Select all that apply.
    1. COCN
    2. CWON
    3. COWN
    4. CWOCN

17. Which type of patient with a colostomy should be given a two-piece appliance that allows frequent pouch changes without skin trauma?
    1. Jewish
    2. Native American
    3. Asian
    4. Muslim

18. Following ileostomy surgery, the stoma is inspected for bleeding and:
    1. edema.
    2. rough edges.
    3. temperature.
    4. color.

19. Following ileostomy surgery, what should the nurse examine when checking the base of the stoma? Select all that apply.
    1. Purulent drainage
    2. Redness
    3. Amount of drainage present
    4. Skin separation
    5. Uneven edges

20. As the body adapts to ileostomy, how often must the pouch be drained?
    1. Every 6 hours
    2. 1–2 times per day
    3. 2–4 times per day
    4. Every 2 hours

21. Postoperative ileostomy patients may experience electrolyte imbalances due to:
    1. passage of liquid stool.
    2. bleeding around the stoma.
    3. poor circulation.
    4. infection.

22. What factors contribute to a prolapsed stoma in a colostomy? Select all that apply.
    1. Increased abdominal pressure
    2. Coughing
    3. Poor blood supply
    4. Parastomal hernia
    5. Poorly attached stoma
    6. Abdominal opening that is too small

23. Place in order, from 1 to 6, the steps for removing the colostomy pouch, cleansing the skin surrounding the stoma, and replacing the pouch around the stoma.
    A. _____   Pat the skin dry.
    B. _____   Apply a skin barrier.
    C. _____   Gently peel the adhesive off the skin.
    D. _____   Apply a protective barrier (sealant).
    E. _____   Wash the stoma and the area around it with water.
    F. _____   Place wafer and pouch around the stoma.

24. What is important to determine from the patient before ostomy surgery? Select all that apply.
    1. Patient's expectations
    2. Training for removing and replacing the pouch
    3. Understanding of the procedure
    4. Fears
    5. Desired information

25. What is the main difference between a continent pouch ileostomy and the ileal-anal pouch anastomosis (IPAA)?
    1. The ileostomy is for urinary incontinence and the IPAA is for fecal incontinence.
    2. The ileostomy requires drainage with a catheter periodically and an IPAA allows anal fecal elimination.
    3. The IPAA has a secured pouch while a catheter is used for an ileostomy.
    4. The ileostomy has a higher incidence of infection than the IPAA.

PART III: CHALLENGE YOURSELF!

F. Getting Ready for NCLEX
Choose the most appropriate answer or select all that apply.

1. The nurse is taking care of a patient following ileostomy surgery. The nurse observes that the color of the stoma is blue. What should the nurse do?
   1. Cleanse skin around the stoma with soap and water.
   2. Apply a protective skin barrier before replacing the pouch.
   3. Notify the health care provider.
   4. Check the pouch hourly to detect leakage.

2. The nurse is taking care of a patient who has had colostomy surgery. What does a small amount of bleeding around the base of a new stoma indicate?
   1. Infection
   2. Tissue injury
   3. Adequate blood supply
   4. Poor circulation

3. A postoperative ileostomy patient becomes confused. What is the nursing intervention for this mental status change?
   1. Check the pouch hourly.
   2. Provide opportunity for the patient to express feelings.
   3. Measure tissue turgor.
   4. Monitor serum electrolytes.

4. A patient has a continent ileostomy. Which foods should this patient avoid initially? Select all that apply.
   1. Pasta
   2. Coffee
   3. Berries
   4. Nuts
   5. Boiled rice
   6. Fresh fruit

5. A nurse notices that the patient's colostomy is not draining properly. What is the appropriate nursing action to take?
   1. Place a gloved finger in the stoma to dilate it.
   2. Use a larger catheter to irrigate.
   3. Inform the health care provider.
   4. Push the catheter in 3 inches.

6. The nurse is taking care of a patient with an ileostomy. The nurse is watching for signs of small bowel obstruction. To reduce the risk of obstruction, what is the appropriate diet for this patient?
   1. Low fiber
   2. Low cholesterol
   3. Soft, bland foods
   4. High residue

7. A patient with an ileostomy 1 week postoperatively has a pulse of 120 bpm, respirations 28/min, temperature of 101°F, and a rigid abdomen. The nurse suspects that this patient has which complication?
   1. Obstruction
   2. Peritonitis
   3. Inflammation
   4. Evisceration of the site

G. Next-Generation NCLEX® Examination-Style Questions

Read the following situations and answer the questions below.

A 47-year-old male client, Mr. C., had a bowel resection and permanent colostomy in the descending colon to remove a malignant tumor. The nurse reviews the physician's progress notes.

Physician's Progress Notes:
6/5/21 0800: A 47-year-old male client had a bowel resection and permanent colostomy in the descending colon to remove a malignant tumor. He is 3 days postoperative. Nurse reports emptying 400 ml loose, brown stool from the colostomy bag. He reports adequate pain control with IV morphine. He has had no nausea and vomiting but has a nasogastric tube attached to low suction. 400 ML noted in the suction canister. He is NPO and is receiving IV fluids at 150 mL/h.
K. Carswell, MD

---

1. The nurse is concerned about the potential for fluid volume deficit for Mr. C. Which are appropriate nursing interventions for this problem? Select all that apply.
   1. Keep accurate intake and output.
   2. Monitor for signs of electrolyte imbalance.
   3. Monitor for signs of hypovolemia.
   4. Prevent fecal matter from contaminating the incision.
   5. Cleanse the skin around the stoma with soap and water.
   6. Monitor for peripheral edema
   7. Irrigate the stoma
   8. Decrease the IV fluid rate

Complete the following sentence by choosing from the list of options below.

2. The client is at highest risk for developing

_____ 1 (Select) related to

_____ 2 (Select).

Options for 1	Options for 2
Fluid volume overload	Pain
Altered body image	Administration of IV fluids
Ineffective breathing pattern	Presence of new stoma
Disturbed sleep pattern	Fecal drainage

A 60-year-old male required a temporary ileostomy. On the first postoperative day he is NPO, receiving intravenous fluids, and has a nasogastric tube in place and set on low intermittent suction. The nurse reviews the physical assessment.

Physical Assessment:
Stoma gray and swollen. Ileostomy pouch contains greenish-brown liquid stool. Large amount of blood at the base of the stoma. Foley catheter in place; urine is light yellow, clear. Bowel sounds not audible.

Vital Signs:

Blood Pressure	88/52 mm Hg
Pulse	112 beats/minute, regular
Respirations	24 breaths/minute
Temperature	98.4°F

---

3. Highlight the assessment findings that require follow-up by the nurse.

Palliative and Hospice Care

Go to http://evolve.elsevier.com/Linton/medsurg/ for additional activities and exercises.

NCLEX CATEGORIES

Psychosocial Integrity

Physiological Integrity: Basic Care and Comfort

PART I: MASTERING THE BASICS

A. Key Terms

Match the definition or description in the numbered column with the appropriate term in the lettered column. Answers may be used more than once.

1. _____ Occurs when the cerebral cortex stops functioning or is irreversibly destroyed

2. _____ Real or potential absence of something or a person that is valued

3. _____ When a cure for a chronic condition is not expected, the goal of this care is to improve quality of life for patients and their families by anticipating, preventing, and treating suffering

4. _____ Embracing palliative care with a focus on quality of life, comfort, and dignity near the end of life

5. _____ Normal response to loss that serves to maintain emotional and physical well-being

6. _____ Refocusing health care toward allowing natural death in a pain- and symptom-controlled environment with psychosocial support

7. _____ Outward part of coping with grief; marked by social customs

8. _____ Total mourning and grief experience

9. _____ Care that includes bereavement care for survivors after the death of the patient

A. Brain death
B. Grief
C. Loss
D. Palliative care
E. Hospice care
F. Mourning
G. Bereavement

Match the physical manifestations of approaching death in the numbered column with the most appropriate term in the lettered column.

10. _____ Rapid, deep breathing with periods of apnea

11. _____ Breathing becomes irregular, gradually slowing down to terminal gasps

12. _____ Grunting and noisy tachypnea

A. Death rattle
B. Cheyne-Stokes breathing
C. "Guppy breathing"

Match the definition in the numbered column with the most appropriate term in the lettered column.

13. _____ The body's cooling after death
14. _____ Discoloration of the skin after death
15. _____ Stiffening of the body after death

A. Rigor mortis
B. Livor mortis
C. Algor mortis

B. Grieving Process

Match the definition or description in the numbered column with the most appropriate stage of grieving in the lettered column. Answers may be used more than once.

1. _____ Patient or family members may become outraged with situations.

2. _____ Person may become somewhat emotionally detached and objective.

3. _____ Patient identifies the loss as inevitable and may want to make plans.

4. _____ Patient refuses to acknowledge the terminal illness.

5. _____ Patient recognizes the terminal stage of illness.

6. _____ Patient seeks to "buy" more time.

7. _____ Defense mechanism that helps the patient and others manage anxiety caused by the threat.

8. _____ Experiences many emotions, including sadness, regret, and fear.

9. _____ Patient begins to accept the reality of impending death.

A. Depression
B. Anger
C. Denial
D. Acceptance
E. Bargaining

Match the description of grief in the numbered column with the appropriate term in the lettered column.

10. _____ Experience of survivor when a person's relationship to the person is not socially recognized

11. _____ Grief that is prolonged, unresolved, or disruptive to the person who experiences it

12. _____ Grief that begins before a death occurs or when the reality that death is inevitable is known

13. _____ Grief that assists the dying person and significant others in accepting the reality of death

A. Uncomplicated grief
B. Complicated grief
C. Disenfranchised grief
D. Anticipatory grief

C. Beliefs About Death

Match the belief about death in the numbered column with the most appropriate age group in the lettered column. Answers may be used more than once.

1. _____ Sees death as inevitable

2. _____ Faces death of parents

3. _____ Examines death as it relates to various meanings, such as freedom from discomfort

4. _____ Sees death as future event

5. _____ Faces death of peers and family members

6. _____ May experience death anxiety

7. _____ Afraid of prolonged health problems

8. _____ Accepts one's own mortality as inevitable

A. Young adult
B. Middle-aged adult
C. Older adult

9. Which are fears associated with terminal illness and dying? Select all that apply.
   1. Fear of pain
   2. Fear of failure
   3. Fear of loneliness
   4. Fear of meaninglessness
   5. Fear of surgery

Match the description in the numbered column with the appropriate term in the lettered column.

10. _____ Patient and family freely discuss the impending death.

11. _____ Patient and family recognize that the patient is ill. They may not understand the severity of the illness and impending death.

12. _____ Patient, family, and health care providers know of the terminal prognosis. Efforts are made to avoid discussing death.

A. Closed awareness
B. Mutual pretense
C. Open awareness

PART II: PUTTING IT ALL TOGETHER

D. Multiple Choice/Multiple Response
Choose the most appropriate answer or select all that apply.

1. Which change occurs preceding death?
   1. Blood pressure rises.
   2. Breathing sounds are quiet.
   3. Pulse slows.
   4. Extremities turn red.

2. Which are associated with the death rattle? Select all that apply.
   1. Suffocation
   2. Mouth breathing
   3. Periods of apnea
   4. Noisy respirations
   5. Accumulation of mucus
   6. Wet-sounding respirations

3. In what parts of the body is livor mortis generally most obvious?
   1. Skin of extremities
   2. Fingers and toes
   3. Face and chest
   4. Back and buttocks

4. What is the last sense to remain intact during the death process?
   1. Vision
   2. Smell
   3. Hearing
   4. Touch

5. Where does the sense of touch decrease first in a dying person?
   1. Face
   2. Abdomen
   3. Arms
   4. Legs

6. Why does the patient who is dying appear to stare?
   1. The blink reflex is lost gradually.
   2. Vision is blurred.
   3. There is decreased lubrication of the eye.
   4. Decreased circulation to the eye occurs progressively.

7. Which body function ceases first in the dying person?
   1. Heartbeat
   2. Respiration
   3. Brain function
   4. Kidney function

8. Which are criteria for determining death? Select all that apply.
   1. Unresponsiveness to external stimuli that would usually be painful
   2. Complete absence of spontaneous breathing
   3. Total lack of reflexes
   4. A flat EEG for 8 hours
   5. Total lack of urinary output

9. Which criterion must be present for brain death to be pronounced and life support disconnected by the health care provider?
   1. All brain function must cease.
   2. Coma or unresponsiveness must be present.
   3. Absence of all brain stem reflexes must be noted.
   4. Apnea must be present.

10. What causes livor mortis after death?
    1. Skin loses elasticity and breaks down easily.
    2. There is a breakdown of red blood cells.
    3. Chemical changes prevent muscle relaxation.
    4. Circulation ceases and the body cools.

11. Which religious group believes that the body should not be shrouded until sacraments have been performed?
    1. Muslims
    2. Orthodox Jews
    3. Protestants
    4. Roman Catholics

12. The durable power of attorney for health care can be used only if the health care provider certifies in writing that the person is:
    1. incapable of making decisions.
    2. brain dead.
    3. unresponsive or in a coma.
    4. lacking reflexes.

13. The Patient Self-Determination Act requires that institutions inform patients about:
    1. rules and regulations about CPR.
    2. the right to have an autopsy.
    3. the right to initiate advance directives.
    4. rules and regulations about the delivery of hospice care.

14. Which statements are true related to assisting patients with a fear of meaninglessness? Select all that apply.
    1. Assure patient that medication will be given promptly, as needed.
    2. Express worth of dying person's life.
    3. Simple presence of person to provide support and comfort.
    4. Holding hands, touching, and listening.
    5. Provide consistent pain control.
    6. Dying person reviews his or her life.
    7. Prayers, thoughts, and feelings provide comfort.

15. Which are common beliefs about death for a 68-year-old person? Select all that apply.
    1. Seldom thinks about death.
    2. Death is temporary and reversible.
    3. Afraid of prolonged health problems.
    4. Faces death of family members and peers.
    5. Sees death as inevitable.
    6. Examines death as it relates to various meanings, such as freedom from discomfort.

16. What are the legal documents that may be completed near the end of life? Select all that apply.
    1. Patient Self-Determination Act
    2. Durable power of attorney
    3. Last will and testament
    4. Directives for health care providers, family members, or surrogates
    5. Tax planning and trust directives
    6. Advance directives
    7. Organ donation wishes
    8. Medical power of attorney

17. Who is responsible for the care of the body after death?
    1. Family members
    2. Clergy
    3. Health care provider
    4. Nurse
    5. Forensic technician

18. What are the signs of impending death? Select all that apply.
    1. Loss of muscle tone
    2. Sensory changes including blurred vision
    3. Abnormal breath sounds
    4. Dying person reviews their life
    5. Abnormal respiratory pattern
    6. Hypotension
    7. Open awareness of the inevitability of death
    8. Bradycardia
    9. Cyanosis and cooling skin

PART III: CHALLENGE YOURSELF!

E. Getting Ready for NCLEX

Choose the most appropriate answer or select all that apply.

1. Place in sequence (from 1 to 5) the Kübler-Ross stages of grieving.
   A. _____ Acceptance
   B. _____ Depression
   C. _____ Bargaining
   D. _____ Denial
   E. _____ Anger

2. The nurse is taking care of a patient who is terminally ill. Which are physical manifestations of approaching death? Select all that apply.
   1. Decreased pain and touch perception
   2. Involuntary blinking of the eyes
   3. Eyelids remain completely open
   4. Cold, clammy skin
   5. Clenched jaw
   6. Difficulty swallowing
   7. Gag reflex stimulated
   8. Drop in blood pressure

3. The nurse is taking care of a dying patient. The patient's family is present at the bedside. A family member asks the nurse which part of the body will stop working first. The nurse tells the family that during the death process, which function stops first?
   1. The heart stops beating.
   2. The body turns cold.
   3. Respirations cease.
   4. Hearing is lost.

4. A 65-year-old patient has cancer and is not expected to recover. He is receiving chemotherapy. His family asks about palliative care. Which primary issues will be addressed if the patient receives palliative care? Select all that apply.
   1. Physical symptoms
   2. Emotional, coping, intellectual, social, and spiritual needs
   3. Efforts made to avoid any discussion of death
   4. Facilitation of patient autonomy
   5. Level of consciousness
   6. Access to information
   7. Issues dealing with the patient's choices

5. A terminally ill patient is experiencing prolonged and unresolved grief. What is the priority nursing intervention for this patient?
   1. Relief of pain
   2. Proper nutrition
   3. Open discussion of feelings
   4. Meditation

6. The nurse is collecting data on a dying patient using an abbreviated assessment. Which data are important to collect as part of a neurologic assessment? Select all that apply.
   1. Color of skin
   2. Level of consciousness
   3. Characteristics of breathing patterns
   4. Reflexes
   5. Pupil response

7. A terminally ill patient is experiencing anticipatory grief. Which is a priority nursing intervention for this patient?
   1. Reassure the patient that everything possible is being done to keep him alive.
   2. Provide reality orientation about environmental surroundings.
   3. Teach the patient about the current treatment and medications he is receiving.
   4. Provide environment that allows the patient to express feelings.

8. The family of a terminally ill patient is concerned about when the patient will be eligible for hospice care under Medicare. What are the requirements for Medicare to offer hospice care? Select all that apply.
   1. Characteristics of breathing patterns
   2. A physician certifies that the patient has a life-limiting condition
   3. Patient has a durable power of attorney
   4. Patient has signed a Do Not Resuscitate order
   5. His or her life expectancy is 6 months or less

9. A terminally ill patient presents a Five Wishes document to the nurse during an assessment. Which patient desires are addressed in this document? Select all that apply.
   1. Decision-making authority
   2. Consent for an autopsy
   3. Comfort measures
   4. Organ donation wishes
   5. Treatment decision
   6. Information to be shared with family
   7. His or her life expectancy is 6 months or less
   8. Medical care

Complementary and Alternative Therapies and Integrative Health Care

Go to http://evolve.elsevier.com/Linton/medsurg/ for additional activities and exercises.

NCLEX CATEGORIES

Psychosocial Integrity

Physiological Integrity: Physiological Adaptation

PART I: MASTERING THE BASICS

A. Key Terms
Match the definition in the numbered column with the most appropriate term in the lettered column.

1. _____ Nonmainstream practices that are used along with conventional therapies

2. _____ Nonmainstream practices incorporated into conventional health care

3. _____ Conventional Western medicine

4. _____ Nonmainstream practices used in place of conventional therapies

A. Allopathic
B. Alternative therapy
C. Complementary therapy
D. Integrative health care

B. Alternative Therapies
Match the descriptions of alternative therapies in the numbered column with the correct terms in the lettered column.

1. _____ Components are quiet, distraction-free setting; a specific, comfortable posture; a focus of attention; and an open attitude

2. _____ Using postures and gentle movement with mental focus, breathing, and relaxation to improve balance, reduce pain, and improve the quality of life

3. _____ Medical practice that treats illnesses with very low doses of substances that create symptoms similar to the condition being treated

4. _____ Medical practice based on the belief that needles inserted in specific locations restore the flow of vital energy called *qi* to treat various conditions

5. _____ Medical practice based on the belief that disease results from an imbalance between two opposing but complementary forces called *yin* and *yang*

6. _____ Originated in India and uses a variety of practices, as well as many potentially unsafe herbals and metals

7. _____ Producing the body's natural relaxation response characterized by slower breathing, lower blood pressure, and feeling of increased well-being

8. _____ Spinal adjustments and other techniques to correct alignment problems, alleviate pain, improve function, and support the body's ability to heal itself

9. _____ Postures, breathing exercises, and meditation that can improve physical fitness, relieve stress, and enhance quality of life

10. _____ The manipulation of soft tissue to stimulate circulation, decrease pain, and promote relaxation

11. _____ Practices that were employed before the advent of modern medicine

A. Chiropractic treatment
B. Massage therapy
C. Meditation
D. Acupuncture
E. Relaxation therapy
F. Tai chi and qigong
G. Traditional or folk medicine
H. Ayurvedic medicine
I. Homeopathic medicine
J. Traditional Chinese medicine
K. Yoga

PART II: PUTTING IT ALL TOGETHER

C. Multiple Choice/Multiple Response

Choose the most appropriate answer or select all that apply.

1. What are the natural products used for health purposes? Select all that apply.
   1. Herbs/botanicals
   2. Guided imagery
   3. Probiotics
   4. Acupuncture
   5. Vitamins and minerals

2. Which statements about dietary supplements are true? Select all that apply.
   1. Manufacturers of dietary supplements are not required to show evidence of safety and efficacy.
   2. Dietary supplements treat illnesses with very low doses of substances that create symptoms similar to the condition being treated.
   3. The labels of DSHEA-approved herbal products must state that the product is not intended to diagnose, treat, cure, or prevent any disease.
   4. Dietary supplements are supported by scientific evidence of their safety and effectiveness.
   5. The Current Good Manufacturing Practices require labels of dietary supplements to correctly state the identity, purity, quality, and strength of the contents.

3. Which are commonly used herbal products? Select all that apply.
   1. Black cohosh
   2. Coenzyme Q-10
   3. Echinacea
   4. Feverfew
   5. Garlic and ginger root
   6. Insulin

4. Which herb-drug interactions are known to cause adverse or interfering effects? Select all that apply.
   1. St. John's wort and oral contraceptives
   2. Garlic and anticoagulant or antiplatelet drugs
   3. Echinacea and immunosuppressants
   4. Kava-kava and warfarin
   5. Probiotics and antibacterial and antifungal drugs
   6. Black cohosh and antihypertensive agents, antidiabetic drugs and estrogens

5. Most mind-body approaches are based on what belief?
   1. Conventional medicine is not effective.
   2. Mind-body approaches are more natural and less expensive.
   3. Illness is caused by lack of balance or harmony within the individual or between the individual and the environment.
   4. Mind-body approaches are safer because they are noninvasive.
   5. Mind-body approaches improve quality of life.

6. Which resources provide factual information about nonmainstream products? Select all that apply.
   1. The National Center for Complementary and Integrative Health (NCCIH)
   2. Search engines such as Google and Yahoo
   3. Cochrane Database of Systematic Reviews
   4. German Commission E
   5. Agency for Safety and Efficacy of Natural Medicines (ASENM)
   6. Office of Dietary Supplements
   7. Natural Medicine Brand Evidence-based Rating system (NMBER)

PART III: CHALLENGE YOURSELF!

D. Getting Ready for NCLEX

Choose the most appropriate answer or select all that apply.

1. When collecting data for the patient assessment, which questions about natural products and nonmainstream therapies should the nurse ask? Select all that apply.
   1. "Do you use any natural products with or in place of prescriptions?"
   2. "Do you use any activities like yoga, exercise, or meditation for health reasons?"
   3. "Did you know natural products can have adverse effects, especially if used with certain prescription medicines?"
   4. "Are you aware that there are many natural products and therapies that can cure your condition?"
   5. "What is the amount of natural products you take and how often do you participate in non-mainstream therapies?"

2. If a patient tells the nurse she is taking probiotics and antibiotics for a urinary tract infection, what should the nurse's response be?
   1. Only take the probiotics, antibiotics are not necessary.
   2. The antibiotics can kill the bacteria and yeasts in the probiotic product.
   3. The patient should immediately stop both medications.
   4. Homeopathy is a better option for urinary tract infections.

3. A patient with arthritis has been prescribed an antiinflammatory medication. The patient wants to take glucosamine instead of the antiinflammatory. This is an example of:
   1. complementary therapy.
   2. conventional therapy.
   3. alternative therapy.
   4. integrative health care.
   5. allopathic practices.
   6. naturopathy.

4. A patient is taking Ayurvedic products purchased over the Internet. What should the nurse advise this patient? Select all that apply.
   1. Many Ayurvedic products contain levels of lead, mercury, and/or arsenic in amounts that may not be acceptable for daily use.
   2. Ayurvedic products are marketed as dietary supplements so their safety and efficacy is not proven.
   3. Women who are pregnant or breastfeeding should not take Ayurvedic products unless approved by their health care provider.
   4. Ayurvedic products may interfere with certain conventional medicines prescribed by their health care provider.
   5. All Ayurvedic medicines must be stopped immediately.
   6. Ayurvedic practitioners are not licensed in the United States.

5. A patient with cancer wants to use a mind-body practice along with chemotherapy and radiation. Which of these is a mind-body approach? Select all that apply.
   1. Yoga
   2. Black cohosh
   3. Chiropractic
   4. Tai chi and qigong
   5. Relaxation therapy
   6. Belladonna injections

6. A patient has asked about having acupuncture treatments for neck and back pain. He has heard that acupuncture can restore the flow of qi. What is qi?
   1. Qi is believed to be the vital energy that flows through the body in channels that form meridians.
   2. Qi is believed to be a patient's psychological balance and ability to cope with illness.
   3. Qi is believed to be the flow of energy to the brain.
   4. Qi is the energy in a patient's bloodstream that travels to all cells.

7. Possible benefits of tai chi to older patients can be: (Select all that apply.)
   1. Improved balance and stability
   2. Healing of back and knee osteoarthritis
   3. Improved quality of life in patients with chronic illness like fibromyalgia
   4. Improved reasoning

8. What are some potentially dangerous herbal remedies that patients should be warned about?
   1. Black cohosh, glucosamine, green tea, and soy
   2. Cranberry juice, flaxseed, and saw palmetto
   3. St. John's wort, sassafras, ephedra, chaparral, borage, calamus, comfrey, germander, life root, and pokeroot
   4. Echinacea, resveratrol, garlic, and gingerroot

9. What is an example of an energy healing? Select all that apply.
   1. Magnet therapy
   2. Yoga
   3. Light therapy
   4. Chiropractic medicine
   5. Healing touch

10. The role of the nurse in relation to nontraditional remedies and therapies include: (Select all that apply.)
    1. Data collection
    2. Discouraging the patient from using nontraditional remedies
    3. Reminding patients to discuss nontraditional remedies, such as Ayurvedic medicine, that they have tried with their health care provider
    4. Mention adverse effects of nontraditional remedies
    5. Have an open mind about nonmainstream practices being a valid choice for some patients
    6. Learn about these therapies and even try some of them him- or herself
    7. Warn patients about expensive therapies that make unusual claims

Neurologic System Introduction

Go to http://evolve.elsevier.com/Linton/medsurg/ for additional activities and exercises.

NCLEX CATEGORIES

Physiological Integrity: Reduction of Risk Potential, Physiological Adaptation

PART I: MASTERING THE BASICS

A. Key Terms

Match the definition in the numbered column with the most appropriate term in the lettered column.

1. _____ A biochemical messenger that stimulates an electrical impulse

2. _____ Affecting the same side

A. Ipsilateral
B. Neurotransmitter

Complete the statements in the numbered column with the most appropriate term in the lettered column. Some terms may be used more than once, and some terms may not be used.

3. Decreased responsiveness accompanied by lack of spontaneous motor activity is _____.

4. A patient who cannot be aroused even by powerful stimuli is _____.

5. The most accurate and reliable indicator of neurologic status is the _____.

6. Excessive drowsiness is _____.

7. If a patient is stuporous but can be aroused, the patient is _____.

8. Unnatural drowsiness or sleepiness is _____.

A. Agitation
B. Level of consciousness
C. Combativeness
D. Somnolence
E. Neuromuscular response
F. Lethargy
G. Comatose
H. Pupillary evaluation
I. Semicomatose
J. Stupor

Match the definition or description in the numbered column with the most appropriate term in the lettered column.

9. _____ Surgery that requires opening the skull

10. _____ Procedure done to repair a skull defect

A. Cranioplasty
B. Craniotomy

11. Which brain dysfunctions are diagnosed using a brain scan? Select all that apply.
    1. Brain abscesses
    2. Tumors
    3. Contusions
    4. Parkinson disease
    5. Vascular occlusions or hemorrhage
    6. Meningitis
    7. Hematomas

B. Anatomy and Physiology of the Nervous System

Match the definition or description in the numbered column with the most appropriate term in the lettered column. Some of the letters may be used more than once.

1. _____   Composed of left and right hemispheres, which are subdivided into specific lobes. It is the largest and most highly developed part of the brain.

2. _____   Includes the midbrain, pons, medulla, and part of the reticular activating system. It controls vital basic functions including respiration, heart rate, and consciousness.

3. _____   The thalamus, hypothalamus, and basal ganglia are other important structures identified with this part of the brain.

4. _____   Composed primarily of water, glucose, sodium chloride, and protein.

5. _____   Carotid and vertebral

6. _____   Two major subdivisions of the autonomic nervous system

7. _____   Functional unit of the nervous system, which conducts electrical impulses from cell to cell

A. Brainstem
B. Cerebral spinal fluid
C. Sympathetic and parasympathetic nervous systems
D. Major cerebral arteries
E. Cerebrum
F. Neuron (nerve cell)
G. Cerebellum

8. Which are neurotransmitters? Select all that apply.
   1. Acetylcholine
   2. Thyroxine
   3. Dopamine
   4. Norepinephrine
   5. Insulin

9. Which responses are controlled by the parasympathetic nervous system? Select all that apply.
   1. Decrease in blood pressure
   2. Decreased heart rate
   3. Increased rate and force of cardiac contractions
   4. Fight-or-flight response
   5. Mediates rest response

10. What functions does the cerebellum coordinate? Select all that apply.
    1. Movement
    2. Higher-order thinking
    3. Balance
    4. Regulation of emotional behavior
    5. Posture

C. Age-Related Changes

1. Which are possible neurologic changes associated with normal aging? Select all that apply.
   1. Nerve cells increase in number.
   2. Brain weight is reduced.
   3. The size of ventricles is reduced.
   4. Increased plaques and tangled fibers are found in nerve tissue.
   5. Pupillary response to light is slower.
   6. Pupil of the eye is larger.
   7. Reaction time increases.

2. What are some of the possible functional abilities affected by aging? Select all that apply.
   1. Vascular occlusion
   2. Tremors in the head, face, and hands
   3. Increased fight-or-flight response
   4. Dizziness
   5. Lack of balance

D. Pathophysiology of Neurologic Diseases
Choose the most appropriate answer or select all that apply.

1. Give an example of a genetic disorder.
   1. Hydrocephalus
   2. Huntington's disease
   3. Encephalitis
   4. Neoplasms

2. What may be the causative agents of meningitis and encephalitis?
   1. Trauma
   2. Degenerative disorder
   3. Viruses or bacteria
   4. Developmental disorder

3. What are examples of some degenerative disorders? Select all that apply.
   1. Alzheimer's
   2. Encephalitis
   3. Multiple sclerosis
   4. Meningitis
   5. ALS (Lou Gehrig's disease)
   6. Parkinson disease

E. Diagnostic Tests and Procedures

Match the intervention or description in the numbered column with the appropriate diagnostic test in the lettered column. Some diagnostic tests may be used more than once.

1. _____ A shampoo is done before the test, and medications such as anticonvulsants and stimulants are withheld 24–48 hours before the test.

2. _____ Tell the patient to lie still on a stretcher while the dye is injected, and radiographs of the head are taken.

3. _____ A cannula is inserted into subarachnoid space at the fourth or fifth lumbar vertebra, which ends at the second lumbar vertebra.

4. _____ Needle electrodes are placed on several points over a nerve and muscles supplied by the nerve.

5. _____ Have the patient void before the procedure to reduce discomfort from the position.

6. _____ Inform the radiologist about any allergies to iodine, shellfish, or contrast media.

7. _____ Patient must remain on one side in a knee-to-chest position.

8. _____ Complementary, computer-assisted radiographic procedure for visualization of cerebral vessels

9. _____ A contrast dye is injected, followed by a series of radiographs.

10. _____ Enhancement of an area may be achieved by injecting contrast medium.

11. _____ This procedure does not expose the patient to radiation. It is a noninvasive examination that involves placing the patient in a strong magnetic field and then applying bursts of radiofrequency waves. Sophisticated technology converts information about the movement of molecules in the tissue into precise, clear images.

12. _____ A puncture is made in the lumbar area between L3 and L4. Radiopaque dye is then injected into the subarachnoid space of the spinal canal. Any obstruction that impedes the flow of the dye can be seen on radiography.

A. Lumbar puncture
B. Myelography
C. Brain scan
D. Cerebral angioplasty
E. Computed tomography (CT)
F. Digital subtraction angiography
G. Magnetic resonance imaging (MRI)
H. Electromyography (EMG)
I. Electroencephalogram (EEG)

F. Drug Therapy

1. What types of drugs are used for neurologic disorders? Select all that apply.
   1. Antiinflammatory agents
   2. Antimicrobials
   3. Stimulants
   4. Analgesics
   5. Diuretics
   6. Beta blockers
   7. Corticosteroids
   8. Anticonvulsants
   9. Chemotherapeutic agents
   10. Dopaminergics
   11. Anticholinergics and cholinergics
   12. Antihistamines

PART II: PUTTING IT ALL TOGETHER

G. Multiple Choice/Multiple Response
Choose the most appropriate answer or select all that apply.

1. To minimize headache following a lumbar puncture, what should be increased?
   1. Calcium
   2. Fluid intake
   3. Potassium
   4. Ambulation

2. The family should be advised that a craniotomy can take as long as:
   1. 2 hours.
   2. 6 hours.
   3. 12 hours.
   4. 24 hours.

3. As intracranial pressure (ICP) increases and perfusion is reduced, oxygen delivery to cerebral tissue is:
   1. increased.
   2. bypassed.
   3. reduced.
   4. stopped.

4. A patient with increased ICP has a "blown pupil." Which describes this condition?
   1. Dilated
   2. Pinpoint
   3. Reacts to light
   4. Unequal to the other pupil

5. The pupils may become dilated and fixed as ICP rises due to pressure on the:
   1. oculomotor nerve.
   2. cerebellum.
   3. hypothalamus.
   4. optic nerve.

6. Which neurons transmit information toward the central nervous system (CNS)?
   1. Sensory
   2. Motor
   3. Efferent
   4. Axon

7. What are the measures used to decrease ICP? Select all that apply.
   1. Positioning
   2. Lumbar puncture
   3. Hyperventilation
   4. Restriction of fluids
   5. Mechanical drainage
   6. Surgery
   7. Drug therapy

8. What evaluations are included in a neurologic assessment? Select all that apply.
   1. Level of consciousness
   2. Pupillary size and response
   3. Coordination
   4. Medical history
   5. Balance
   6. Sensory function
   7. Family history
   8. Reflexes

9. What are the possible risks for a patient who has had a craniotomy performed? Select all that apply.
   1. Increased ICP
   2. CSF leak
   3. Dehydration
   4. Meningitis
   5. Seizures
   6. Paralysis
   7. Impaired speech, vision, and hearing
   8. Incontinence
   9. Memory loss
   10. Confusion

10. Which priority measures are indicated for patients with increased ICP? Select all that apply.
    1. Raise the head of the bed 90 degrees.
    2. Increase fluids and monitor carefully.
    3. Monitor for changes in level of consciousness.
    4. Check pupillary reactivity.
    5. Administer antimicrobials after cerebral spinal fluid sample is obtained.

11. Which drugs are commonly used in the treatment of patients with increased ICP? Select all that apply.
    1. Hyperosmolar agents (mannitol)
    2. Corticosteroids
    3. Diuretics (furosemide)
    4. Antihypertensives
    5. Barbiturates

12. Which are characteristics of reflexes in the older patient?
    1. Jerky
    2. Tremors present
    3. Slower
    4. Remain intact
    5. Hyperreflexive

PART III: CHALLENGE YOURSELF!

H. Getting Ready for NCLEX

Choose the most appropriate answer or select all that apply.

1. A nurse is caring for a patient who was a victim of a violent crime and has experienced a head injury. She is lying very still and does not respond when spoken to or when shaken by the shoulder. The nurse squeezes her trapezius muscle and the patient responds to the painful stimuli. What is the term that describes her level of consciousness?
    1. Somnolent
    2. Comatose
    3. Lethargic
    4. Semicomatose

2. Disturbances in glucose metabolism and electrolyte imbalances can lead to deterioration in which two neurologic functions?
    1. Tissue perfusion
    2. Pupil stability
    3. Thought processes
    4. Level of consciousness

3. Indicate the correct sequence (1–5) of steps to perform a Romberg test. After asking the patient to stand with arms at his or her side and eyes closed, the following coordination of movements should be evaluated:

    _____ Ask the patient to touch his or her nose with the index finger, first with the eyes open and then with the eyes closed.

    _____ Hold up one of your fingers and instruct the patient to touch it with his or her index finger.

    _____ Alternate tapping with the heel and then the toes of one foot and then the other foot.

    _____ Ask the patient to run the heel of one foot down the shin of the other leg and then repeat with the opposite heel.

    _____ Ask the patient to pat his or her knees with the palms of the hands and then with the backs of the hands in a rapid, alternating pattern.

4. The nurse is taking care of a patient with a suspected brain tumor. What diagnostic procedure may be performed to confirm the diagnosis? Select all that apply.
    1. EEG
    2. EMG
    3. Lumbar puncture
    4. Myelography
    5. CT
    6. Brain scan

I. Nursing Assessment

Answer the following questions regarding information for an assessment of a patient with a neurologic disorder. Choose the most appropriate answer or select all that apply.

1. What should the nurse evaluate when asking the patient about his or her present health? Select all that apply.
    1. The patient's age
    2. Reason for seeking medical care
    3. The patient's speech, behavior, coordination, alertness, and comprehension
    4. Responses to yes/no questions
    5. Ability to respond verbally and nonverbally
    6. Past neurologic disorders
    7. Appropriateness of verbal responses, facial expressions, and physical reactions
    8. Family history of neurologic disorders
    9. Fluency and word recall

2. Which conditions during the review of the patient's systems are especially important to note? Select all that apply.
   1. Weakness
   2. Impaired movement
   3. Pain (especially headache)
   4. Dysphagia
   5. Bowel or bladder incontinence
   6. Dates of immunizations
   7. Visual disturbances
   8. Orientation to person, place, and time
   9. Mental or emotional changes
   10. Altered sensation
   11. Vital signs

3. If a patient's ICP is not being monitored, what neurologic checks should be conducted frequently during an assessment? Select all that apply.
   1. Evaluating level of consciousness
   2. Pupil appearance and response to light
   3. Moisture content of membranes
   4. The patient's ability to follow commands
   5. Whether the patient is combative when responding
   6. Movement and sensation of extremities
   7. Vital signs

4. What score would a patient in a coma receive on the Glasgow Coma Scale?
   1. 15 or above
   2. 7 or less
   3. A score indicating lethargy
   4. 115

5. What are the four major components of a routine neurologic examination performed when the patient is stable and can provide valuable information regarding the overall integrity of the CNS? Select four that apply.
   1. Level of consciousness
   2. Pupillary evaluation
   3. Bowel or bladder incontinence
   4. Neuromuscular response
   5. Mental or emotional changes
   6. Vital signs

Neurologic Disorders

Go to http://evolve.elsevier.com/Linton/medsurg/ for additional activities and exercises.

NCLEX CATEGORIES

Safe and Effective Care Environment: Safety and Infection Control

Health Promotion and Maintenance

Psychosocial Integrity

Physiological Integrity: Reduction of Risk Potential, Physiological Adaptation

PART I: MASTERING THE BASICS

A. Types of Headaches and Seizures
Match the definition in the numbered column with the most appropriate term in the lettered column.

1. _____ Causes intense unilateral pain and usually begins in temple or eyes

2. _____ Frequently occurs in a series followed by an extended period with no symptoms

3. _____ Can last for days or even years and the location of the pain can vary

4. _____ Can be simple or complex but either can progress to involve the entire brain

5. _____ Involves the entire brain from the onset and patient usually loses consciousness

6. _____ Continuous or repeated seizures that can cause brain damage

7. _____ Sensation such as dizziness, eye or hearing disruption, etc., that can occur prior to a seizure

A. Aura
B. Cluster
C. Generalized
D. Migraine
E. Focal seizure
F. Status epilepticus
G. Tension

B. Types of Head Injuries
Match the definition in the numbered column with the most appropriate term in the lettered column.

1. _____ Describes the signs and symptoms that a person may experience after a mild TBI

2. _____ Head trauma in which there is actual bruising and bleeding in the brain tissue

3. _____ A collection of blood, usually clotted, which may be classified as subdural or epidural

A. Contusion
B. Hematoma
C. Concussion

4. Which are common scalp injuries? Select all that apply.
   1. Lacerations
   2. Fissures
   3. Contusions
   4. Abrasions
   5. Hematomas
   6. Tumors

5. Which are neurotransmitters? Select all that apply.
   1. Acetylcholine
   2. Thyroxine
   3. Myosin
   4. Norepinephrine
   5. Insulin

C. Common Neurologic Disorders

Match the statements in the numbered column with the most appropriate term in the lettered column.

1. _____ Inflammation of the coverings of the brain and spinal cord caused by either viral or bacterial organisms

2. _____ Inflammation of brain tissue usually caused by a virus

3. _____ A rapidly progressing disease that affects the motor component of the peripheral nervous system

4. _____ A progressive degenerative disorder that results in an eventual loss of coordination and control over involuntary motor movement

5. _____ A chronic, progressive disease in which the amount of acetylcholine available at the neuromuscular junction is reduced

6. _____ A degenerative neurologic disease; also known as *Lou Gehrig's disease*

7. _____ A chronic, progressive, degenerative disease attacking the myelin sheath, disrupting motor pathways of the CNS

A. Meningitis
B. Parkinson disease
C. Guillain-Barré syndrome
D. Encephalitis
E. Multiple sclerosis (MS)
F. Amyotrophic lateral sclerosis (ALS)
G. Myasthenia gravis

Match the definition in the numbered column with the most appropriate neurologic disease in the lettered column.

8. _____ Characterized by intense pain along the distribution of one of the three branches of the fifth cranial nerve

9. _____ Acute paralysis of the seventh cranial nerve

10. _____ Paralysis associated with a loss of motor coordination caused by cerebral damage

11. _____ Progressive muscle weakness, fatigue, pain, and respiratory problems years after the initial infection, illness, and recovery

A. Cerebral palsy
B. Bell's palsy
C. Postpolio syndrome
D. Trigeminal neuralgia

D. Clinical Manifestations of Parkinson Syndrome

Refer to the figure (Figure 22.4 from the book). Match the description of symptoms of Parkinson disease in the numbered column with the most appropriate term in the lettered column. Some terms may not be used.

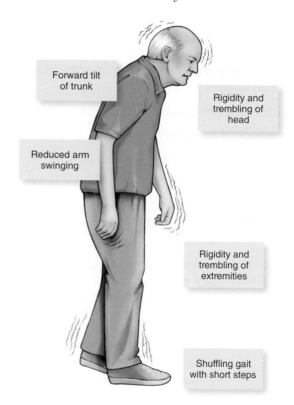

1. _____ Trembling, shaking type of movement usually seen in upper extremities

2. _____ Stiffness

3. _____ Extremely slow movements

4. _____ Movement of thumb against fingertips

A. Bradykinesia
B. Tremor
C. Bradycardia
D. Rigidity
E. Pill-rolling
F. Dementia

5. What are the three major symptoms (major triad) of Parkinson syndrome? Select three that apply.
   1. Aching
   2. Monotone voice
   3. Tremors at rest
   4. Rigidity
   5. Slumped posture
   6. Bradykinesia

6. What is characteristic of the tremors of a patient with Parkinson syndrome?

7. What are the two main goals for the patient with Parkinson disease?

E. Drug Therapy
Match the uses of drugs in the numbered column with names of drugs used for multiple sclerosis (MS) in the lettered column.

1. _____ Drug used during period of exacerbation

2. _____ Drug used to encourage remission

3. _____ Drug used to modulate the immune response and the course of MS

4. _____ Drug used to treat the spasticity experienced by MS patients

A. Betaseron (interferon beta-1b)
B. Prednisone
C. Baclofen
D. Adrenocorticotropic hormone (ACTH)

F. Divisions of Trigeminal Nerve
Refer to Figure 22.7 to answer questions 1–3.

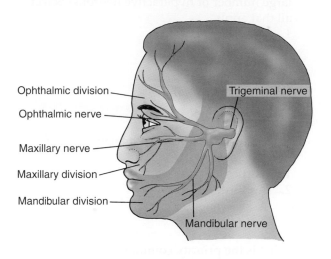

1. What disease is characterized by intense pain along one of the three branches of the trigeminal nerve?

2. What is the main focus of nursing care for the patient with trigeminal neuralgia?

3. What other problems does this patient have due to nerve involvement? Select all that apply.
   1. Imbalanced nutrition
   2. Social isolation
   3. Increased intracranial pressure (ICP)
   4. Hypertension
   5. Ineffective tissue perfusion

PART II: PUTTING IT ALL TOGETHER

G. Multiple Choice/Multiple Response
Choose the most appropriate answer or select all that apply.

1. A type of headache in which the pain is usually unilateral and has a warning is called:
   1. cluster.
   2. migraine.
   3. tension.
   4. sinus.

2. A patient is having frequent seizure activity. As a result, which are used excessively by the large number of hyperactive neurons? Select all that apply.
   1. Calcium
   2. Potassium
   3. Oxygen
   4. Glucose
   5. Sodium
   6. Acetylcholine

3. What is used in the initial management of bacterial meningitis?
   1. Corticosteroids
   2. Antihistamines
   3. Anticholinergics
   4. Antimicrobials

4. What is the priority common source of anxiety for many patients with Guillain-Barré syndrome?
   1. Loss of verbal communication
   2. Lowered self-esteem
   3. Deficient knowledge
   4. Decreased sensation in feet

5. To reduce the symptoms of Parkinson disease, what is L-dopa converted to as it crosses the blood-brain barrier?
   1. Epinephrine
   2. Dopamine
   3. Norepinephrine
   4. Acetylcholine

6. The nurse is taking care of a patient with myasthenia gravis. Which are signs and symptoms that the nurse would expect to see in the health history of this patient? Select all that apply.
   1. Muscle weakness
   2. Diplopia
   3. Breathing difficulties
   4. Loss of balance
   5. Fever and chills

7. Which priority measures are indicated for patients with increased ICP? Select all that apply.
   1. Raise the head of the bed 90°.
   2. Increase fluids and monitor carefully.
   3. Monitor for changes in the level of consciousness.
   4. Check pupillary reactivity.
   5. Administer antimicrobials after the cerebral spinal fluid sample is obtained.

8. What physical therapy programs are most helpful for patients with Parkinson disease? Select all that apply.
   1. Crutch walking
   2. Massage
   3. Cold compresses
   4. Exercise
   5. Gait retraining

9. What are ways to improve mobility for a patient with Parkinson disease? Select all that apply.
   1. Scoot to the edge of a chair before trying to stand.
   2. March in place before starting to walk.
   3. Use cotton sheets to make it easier to move in and out of bed.
   4. Practice lifting the foot as if to step over an object on the floor to initiate walking.
   5. Shift position in wheelchair every hour to build strength for walking.

10. What are the findings a nurse would expect to see when doing a physical examination of a patient with ALS? Select all that apply.
    1. Muscle atrophy
    2. Paralysis
    3. Improvement with rest
    4. Abnormal reflexes

PART III: CHALLENGE YOURSELF!

H. Getting Ready for NCLEX
Choose the most appropriate answer or select all that apply.

1. What is the priority cause of nutritional problems in patients with ALS?
   1. Oropharyngeal muscle weakness
   2. Paralysis of respiratory muscles
   3. Dysphagia
   4. Progressive illness of patient

2. What health promotion interventions should be performed for patients with meningitis and those who will be interacting with them? Select all that apply.
   1. Patient should remain calm to prevent seizures.
   2. Patient should receive vaccination to prevent pneumonia and/or influenza.
   3. Prophylactic antibiotics should be administered to those interacting with the patient.
   4. Anyone who has had contact with the patient should be quarantined for 48 hours.

I. Next-Generation NCLEX® Examination-Style Questions

A 70-year-old male who lives alone has a history of generalized tonic-clonic seizures. The nurse reviews the client's health history.

> Health History:
> A 70-year-old male who lives alone has a history of generalized tonic-clonic seizures. He has been taking carbamazepine (Tegretol), but recently ran out of his prescription. While mowing the lawn he suddenly collapsed, and began to display muscle stiffness in the arms, legs, chest and back followed by muscle jerking and twitching. His neighbor witnessed the seizure.

1. Based on the client information provided, what actions should the neighbor have taken to manage the seizure? Select all that apply.
   1. Remove any objects that could cause harm.
   2. Place a tongue blade between the client's teeth.
   3. Turn the client to one side.
   4. Perform a sternal rub to arouse the client.
   5. Note the time the seizure began and how it progressed.
   6. Restrain the client.
   7. Begin CPR.

A 35-year-old female client goes to her primary care physician with complaints of fatigue, weakness, and tingling in her right upper extremity. The nurse reviews the client's health history and physician's progress notes.

> Health History:
> A 35-year-old female client presents with complaints of fatigue, weakness, and tingling in her right upper extremity. She states that she has been having frequent visual disturbances with no significant medical history. Client reports falling last week due to impaired balance.
>
> Physician's Progress Notes:
> 7/5/21 0900: MRI of the brain and spinal cord reveals plaques characteristic of multiple sclerosis. *L. Lyons, MD*

Complete the following sentence by choosing from the list of options below.

2. The client is most at risk for _____ (1), related to _____ (2).

Options for 1	Options for 2
Constipation	Neurologic impairment
Injury	Dehydration
Ineffective breathing pattern	Fatigue
Acute pain	Muscle deterioration

Cerebrovascular Accident

chapter
23

Go to http://evolve.elsevier.com/Linton/medsurg/ for additional activities and exercises.

NCLEX CATEGORIES

Safe and Effective Care Environment:
Coordinated Care, Safety and Infection Control

Health Promotion and Maintenance

Psychosocial Integrity

Physiological Integrity: Pharmacological Therapies, Reduction of Risk Potential, Physiological Adaptation

PART I: MASTERING THE BASICS

A. Key Terms

Match the definition in the numbered column with the most appropriate term in the lettered column.

1. _____ Inability to speak clearly because of neurologic damage that affects the muscles of speech

2. _____ Drooping of the upper eyelid

3. _____ Difficulty understanding written or spoken words

4. _____ Double vision

5. _____ Defect in use of language: speech, reading, writing, or word comprehension

6. _____ Loss of one side of the field of vision; loss is on the side opposite the brain lesion

7. _____ Partial inability to initiate coordinated voluntary motor acts

8. _____ Difficulty speaking and writing

9. _____ Difficulty swallowing

10. _____ Paralysis of one side of the body

11. _____ Difficulty initiating speech

A. Hemiplegia
B. Nonfluent aphasia
C. Dyspraxia
D. Dysarthria
E. Ptosis
F. Homonymous hemianopsia
G. Expressive aphasia
H. Aphasia
I. Dysphagia
J. Diplopia
K. Receptive aphasia

Match the definition or description in the numbered column with the most appropriate term in the lettered column. Some terms may be used more than once, and some terms may not be used.

12. _____ An important warning condition for a possible later stroke

13. _____ The common name for cerebrovascular accident; interruption of blood flow to part of the brain

14. _____ A hemorrhage that can be caused by rupture of an aneurysm

15. _____ Improves blood flow by dilating the narrowed artery with a balloon that is inserted into the artery

16. _____ Opening an obstructed blood vessel and removing the plaque

17. _____ Set of neurologic signs and symptoms caused by impaired blood flow to the brain that lasts for more than 24 hours

A. Subarachnoid
B. Transient ischemic attack (TIA)
C. Angioplasty
D. Stroke
E. Endarterectomy
F. Atherosclerosis

B. Acute Phase

1. How long does the acute phase of a stroke usually last after onset?
   1. 2–3 hours
   2. 24–48 hours
   3. 4–5 days
   4. 7 days

Match the definition or description in the numbered column with the most appropriate term in the lettered column. Some terms may be used more than once.

2. _____ Continuous cardiac monitoring is necessary after a stroke to identify possible changes

3. _____ Priority treatment to prevent extension of affected area

4. _____ Can potentially worsen stroke outcome if not normalized

5. _____ May worsen brain tissue damage

6. _____ Occurs in the absence of having a history of diabetes

7. _____ Dehydration may be a cause and may lead to decrease of blood flow to brain

8. _____ Can be managed with acetaminophen

A. Hypertension
B. Oxygenation
C. Hyperthermia
D. Hyperglycemia
E. Arrhythmia

Match the criteria in the numbered column with the tissue plasminogen activator (t-PA) (alteplase [Activase, Activase rt-PA]) screening list in the lettered column. Some list items may be used more than once.

9. _____ Extend IV r-tPA treatment 3 hours to 4.5 hours from symptom onset

10. _____ Onset of stroke is less than 3 hours

11. _____ Patient has seizure at time of stroke

12. _____ Elevated blood pressure

13. _____ Recent gastrointestinal hemorrhage

A. Inclusion criteria
B. Exclusion criteria
C. Relative exclusion criteria

C. Types of Stroke

Match the definition in the numbered column with the most appropriate term in the lettered column.

1. _____ Caused by cerebral arterial wall rupture

2. _____ Caused by obstruction of blood vessel by plaque, blood clot, or both

3. _____ Caused by obstruction forming in blood vessel of the brain

A. Thrombotic stroke
B. Embolic stroke
C. Hemorrhagic stroke

PART II: PUTTING IT ALL TOGETHER

D. Multiple Choice/Multiple Response

Choose the most appropriate answer or select all that apply.

1. One of the most important needs of the acute stroke patient is to be turned and repositioned at least every:
   1. 2 hours.
   2. 4 hours.
   3. 8 hours.
   4. 12 hours.

2. Turning and repositioning the stroke patient will reduce the incidence of:
   1. hypertension.
   2. skin breakdown.
   3. headache.
   4. cerebral edema.

3. Which of the following are signs and symptoms in a patient who has just been admitted with a stroke? Select all that apply.
   1. Headache
   2. Numbness
   3. One-sided weakness
   4. Seizures
   5. Wound infection
   6. Speech problems

4. Which diagnostic test shows narrowing of cerebral blood vessels?
   1. Computed tomography (CT) scan
   2. Magnetic resonance imaging (MRI)
   3. Electroencephalogram (EEG)
   4. Noninvasive vascular studies

5. Which of the following are the possible causes of constipation in the patient with a stroke? Select all that apply.
   1. Infection
   2. Cerebral edema
   3. Immobility
   4. Dehydration
   5. Drug therapy

6. The main focus of the rehabilitation phase following a stroke is to:
   1. cure the disease process.
   2. assist the patient into remission.
   3. prevent another stroke from occurring.
   4. return the patient to the highest functional level possible.

7. What is the most frequent cause of death following a stroke?
   1. Kidney failure
   2. Pneumonia
   3. Seizure
   4. Heart attack

8. The nurse is teaching a class at a community health clinic about risk factors for stroke. Which are common modifiable risk factors for a stroke? Select all that apply.
   1. High blood pressure
   2. Atrial fibrillation
   3. Thyroid problems
   4. Physical inactivity
   5. Lack of calcium in diet

9. What is a priority problem immediately following a stroke?
   1. Oxygenation
   2. Hydration
   3. Nutrition
   4. Thermoregulation

10. What is a common sensory-perceptual problem in a patient with a stroke?
    1. Weakness
    2. Paralysis
    3. Diplopia
    4. Dysphagia

11. A patient who does not feel pressure or pain due to lost sensation following a stroke is at risk for:
    1. aphasia.
    2. paralysis.
    3. injury.
    4. infection.

12. A patient is experiencing an acute ischemic stroke. To improve chances for recovery, the patient should receive tissue plasminogen activator (tPA or IV rtPA) within a time span of: (Select all that apply.)
    1. 60–90 minutes.
    2. 2–2.5 hours.
    3. 3–4.5 hours.
    4. 6–8 hours.

13. Which term is used to describe speech impaired to the point that the person has almost no ability to communicate?
    1. Global aphasia
    2. Expressive aphasia
    3. Receptive aphasia
    4. Nonfluent aphasia

14. Which of the following are signs or symptoms of a stroke? Select all that apply.
    1. Sudden, severe headache with no known cause
    2. Sudden trouble seeing
    3. Tremors of extremities at rest
    4. Rigidity of movement
    5. Sudden trouble speaking
    6. Numbness or weakness of the face, arm, or leg

15. According to the NIH stroke scale, which variables are assessed in a patient who has had a CVA? Select all that apply.
    1. Level of consciousness
    2. Visual fields
    3. Motor function
    4. Language
    5. Blood pressure
    6. Sensory comparison side to side
    7. Temperature
    8. Pupillary reaction

PART III: CHALLENGE YOURSELF!

E. Getting Ready for NCLEX

Choose the most appropriate answer or select all that apply.

1. The nurse is taking care of a patient recently admitted with a stroke. Which of the following factors create problems related to physical mobility for this patient? Select all that apply.
   1. Edema
   2. Dyspraxia
   3. Hypertension
   4. Visual field disturbances
   5. Hemiplegia

2. You are assisting the nurse with teaching an in-service program about medications used to treat strokes. You plan to include the drugs and their uses in your talk. Match the uses of drugs in the numbered column with the drugs used for treatment of stroke in the lettered column.
   1. _____ Used to treat cerebral edema
   2. _____ Used to treat hemorrhagic stroke by dilating and preventing spasms in cerebral blood vessels
   3. _____ Used to reduce intracranial pressure (ICP) by reducing cerebral inflammation
   4. _____ Used to decrease chance of thrombosis and prevent recurrence of strokes caused by thrombi
   5. _____ Used to dissolve clots that cause acute ischemic stroke
   6. _____ Used to treat seizures, if seizures are present with stroke
   A. Anticonvulsants, such as phenytoin and phenobarbital
   B. Platelet aggregation inhibitors, such as aspirin
   C. Hyperosmotic agents, such as mannitol
   D. Calcium channel blockers, such as nimodipine
   E. Tissue plasminogen activator (t-PA) and recombinant tissue plasminogen activator (rt-PA)
   F. Corticosteroids

3. According to *Healthy People 2030*, what is the role of the nurse in stroke prevention and treatment? Select all that apply.
   1. Spread the word about risk factors for and warning signs of stroke.
   2. Participate in stroke and blood pressure screenings.
   3. Engage in and promote physical activity.
   4. Assist patients to locate antismoking campaigns.
   5. Encourage yearly eye exams.
   6. Help increase the number of adult stroke survivors who receive adequate care and are screened for depression.

4. How does the nurse identify whether a patient has right or left brain damage after suffering from a stroke? Match the type of damage in the numbered column with the side affected (R = right brain damage; L = left brain damage). (See Figure 23.3 in the book.)
   1. _____ Impaired judgment
   2. _____ Left-sided neglect
   3. _____ Impaired language and math comprehension
   4. _____ May deny or diminish problems
   5. _____ Impaired right/left discrimination
   6. _____ Slow performance, cautious
   7. _____ Paralyzed right side
   8. _____ Short attention span
   9. _____ Difficulty with concept of time
   10. _____ Speech impairment

5. The initial assessment of a patient suspected of having an acute stroke is directed at determining the type and extent of stroke. According to the Cincinnati Pre-hospital Stroke Scale, what is an abnormal finding when the patient is asked to show teeth or smile?

6. The nurse is monitoring a newly admitted patient with a possible stroke. What is an abnormal finding when the patient is asked to close both eyes and hold both arms straight out for 10 seconds?

7. When administering the Cincinnati Pre-hospital Stroke Scale, what are abnormal findings that may indicate the patient is having a stroke when the patient is asked to repeat a simple phrase such as, "You can't teach an old dog new tricks"? Select all that apply.
   1. Uses correct words, but speaks slowly
   2. Slurs words
   3. Uses the wrong words
   4. Speaks with a lisp
   5. Unable to speak

8. A female patient with a stroke describes a "feeling of lost sensation in my right leg." She says she does not feel pressure or pain in her right leg. The priority problem for this patient is:
   1. potential for injury.
   2. potential for infection.
   3. impaired mobility.
   4. inadequate nutrition.

9. In the acute phase following a stroke, if the patient has homonymous hemianopsia, the environment is arranged so that the important items are available on the:
   1. unaffected side.
   2. affected side.
   3. left side.
   4. right side.

F. Next-Generation NCLEX® Examination-Style Questions

Read the following situations and answer the questions 1-3. For more information, refer to Nursing Care Plan, Patient with a Stroke, in your book.

An obese 78-year-old male client was admitted with weakness on the right side and slurred speech. The nurse reviews the health history, physical assessment, and vital signs.

Health History:
Obese 78-year-old male client admitted with weakness on the right side and slurred speech. He has had type 2 diabetes mellitus for 10 years and takes an oral hypoglycemic drug. He had a myocardial infarction at age 75. He has no changes in vision, good hearing, no headaches, and no loss of bowel or bladder control. He is right-handed. He was unable to stand when he awoke this morning. He had difficulty swallowing a glass of water. He is a retired construction worker; his hobbies are watching television.

Physical Assessment:
5/3/21 0800: Client acknowledges that he is in the hospital but is uncertain about day or date and time. Unable to find the right words when responding to questions. Pupils equal and reactive to light. Ptosis of right eyelid is noted. Hand grips; voluntary movements; and reflexes of leg, arm, and hand are normal on left side but diminished on right side. Leans toward right side when not supported.

Vital Signs:

Blood Pressure	210/140 mm Hg
Pulse	96 beats/minute
Respirations	22 breaths/minute
Temperature	97°F

1. Highlight the risk factors for stroke that are evident in the history of this patient.

2. Which of the following are caused by effects of the stroke on this patient? Select all that apply.
   1. Impairments in speech
   2. Motor function
   3. Bladder control
   4. Personality changes
   5. Emotional lability
   6. Visual disturbances

Mr. Jones is a 70-year-old African American male client admitted with right-sided facial drooping and slurred speech. The nurse reviews the client's health history.

Health History:
70-year-old African American male client admitted with right-sided facial drooping and slurred speech. He has a medical history of TIA 6 months ago and hypertension. He smokes 1/2 pack of cigarettes per day with a 20-year pack history. His wife cooks him bacon and eggs for breakfast every morning. He is a retired school teacher and spends his days lounging in his recliner.

3. Using the health history, highlight the nonmodifiable risk factors related to stroke.

Spinal Cord Injury

Go to http://evolve.elsevier.com/Linton/medsurg/ for additional activities and exercises.

NCLEX CATEGORIES

Safe and Effective Care Environment: Safety and Infection Control

Health Promotion and Maintenance

Psychosocial Integrity

Physiological Integrity: Basic Care and Comfort, Reduction of Risk Potential, Physiological Adaptation

PART I: MASTERING THE BASICS

A. Key Terms
Match the definition in the numbered column with the most appropriate term in the lettered column.

1. _____ Loss of motor and sensory function in all four extremities due to damage to the spinal cord

2. _____ Soft, in relation to muscle; lacking tone

3. _____ Abnormally exaggerated response of the autonomic nervous system to a stimulus

4. _____ Loss of motor and sensory function due to damage to the spinal cord that spares the upper extremities, but depending on the level of the damage, affects the trunk, pelvis, and lower extremities

5. _____ Increased muscle tone characterized by sudden, involuntary muscle spasms

6. _____ Surrounded with a sheath

A. Paraplegia
B. Myelinated

C. Tetraplegia
D. Flaccid
E. Spasticity
F. Autonomic dysreflexia

Match the statements in the numbered column with the most appropriate term in the lettered column. Some terms may be used more than once.

7. _____ Removal of all or part of the posterior arch of the vertebra

8. _____ The placement of a piece of donor bone, commonly taken from the hip, into the area between the involved vertebrae

9. _____ The surgical procedure done to alleviate compression of the spinal cord or nerves

A. Spinal fusion
B. Laminectomy

B. Spinal Cord Injury

1. What spinal areas are most vulnerable to injury? Select two locations.
   1. Cervical
   2. Thoracic
   3. Lumbar
   4. Sacral

2. After establishing a patent airway, what is the greatest priority in the acute phase of a spinal cord injury?
   1. Immobilize the patient.
   2. Apply pneumatic stockings to lower extremities.
   3. Prevent complications of immobility.
   4. Take vital signs.

3. During the acute phase, what procedure may be done to decrease pressure on the spinal cord?
   1. Placement of halo device
   2. Laminectomy
   3. Placement of Crutchfield tongs
   4. Lumbar puncture

4. Explain why the traditional head-tilt/chin-lift method of opening the airway is inappropriate in spinal cord–injured patients.

PART II: PUTTING IT ALL TOGETHER

C. Multiple Choice/Multiple Response
Choose the most appropriate answer or select all that apply.

1. The halo device is used to provide immobilization and alignment of the:
   1. cervical vertebrae.
   2. thoracic vertebrae.
   3. lumbar vertebrae.
   4. sacral vertebrae.

2. Prompt intervention following autonomic dysreflexia must be directed toward severe:
   1. hypertension.
   2. hypotension.
   3. infection.
   4. lung compromise.

3. Patients with skull tongs are maintained on:
   1. bedrest with ambulation 3 times a day.
   2. isolation precautions.
   3. high-roughage diets.
   4. strict bedrest.

4. Following an ileus, the patient will be given oral fluids and food when:
   1. the swallow reflex returns.
   2. the patient is no longer anorexic.
   3. bladder continence returns.
   4. peristalsis returns.

5. After a spinal cord injury, what methods are used to assess sensory function? Select all that apply.
   1. Movement
   2. Muscle strength
   3. Self-concept
   4. Eye movement

6. Which type of spinal cord injury will result in a loss of motor control below the waist?
   1. C4
   2. C7
   3. T4
   4. T10

7. Which action is indicated in the management of spasticity in the spinal cord–injured patient?
   1. Increase tactile stimuli.
   2. Administer antihypertensive medications.
   3. Perform passive ROM exercises at least 4 times a day.
   4. Turn and reposition the patient at least every 4 hours.

8. Injuries at or above C5 may result in instant death because the:
   1. innervation to the phrenic nerve is interrupted.
   2. sympathetic innervation to the heart is blocked.
   3. sensory nerves to the brain are interrupted.
   4. saphenous nerve can no longer transmit impulses.

9. The spinal cord–injured patient may have difficulty maintaining body temperature within a normal range because the:
   1. hypothalamus can no longer regulate temperature.
   2. regulatory mechanisms of vasoconstriction and sweating are lost.
   3. peripheral nerves to the skin are interrupted.
   4. skin is not able to lose heat through evaporation.

10. At the scene of an accident involving a patient with spinal cord injury, emergency personnel will apply a hard cervical collar around the patient's neck to immobilize the:
    1. skull.
    2. spinal column.
    3. brain.
    4. upper part of the body.

11. Which type of traction, applied to a fiberglass jacket, is used to immobilize and align the cervical vertebrae and relieve compression of nerve roots?
    1. Philadelphia collar
    2. Gardner-Wells tongs
    3. Crutchfield tongs
    4. Halo device

12. Which condition is an exaggerated sympathetic response to stimuli, such as bladder distention, that produces severe hypertension with the potential for seizures and stroke?
    1. Spinal cord injury
    2. Autonomic dysreflexia
    3. Meningitis
    4. Amyotrophic lateral sclerosis

13. As spinal shock begins to subside and reflex activity returns, the patient with a spinal cord injury is at risk for:
    1. respiratory arrest.
    2. autonomic dysreflexia.
    3. ileus.
    4. coma.

14. Which of the following statements are true about spinal shock? Select all that apply.
    1. Reflex activity below the level of the injury temporarily ceases
    2. Immediate, transient response to injury
    3. Paralysis is flaccid during this time
    4. Exaggerated response of the autonomic nervous system in patients whose injury is at or above the T6 level
    5. Resolution of spinal shock occurs when spastic, involuntary movement of extremities ceases

15. What is the reason most spinal cord–injured patients can maintain bowel function?
    1. Most spinal cord injuries occur above the T6 level.
    2. Peristalsis is interrupted by most spinal cord injuries, but responds to fecal mass.
    3. The bowel musculature has its own neural center that responds to fecal distention.
    4. The bowel function is not affected by spinal cord injuries.

16. What are some of the problems associated with spasticity? Select all that apply.
    1. Muscle briefly displays increased resistance followed by sudden relaxation
    2. Incontinence
    3. Reflexes become hyperactive
    4. Impaired temperature regulation

17. What are the main reasons a patient with spinal cord injury may have difficulty coping? Select all that apply.
    1. Disturbed sensory perception
    2. Impaired ADLs
    3. Overwhelming losses
    4. Limited potential for recovered function
    5. Lack of sensory function

18. What are the main reasons a spinal cord–injured patient is at risk for injury? Select all that apply.
    1. Involuntary muscle spasms
    2. Lack of motor function
    3. Lack of sensory function
    4. Involvement of intercostal muscles
    5. Orthostatic hypotension

PART III: CHALLENGE YOURSELF!

D. Getting Ready for NCLEX
Choose the most appropriate answer or select all that apply.

1. The nurse is taking care of a patient who is maintained in cervical traction while on a conventional bed. Which is the best method for changing positions of this patient?
   1. Assisted ambulation
   2. ROM exercises
   3. Logrolling
   4. Grasping the muscles

2. When the spinal cord–injured patient has spasticity, to what is nursing management directed? Select all that apply.
   1. Prevention of infection
   2. Prevention of muscle atrophy
   3. Prevention of contracture
   4. Prevention of dyspnea
   5. Prevention of inadequate coping

3. During the time of flaccid paralysis, the nurse must be diligent in performing:
   1. active ROM exercises.
   2. passive ROM exercises.
   3. coughing and deep-breathing exercises.
   4. early ambulation.

4. The nurse is caring for a postoperative laminectomy patient. Which finding is reported to the health care provider?
   1. WBC of 7000/mm^3
   2. Blood pressure 125/80 mmHg
   3. Clear drainage from incision site
   4. Respirations of 18/min

5. When the nurse is taking care of a postoperative laminectomy patient, what nursing interventions are implemented to promote tissue perfusion? Select all that apply.
   1. Maintain elastic stockings on lower extremities.
   2. Assist the patient with ROM exercises.
   3. Administer analgesics for pain relief.
   4. Follow strict hand hygiene technique.
   5. Assess for urinary distention.

6. Which of the following emotions or actions the spinal cord–injured patient may have during the initial acute phase of adaptation? Select all that apply.
   1. Rage
   2. Depression
   3. Verbal abuse
   4. Shock
   5. Disbelief
   6. Denial

7. After the period of reaction for the spinal cord–injured patient subsides, the nurse should focus interventions related to altered self-concept on:
   1. patient's independence and control.
   2. protecting patient from harm.
   3. patient's expression of anger and bargaining.
   4. reassuring patient about body image.

8. Which are safety measures the nurse should take while caring for a spinal cord–injured patient who is experiencing spastic paralysis? Select all that apply.
   1. Secure the patient with a protective strap across the chest.
   2. Avoid stimulation of the spastic extremity.
   3. Grasp the muscle when performing ROM exercises or positioning the patient.
   4. Support joints above and below the affected muscle group with palms of hands.
   5. Raise the head of the bed to a 45° angle.

9. The patient with spinal cord injury has a potential for injury. What nursing measures will help prevent venous thromboembolism in this patient? Select all that apply.
   1. Pressure stockings
   2. Sequential compression devices when patient is up walking
   3. Administer injections above the level of paralysis
   4. Use of an incentive spirometer
   5. Apply firm pressure to the diaphragm when assisting with breathing exercises

10. The patient with spinal cord injury is experiencing a sudden pounding headache, facial flushing, and increased blood pressure. What is the priority nursing action to take for this patient?
    1. Check the indwelling catheter for occlusion.
    2. Remove any fecal impaction.
    3. Raise the patient's head to a 45° angle.
    4. Perform passive ROM exercises.

11. Which are health promotion considerations to teach a spinal cord–injured patient who is being discharged from the hospital regarding skin care? Select all that apply.
    1. Bathe in tepid water with mild soap; dry thoroughly.
    2. Wear cotton undergarments.
    3. Eat a balanced diet with high amounts of potassium and calcium.
    4. When in bed, turn at least every 2 hours.
    5. Sit up in a chair at least twice a day.

12. A patient is in the acute phase of a spinal cord injury. A problem noted by the nurse is that the patient has potential complications related to immobility. Which goal is the desired outcome for this patient's problem?
    1. Absence of complications of immobility
    2. No signs of autonomic dysreflexia
    3. Adequate oxygenation
    4. Pin site is free of infection

E. Case Study
Read the situation below and answer questions 1-3.

A patient had a lumbar laminectomy 1 day ago to relieve pressure on spinal nerves. Postoperatively, the nurse identified the following problems in this patient: potential for injury, inadequate circulation, pain, difficulty voiding, constipation, and impaired mobility.

1. Which finding, if observed by the nurse, should be reported to the health care provider?
   1. Decreased pulse
   2. Fever of 100°F
   3. Clear drainage from incision
   4. Blood pressure of 110/70 mmHg

2. Which intervention may help relieve the patient's pain?
   1. Wear pressure stockings
   2. Keep the bed flat (or with head slightly elevated)
   3. Take measures to promote voiding
   4. Encourage the patient to gradually increase ambulation

3. Which problems of this patient need to be addressed first? Select three priority problems for this patient.
   1. Potential for injury
   2. Constipation
   3. Pain
   4. Impaired mobility
   5. Inadequate circulation
   6. Difficulty voiding

F. Next-Generation NCLEX® Examination-Style Questions

Read the situations below and answer the questions.

A 45-year-old female client admitted to the hospital for a T6 spinal cord injury is lying in bed. The nurse reviews the physical assessment and vital signs.

Physical Assessment Findings:
Patient presents with diaphoresis, facial flushing, and complaints of headache 9/10 on numeric scale. Foley catheter in place. No urine in bag

Vital Signs:

Blood Pressure	188/90 mmHg
Pulse	56 beats/minute
Temperature	100°F

1. Based on the client information provided, what would be the nurse's first action?
   1. Administer antihypertensives
   2. Apply a cool towel to the client's neck
   3. Check for foley catheter occlusion
   4. Administer acetaminophen
   5. Elevate the head of bed 45°
   6. Administer IV fluids
   7. Call a code blue
   8. Encourage the client to use the incentive spirometer

A 38-year-old male client is admitted to the surgical unit following a spinal laminectomy. The nurse reviews the physical assessment and vital signs.

Physical Assessment:
Client is alert and oriented times 3, rates his pain 5/10 on a numeric scale, and his dressing is clean dry and intact. Peripheral pulses are equal and strong. Strength is equal in all four extremities.

Vital Signs:

Blood Pressure	120/72 mmHg
Pulse	70 beats/minute
Respirations	18 breaths/minute
Temperature	98.6°F

2. Based on the client information provided, what should be included in the nursing care? Select all that apply.
   1. Maintain elastic stockings on lower extremities to prevent deep vein thrombosis (DVT).
   2. Maintain the bed at 90° to reduce strain on the operative site.
   3. Encourage range-of-motion exercises 4 times a day.
   4. Encourage position changes every 4 hours.
   5. Encourage deep-breathing exercises every 2 hours.
   6. Restrict fluid intake.
   7. Auscultate breath sounds every 2–4 hours.
   8. Have the patient perform incentive spirometry every 2 hours while awake.
   9. Encourage bedrest to reduce spasms.

Respiratory System Introduction

Go to http://evolve.elsevier.com/Linton/medsurg/ for additional activities and exercises.

NCLEX CATEGORIES

Safe and Effective Care Environment:
Coordinated Care, Safety and Infection Control

Health Promotion and Maintenance

Psychosocial Integrity

Physiological Integrity: Basic Care and Comfort, Pharmacological Therapies, Reduction of Risk Potential, Physiological Adaptation

PART I: MASTERING THE BASICS

A. Key Terms
Match the statement in the numbered column with the most appropriate term in the lettered column. Some terms may be used more than once.

1. _____   The term for nosebleed
2. _____   Abnormal sounds associated with cardiac and pulmonary conditions
3. _____   High-pitched sound of air passing through a passageway narrowed by disease
4. _____   Appearance of bluish color on the lips, nose tip, gums, or under the tongue related to inadequate tissue oxygenation
5. _____   Dry, rattling sound caused by partial bronchial obstruction
6. _____   The term for shortness of breath
7. _____   Difficulty breathing while in a lying position
8. _____   Low oxygen level in the blood

A. Crackles
B. Cyanosis
C. Dyspnea
D. Epistaxis
E. Hypoxia
F. Orthopnea
G. Rhonchus
H. Wheezes

B. Structure of the Respiratory System
Refer to Figure 25.1, and label the structures of the nose and throat (A–J) by using the terms (1–10) below.

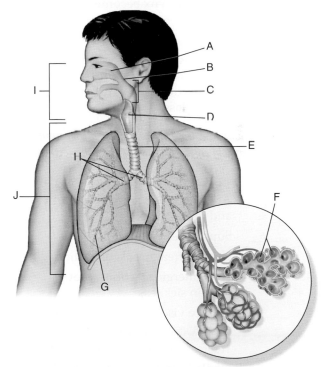

1. _____   Nasal cavity
2. _____   Upper respiratory tract
3. _____   Pharynx
4. _____   Lower respiratory tract
5. _____   Trachea

6. _____ Left and right primary bronchi
7. _____ Bronchioles
8. _____ Alveoli
9. _____ Nasopharynx
10. _____ Larynx

C. Age-Related Changes

1. Which are age-related changes of the nose, throat, and sinuses? Select all that apply.
   1. Decreased nasal obstruction
   2. Cartilage of the external nose hardens
   3. Increased, more serious side effects of nasal decongestants
   4. Production of mucus increases
   5. Mucous membrane becomes thinner
   6. Sense of smell declines
   7. Occurrence of epistaxis (nosebleed) increases
   8. Esophageal sphincter may weaken, causing gastric contents to flow back into the throat when patient lies down
   9. Tissues of the larynx become less elastic

D. Drug Therapy

The nurse is assisting with an in-service program on the actions and uses of medications for treating upper respiratory infections. The nurse uses the exercise below in the class.

Match the actions and uses of the drugs in the numbered column with the classification of drugs in the lettered column.

1. _____ Anesthetic effect on nasopharnyx and oropharnyx
2. _____ Suppresses cough reflex
3. _____ Used to treat nasal congestion
4. _____ Treat allergic reactions, prevent motion sickness
5. _____ Reduce viscosity and elasticity of mucus
6. _____ Treats acute bronchial constriction
7. _____ Inhaled drug causes bronchodilation

A. Decongestants
B. Anticholinergics
C. Antihistamines
D. Antitussives
E. Mucolytics
F. Topical anesthetics
G. Corticosteroids oral

PART II: PUTTING IT ALL TOGETHER

E. Multiple Choice/Multiple Response

Choose the most appropriate answer or select all that apply.

1. Inspection and palpation of the neck may reveal enlarged:
   1. lymph nodes.
   2. tonsils.
   3. adenoids.
   4. vocal cords.

2. Following laryngoscopy, the patient takes nothing by mouth until:
   1. respirations are normal.
   2. vomiting has stopped.
   3. the gag reflex returns.
   4. 24 hours after surgery.

3. Before suctioning a patient, it is important to:
   1. administer antiemetics as prescribed.
   2. ambulate the patient.
   3. oxygenate the patient.
   4. administer antibiotics as prescribed.

4. Which is a key point to remember when suctioning a patient?
   1. Keep the vent closed when inserting the catheter.
   2. Apply suction continuously as the catheter is withdrawn.
   3. Suction for no longer than 30 seconds.
   4. Use sterile procedure.

5. When providing tracheostomy care to a patient, which is the appropriate intervention?
   1. Use standard precautions.
   2. Suction the tracheostomy after removing the old dressings.
   3. Use a sterile solution of iodine to clean the inner cannula.
   4. Cut a new pad to fit around the tracheostomy site.

6. Which are common problems the nurse monitors in a patient who has had nasal surgery? Select all that apply.
   1. Bradycardia
   2. Dyspnea
   3. Pain
   4. Bleeding
   5. Anxiety
   6. Hypertension
   7. Pallor

7. The patient who has had nasal surgery may be at risk for cardiac irregularities because of:
   1. blood loss from nasal passageways.
   2. nasal packing.
   3. airway obstruction.
   4. facial bruising.

8. What is the priority problem for a patient following nasal surgery?
   1. Hemorrhage
   2. Infection
   3. Hypertension
   4. Confusion

9. Laxatives or stool softeners may be prescribed for patients after nasal surgery to prevent:
   1. diarrhea.
   2. vomiting.
   3. hypertension.
   4. straining.

10. Which is the best position for patients after nasal surgery to help control swelling?
    1. Lying flat in bed
    2. Semi Fowler to high Fowler
    3. Side lying
    4. Supine

11. When the nasal cavity is packed following surgery, the patient is breathing through the mouth. Which of the following are measures that help decrease dryness of the mucous membranes? Select all that apply.
    1. Frequent oral hygiene
    2. Humidifiers
    3. Oral fluids high in vitamin C
    4. Ice packs

12. Patients may experience altered self-concept following nasal surgery due to:
    1. airway obstruction.
    2. blood loss.
    3. hypovolemia.
    4. facial bruises.

13. Suctioning is limited to 10 seconds because prolonged suctioning may lead to:
    1. hypoxia.
    2. hypertension.
    3. increased intracranial pressure.
    4. bradycardia.

14. Gently closing one naris at a time and instructing the patient to breathe through the other naris is a way to assess:
    1. lung sounds.
    2. aphonia.
    3. sense of smell.
    4. patency of the nostrils.

15. Normally, the frontal and maxillary sinuses are filled with what?
    1. Fluid
    2. Air
    3. Polyps
    4. Cysts

PART III: CHALLENGE YOURSELF!

F. Getting Ready for NCLEX
Choose the most appropriate answer or select all that apply.

1. The nurse is developing a smoking cessation group for high-school students. Which cultural group has the highest incidence of smoking?
   1. non-Hispanic American Indians
   2. non-Hispanic whites
   3. Latinos
   4. African Americans

2. What sounds indicate a potential problem when auscultating the lungs? Select all that apply.
   1. Wheezes
   2. Hyperpnea
   3. Rhonchi
   4. Crackles
   5. Vesicular breath sounds
   6. Pleural friction rub

3. A throat culture is recommended when a patient is suspected of having which condition? Select all that apply.
   1. Epiglottitis
   2. Neisseria meningitidis
   3. Streptococcal sore throat
   4. Asthma

4. When administering drugs by the nasal route, what are some of the procedures the nurse should follow? Select all that apply.
   1. The patient's head must be titled forward.
   2. Ask the patient to blow his or her nose first.
   3. Do not allow the dropper to touch the nose.
   4. Discard unused solution rather than returning it to the bottle.
   5. Do not allow the patient to expectorate any of the solution once it is administered.
   6. The patient should not feel medication running down the throat.

5. When caring for patients on mechanical ventilation, what should the nurse be aware of? Select all that apply.
   1. Ensure that high- and low-pressure alarm settings are activated.
   2. Determine settings based on patient response.
   3. Have a manual resuscitator and O_2 source readily available.
   4. Water should be present within the tubing.
   5. Monitor vital signs and breath sounds.
   6. Inform patient he or she will be unable to speak while being intubated.

6. The nurse may assist the patient, who is at risk for pneumonia and atelectasis, after a thoracotomy to improve gas exchange by elevating the head of the bed by how many degrees?
   1. 10–15
   2. 20–40
   3. 45
   4. No elevation required

G. Case Study

Health history: A 45-year-old man has had chronic sinusitis for 3 years resulting in numerous sick days.

His symptoms included fatigue, difficulty breathing, and postnasal drainage. The symptoms would usually last from 10 to 12 weeks and recently he was beginning to have severe headaches and an elevated temperature. Upon physical examination several polyps that were obstructing his passageways were identified, and the patient was admitted for endoscopic surgery to remove the polyps.

Refer to the section Nursing Care of the Patient Having Nasal Surgery in the book to answer the following questions.

1. What is the most important priority for the nurse after a patient has nasal surgery?

2. List different methods to monitor for excessive blood loss after nasal surgery.

3. What were the patient's signs and symptoms listed in the health history that indicated a need for surgery?

   1. _____

   2. _____

4. Which methods should the nurse use to reduce or prevent hemorrhaging after nasal surgery? Select all that apply.
   1. Prevent patient from blowing nose.
   2. Offer laxatives to prevent straining.
   3. Position the patient so that his head is elevated to a 45-degree angle.
   4. Avoid aspirin and aspirin products.
   5. Prevent patient from standing.
   6. Encourage patient to drink citrus juices.

5. After surgery, what is the best position for the patient to reduce swelling?

Upper Respiratory Disorders

Go to http://evolve.elsevier.com/Linton/medsurg/ for additional activities and exercises.

NCLEX CATEGORIES

Safe and Effective Care Environment:
Coordinated Care, Safety, and Infection Control

Health Promotion and Maintenance

Psychosocial Integrity

Physiological Integrity: Basic Care and Comfort, Pharmacological Therapies, Reduction of Risk Potential, Physiological Adaptation

PART I: MASTERING THE BASICS

A. Key Terms
Match the statement in the numbered column with the most appropriate term in the lettered column. Some terms may be used more than once.

1. _____ Nosebleeds that can be minor or severe

2. _____ Most common in children and can be caused by bacteria or virus

3. _____ Substances that are everywhere, such as dust and dander, that can cause a reaction

4. _____ Infection that usually begins in the nasal passages and is caused by bacteria or a virus and occasionally fungus

5. _____ Surgical procedure to treat cancer of the larynx

6. _____ Drugs used to treat allergic rhinitis and are primarily intranasal corticosteroids

7. _____ Commonly referred to as "hay fever," classified as intermittent (seasonal) or persistent (perennial)

8. _____ Also known as the *common cold*

9. _____ An inflammation of the larynx that can be caused by sinus infections or irritants

10. _____ A drug that helps relieve (but not cure) symptoms of rhinitis

11. _____ Swollen masses of sinus or nasal mucosa and connective tissue that extend into the nasal passages

A. Allergen
B. Antihistamine
C. Coryza
D. Decongestant
E. Epistaxis
F. Laryngectomy
G. Laryngitis
H. Polyps
I. Rhinitis
J. Sinusitis
K. Tonsillitis

B. Sleep Apnea

Refer to Figure 26.1 in the book to answer questions 1–3.

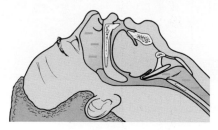

A

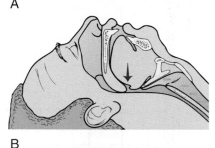

B

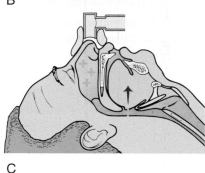

C

1. _____   Which figure shows the nasal continuous positive airway pressure (CPAP) in place?

2. _____   Which figure shows a patient predisposed to obstructive sleep apnea (OSA) with a small pharyngeal airway?

3. _____   Which figure shows the relaxation of the pharyngeal muscles, allowing the airway to close, resulting in repeated apneic episodes?

4. Which are symptoms of OSA? Select all that apply.
   1. Sore throat
   2. Epistaxis
   3. Irritable and sleepy during the day
   4. Impaired concentration and memory
   5. Muscle aches
   6. Loud snoring
   7. Hypotension
   8. Cardiac dysrhythmias

5. Which diagnostic test is done to confirm OSA?
   1. Laryngoscopy
   2. Bronchoscopy
   3. Polysomnography
   4. Blood gases

C. Laryngectomy Key Terms

Complete the statement in the numbered column with the most appropriate term in the lettered column.

1. Following laryngectomy, many patients are able to learn to control and use air to produce sounds, which is called _____.
2. Following laryngectomy, some patients use an electronic device to produce sound, which is called a(n) _____.
3. A procedure used for small tumors of the larynx is _____.
4. Surgery in which the voice is preserved is _____.

A. Laser surgery
B. Artificial larynx
C. Esophageal speech
D. Supraglottic laryngectomy

D. Pharyngitis

Indicate for each characteristic below whether it refers to (A) viral pharyngitis, (B) bacterial pharyngitis, or (C) both.

1. _____   Usually caused by strep throat
2. _____   Tonsillar exudate
3. _____   Most common form of pharyngitis
4. _____   Enlarged tonsils
5. _____   Abrupt onset of symptoms
6. _____   Diagnosis includes throat culture
7. _____   Fever
8. _____   Treatment focuses on symptoms
9. _____   Treated with antibiotics
10. _____   Complications are less likely

PART II: PUTTING IT ALL TOGETHER

E. Multiple Choice/Multiple Response

Choose the most appropriate answer or select all that apply.

1. For patients with throat disorders, for what does the nurse inspect the mucous membranes of the throat and tonsils? Select all that apply.
   1. Cyanosis
   2. Lesions
   3. Pallor
   4. Redness
   5. Drainage
   6. Swelling

2. During severe epistaxis, the patient's vital signs are monitored to detect signs of:
   1. hypokalemia.
   2. hypernatremia.
   3. hypovolemia.
   4. inadequate circulation.

3. Serious neurologic complications should be suspected in patients with sinusitis if the patient develops what?
   1. Tachycardia and restlessness
   2. High fever and seizures
   3. Confusion and cyanosis
   4. Dyspnea and anxiety

4. Desensitizing injections or "allergy shots" are composed of dilute solutions of what?
   1. Allergens
   2. Histamines
   3. Antihistamines
   4. Plasma

5. A major deviated septum may obstruct the nasal passage and block what?
   1. Sinus drainage
   2. Eustachian tube drainage
   3. Pharyngeal drainage
   4. Jugular vein drainage

6. Patients with a deviated septum may complain of epistaxis, sinusitis, and:
   1. palpitations.
   2. headaches.
   3. insomnia.
   4. sweating.

7. Patients with severe epistaxis may be at high risk for infection due to:
   1. possible airway obstruction.
   2. nasal packing.
   3. hypotension.
   4. hypovolemia.

8. The two major problems that may develop in the postoperative phase of tonsillectomy are respiratory distress and:
   1. infection.
   2. hemorrhage.
   3. hypersensitivity reaction.
   4. cardiac dysrhythmia.

9. Following a tonsillectomy, a treatment that may be applied to the neck to decrease swelling and pain is:
   1. a heating pad.
   2. a TENS unit.
   3. antibiotic ointment.
   4. an ice collar.

10. A postoperative tonsillectomy patient is ready to be discharged. Which symptoms should be reported to the health care provider if the nurse observes them?
    1. Bleeding
    2. Earache
    3. White patches in the throat (surgical site)
    4. Sore throat

11. Which treatment is usually prescribed to reduce irritation of the larynx in patients with laryngitis?
    1. Surgery
    2. Voice rest
    3. Intravenous fluids
    4. Application of heat

12. What is the correct term for benign masses of fibrous tissue that result primarily from overuse of the voice or following infections?
    1. Nodules
    2. Myomas
    3. Fibromas
    4. Tumors

13. The only symptom of laryngeal nodules is:
    1. pain.
    2. fever.
    3. dysphagia.
    4. hoarseness.

14. Which is the term for a swollen mass of mucous membrane attached to the vocal cord?
    1. Nodule
    2. Tumor
    3. Cancer
    4. Polyp

15. Individuals who both smoke and use alcohol are at particularly high risk for:
    1. tonsillitis.
    2. pneumonia.
    3. cancer of the larynx.
    4. nasal polyps.

16. What is the most common site of metastasis in a patient with laryngeal cancer?
    1. Liver
    2. Colon
    3. Lung
    4. Brain

17. Total laryngectomy causes permanent loss of the:
    1. voice.
    2. cough.
    3. sternocleidomastoid muscle movement.
    4. swallow reflex.

18. A total laryngectomy involves removal of the entire larynx, vocal cords, and:
    1. pharynx.
    2. epiglottis.
    3. tonsils.
    4. esophagus.

19. In the immediate postoperative period after total laryngectomy, the nurse's assessment focuses on comfort, circulation, and:
    1. fluid balance.
    2. oxygenation.
    3. infection.
    4. hypovolemia.

20. Which position promotes maximal lung expansion in the patient with a laryngectomy?
    1. Semi-prone
    2. Flat
    3. Semi-Fowler
    4. Side-lying

21. To prevent pooling of secretions in the lungs of patients with laryngectomies, which should the nurse encourage?
    1. Coughing and deep breathing
    2. Increased fluid intake
    3. Early ambulation
    4. Avoidance of dusty places

22. Which herb is used to boost the immune system and is taken by some to decrease the severity of a cold?
    1. Ginseng
    2. Ephedra
    3. Echinacea
    4. St. John's wort

23. To decrease the patient's reaction to offending allergens, the allergist may recommend injections for what purpose?
    1. Provide desensitization
    2. Treat tissue injury
    3. Increase immunity
    4. Prevent inflammation

24. Which are true statements about sinusitis? Select all that apply.
    1. Pain or a feeling of heaviness over the frontal or maxillary area is a common symptom.
    2. Toothache-like pain is a common symptom of sinusitis that involves the frontal sinus.
    3. Complications of sinusitis include brain abscess and meningitis.
    4. Most sinus infections are caused by a virus.
    5. With sinusitis, the throat appears red and tonsils may be enlarged.

25. Which are true statements about pharyngitis? Select all that apply.
    1. Pharyngitis is treated with rest, fluids, analgesics, and throat gargles.
    2. A soft or liquid diet may be prescribed because of nausea.
    3. A treatment that may be prescribed is humidification.
    4. The recommended daily fluid intake for patients with pharyngitis is 1000–1500 mL.
    5. Hospitalization is usually required while nasal packing is in place.

26. Which are complications of bacterial pharyngitis that may occur after the throat infection? Select all that apply.
    1. Acute glomerulonephritis
    2. Meningitis
    3. Sinusitis
    4. Brain abscess
    5. Rheumatic fever

PART III: CHALLENGE YOURSELF!

F. Getting Ready for NCLEX
Choose the most appropriate answer or select all that apply.

1. The nurse is teaching a community health class on tonsillitis. Which are true statements about patients with tonsillitis that should be included in the presentation? Select all that apply.
   1. Tonsillitis is not contagious.
   2. A patient with tonsillitis usually reports a sore throat, difficulty swallowing, fever, chills, and muscle aches.
   3. If swollen tissue blocks the eustachian tubes in patients with tonsillitis, there may also be pain in the lungs.
   4. An elevated white blood cell count in patients with tonsillitis suggests a viral infection.
   5. The medical treatment of tonsillitis usually includes the use of antibiotics.

2. A patient is experiencing epistaxis. Which common problems for this patient are likely to be present? Select all that apply.
   1. Potential airway obstruction related to increased pulmonary secretions or weak cough
   2. Decreased cardiac output related to hypovolemia secondary to hemorrhage
   3. Potential for injury related to pressure (of packing, balloon) and possible airway obstruction
   4. Potential for infection related to the presence of nasal packing

3. Two patients have walked into the clinic, one with facial trauma and one with a nasal fracture. The recommended initial treatment for these two patients is application of:
   1. an ice pack.
   2. a warm compress.
   3. direct pressure.
   4. heat.

4. The nurse is taking care of a postoperative tonsillectomy patient. Which are early signs of inadequate oxygenation in this patient? Select all that apply.
   1. Cyanosis
   2. Pallor
   3. Numbness
   4. Confusion
   5. Restlessness
   6. Increased pulse rate

5. Your patient has had a tonsillectomy. Which foods should be avoided in this patient following the surgery?
   1. Frozen liquids
   2. Ice cream
   3. Applesauce
   4. Citrus juices

6. The nurse is taking care of a patient who has had a laryngectomy. The nurse monitors the need for suctioning by observing what? Select all that apply.
   1. Increased pulse
   2. Swelling
   3. Pain
   4. Restlessness
   5. Audible or visible mucus

7. The nurse is taking care of a patient who has had a laryngectomy. Which are factors that affect the respiratory status of this patient? Select all that apply.
   1. Nutrition
   2. Verbal communication
   3. Humidification
   4. Personal hygiene
   5. Positioning
   6. Fluid intake

8. An older adult has pharyngitis. Why must fluids be increased slowly in older adults?
   1. They do not adjust well to sudden changes in blood volume.
   2. They have decreased kidney function.
   3. They may develop cardiac edema if the fluids are given too rapidly.
   4. The esophagus is more narrow.

G. Next-Generation NCLEX® Examination-Style Questions

Refer to the health history and answer the questions below.

Health history:
A 20-year-old college student has had tonsillitis three times this year, resulting in absences from school. Symptoms included sore throat, dysphagia, fever and chills, muscle aches, and headache. She was admitted for tonsillectomy, which was performed under anesthetic this morning. Postoperatively, she complained of throat pain. She has a small amount of sanguineous drainage. Physical examination: Blood pressure 110/88 mm Hg, pulse 100 bpm, respiration 18 breaths per minute, temperature 98°F.

---

1. Highlight the patient's signs and symptoms listed in the health history that indicate a need for a tonsillectomy?
2. Based on the client information provided, which three nursing interventions should the nurse perform first?
   1. Monitor patient for tachycardia and restlessness
   2. Apply oxygen
   3. Advise the patient not to cough or clear throat
   4. Provide the client with ice chips
   5. Administer antibiotics
   6. Change the surgical dressing
   7. Inspect the drainage for bleeding

Read the situation below and answer the question.
A 15-year-old female client presents to the Emergency Department with uncontrolled bleeding of the nose. The nurse reviews the medical history, nurse's notes, and vital signs.

Medical History:
Asthma
Tonsilitis 2 years ago

Nurse's Notes:
0800: Client presents with uncontrolled bleeding of the nose. Mother states she has applied two towels to the area to try to contain the blood without success. Client is alert and oriented times 3 and appears restless. *Sally Johnson, RN*

Vital Signs:

Blood Pressure	90/50 mm Hg
Pulse	110 beats/minute
Respirations	22 breaths/minute

Use the client data to complete the following sentence by choosing from the list of options below.

The client is most at risk for _____(1)

related to _____(2) secondary to

_____(3).

Options for 1	Options for 2	Options for 3
Impaired gas exchange	Hypovolemia	Hemorrhage
Decreased cardiac output	Restlessness	Asthma
Ineffective airway clearance	Hypoxia	Tonsillitis
Impaired peripheral tissue perfusion	Dyspnea	Airway obstruction

Acute Lower Respiratory Tract Disorders

chapter
27

Go to http://evolve.elsevier.com/Linton/medsurg/ for additional activities and exercises.

NCLEX CATEGORIES

Safe and Effective Care Environment: Safety and Infection Control

Health Promotion and Maintenance

Psychosocial Integrity

Physiological Integrity: Pharmacological Therapies, Reduction of Risk Potential, Physiological Adaptation

PART I: MASTERING THE BASICS

A. Key Terms
Match the definition in the numbered column with the most appropriate term in the lettered column.

A. Atelectasis
B. Hemothorax
C. Hypercapnia
D. Pneumothorax
E. Acute bronchitis
F. Embolus
G. Empyema
H. Flail chest
I. Hemoptysis
J. Pleurisy

1. _____   Inflammation in the lower respiratory system, usually viral
2. _____   The presence of purulent exudate in the pleural cavity
3. _____   Presence of air in the pleural cavity that causes the lung on the affected side to collapse
4. _____   Injury in which two adjacent ribs on the same side of the chest are each broken into two or more segments
5. _____   Accumulation of blood in the pleural space
6. _____   Inflammation of the pleura
7. _____   Coughing up blood
8. _____   Collapsed alveoli
9. _____   Foreign substance, usually blood clots, carried through the bloodstream
10. _____   Excess carbon dioxide in the blood

B. Signs and Symptoms
Match the signs and symptoms in the numbered columns with the acute lower respiratory disorders in the lettered column. Some items may be used more than once and some signs and symptoms may have more than one answer.

1. _____   Diffuse crackles
2. _____   Cyanosis of the mouth
3. _____   Sputum production
4. _____   Paradoxical movement of the chest
5. _____   High fever
6. _____   Tachypnea
7. _____   Asymmetric chest wall movement
8. _____   Visible bone fragments
9. _____   Pain on one side of the chest
10. _____   Unilateral calf or thigh pain
11. _____   Hemoptysis
12. _____   General body aches and pains
13. _____   Orthopnea
14. _____   Wheezing or rhonchi
15. _____   Anxiety

A. Acute bronchitis
B. Influenza
C. Pneumonia
D. Pleurisy
E. Chest trauma
F. Pneumothorax
G. Rib fractures
H. Flail chest
I. Pulmonary embolus
J. Acute respiratory distress syndrome

C. Medical Diagnosis and Treatment

Choose the most appropriate answer or select all that apply.

1. What are beta-2 agonists used for in the treatment of acute bronchitis?
   1. Infection control
   2. Eliminate fatigue
   3. Relieve chest tightness
   4. Reduce cough

2. What are the most common tests for diagnosing influenza?
   1. Rapid molecular assays
   2. Rapid respiratory diagnostic tests
   3. Rapid cell culture
   4. Rapid influenza diagnostic tests

3. Which drugs are effective in the treatment of influenza? Select all that apply.
   1. Echinacea
   2. Acetaminophen
   3. Oral oseltamivir
   4. Baloxavir
   5. Zinc

4. When a patient presents with pneumonia symptoms, which methods are used in confirming the diagnosis? Select all that apply.
   1. Gram stain
   2. Pneumococcal urinary antigen
   3. Molecular assays
   4. Stool culture

5. Why is a vented dressing necessary when treating a patient with chest trauma?
   1. Prevents viral pneumonia
   2. Pain reduction
   3. Allows air to enter the chest
   4. Prevents a tension pneumothorax

6. How is accumulated air or fluid aspirated from the patient being treated for a pneumothorax? Select all that apply.
   1. Insertion of 18-gauge needle into pleural space to aspirate accumulated air or fluid before insertion of a chest tube
   2. Insert chest tube immediately, forgoing the needle procedure
   3. Chest tube is inserted surgically while the patient is anesthetized
   4. A chest pump is used to remove air or fluids until the patient is stabilized

7. What methods are used to confirm a diagnosis of pulmonary emboli? Select all that apply.
   1. Chest x-ray
   2. Arterial blood gas analysis
   3. Listening to the chest for fine crackles
   4. Ventilation-perfusion scan
   5. Electrocardiogram
   6. D-dimer blood test

8. Why is heparin used in the treatment of pulmonary emboli? Select all that apply.
   1. Dissolves the blood clots
   2. Slows heart rate
   3. Prevents more emboli from forming
   4. Blocks extension of existing emboli

9. What methods are used for the treatment of the patient with acute respiratory distress syndrome? Select all that apply.
   1. t-PA given intravenously
   2. Intubation
   3. Mechanical ventilation
   4. IPPB therapy
   5. Drug therapy may be required
   6. Sedation may be required

D. Patient Problems

Match the goals or objectives in the numbered column with the patient problems in the lettered column. Items may be used more than once.

1. _____ Calm demeanor
2. _____ Moist mucous membranes
3. _____ Pulse and blood pressure consistent with patient norms
4. _____ Clear breath sounds without wheezes or crackles
5. _____ Relaxed appearance
6. _____ Normal arterial blood gases, heart rate, and respiratory rate

7. _____ Normal white blood cell count
8. _____ Stable body weight
9. _____ Patient statement of reduced anxiety
10. _____ Normal breath sounds

A. Inadequate oxygenation
B. Inadequate nutrition
C. Potential for fluid volume deficit
D. Pain
E. Fear
F. Inadequate circulation
G. Potential for infection
H. Anxiety
I. Airway obstruction

PART II: PUTTING IT ALL TOGETHER

E. Multiple Choice/Multiple Response
Choose the most appropriate answer or select all that apply.

1. Who is at greatest risk for having aspiration pneumonia?
   1. Chronically ill patients
   2. Patients with tube feedings
   3. Immunosuppressed patients
   4. Smokers

2. For a patient with influenza, which type of drugs must be started soon after the onset of symptoms and continued for 10 days?
   1. Antimicrobials
   2. Antifungals
   3. Antivirals
   4. Corticosteroids

3. At what age is it recommended that individuals begin getting a yearly influenza vaccination?
   1. 12 years
   2. 6 months
   3. 65 years
   4. 1 year

4. Indicate which are (A) penetrating injuries to the chest, or (B) nonpenetrating injuries to the chest.
   1. _____ Gunshot
   2. _____ Automobile accidents
   3. _____ Falls
   4. _____ Stabbing
   5. _____ Blast injuries

5. Which condition indicates a medical emergency?
   1. Pneumothorax
   2. Acute bronchitis
   3. Pleurisy
   4. Pneumonia

6. When fine crackles are revealed during auscultation of the lungs, which disorder may be suspected?
   1. Pneumonia
   2. Chest trauma
   3. ARDS
   4. Pleurisy

7. Aerosol therapy may be used to improve which patient problem?
   1. Inadequate circulation
   2. Inadequate nutrition
   3. Airway obstruction
   4. Potential for infection

8. A patient at risk for inadequate oxygenation should be placed in a semi-Fowler position for which reason?
   1. Decrease pressure of abdominal organs on the diaphragm
   2. Enable patient to improve fluid intake more easily
   3. Improve ability to cough and expectorate
   4. Allows patient more freedom of movement

9. If the patient has a weak cough and is unable to expectorate sufficiently, what may be required?
   1. Spirometry
   2. A lung scan
   3. An MRI
   4. Suctioning

10. An obese female patient who undergoes bilateral knee replacement surgery is at risk for which disorder?
    1. Pleurisy
    2. Pulmonary emboli
    3. Bronchospasm
    4. Tachycardia

11. Which is a symptom of hypoxemia?
    1. Lethargy
    2. Low hemoglobin
    3. Excess CO_2 in the blood
    4. Increased white blood cell count

12. Ventilators are most commonly required for patients with:
    1. oxygen toxicity.
    2. tachycardia.
    3. hypoxemia.
    4. hyperventilation.

13. The seasonal flu vaccine protects from all except which type of flu?
    1. H1N1
    2. B viruses
    3. C viruses
    4. H3N2

14. If necessary, how is accumulated fluid removed from a patient with pleurisy?
    1. Postural drainage
    2. Splint rib cage
    3. Administer antitussives
    4. Thoracentesis

15. When treating a patient with a chest trauma who has been impaled, how should the impaled object be managed?
    1. Prepare patient for surgical removal of object.
    2. Remove slowly after applying topical drugs for numbness and infection prevention.
    3. Leave in place and stabilize with dressings.
    4. Adjust patient's position to prevent discomfort and calm anxiety.

16. Why is it necessary to monitor the blood gases of a patient with a pneumothorax?
    1. To test for hypoxemia and hypercapnia
    2. To ensure white blood cell count remains stable
    3. To measure blood pH
    4. To inspect for mediastinal shift

17. When treating a patient with broken ribs, what is the primary problem?
    1. Impaired mobility
    2. Inadequate circulation
    3. Inadequate oxygenation
    4. Potential for infection

18. For the patient with a chest trauma, what are the best ways to decrease anxiety? Select all that apply.
    1. Promptly respond to patient's needs.
    2. Request a prescription for antianxiety drugs from health care provider.
    3. Provide simple explanations.
    4. Acknowledge the patient's concerns.
    5. Cover the patient with a warm blanket.

PART III: CHALLENGE YOURSELF!

F. Getting Ready for NCLEX
Choose the most appropriate answer or select all that apply.

1. The nurse is teaching a health class to a group of older community members on how to continue home care after being treated for pneumonia. Which items are related to pneumonia self-care? Select all that apply.
    1. Avoid others who have colds or infections.
    2. Take deep breaths every 1–2 hours.
    3. Ensure you are getting plenty of fluids.
    4. Avoid aspirin.
    5. Use a soft toothbrush and electric razor.
    6. Take all medicines as prescribed.

2. The nurse is caring for a patient with fractured ribs. The patient has difficulty breathing due to:
    1. increased sputum production.
    2. ineffective cough.
    3. pain.
    4. atelectasis.

3. Which are the best outcomes for a patient with fractured ribs? Select all that apply.
    1. Vital signs within normal range
    2. Absence of dyspnea
    3. Increased cardiac output
    4. Breath sounds clear to auscultation
    5. Fluid intake increased

4. A patient was in a car accident and is admitted to the hospital with four fractured ribs. What is the priority nursing intervention for this patient?
    1. Breathing exercises to prevent pulmonary complications.
    2. Provide a calm environment.
    3. Manage pain; administer analgesics as prescribed.
    4. Institute a plan to balance rest and activity.

5. The patient with a pulmonary embolism is going home from the hospital with a prescription for Coumadin, following a week of heparin therapy in the hospital. What are the key points for discharge teaching? Select all that apply.
   1. Use a soft toothbrush.
   2. Avoid constricting clothing.
   3. Place a pillow under both knees when sitting.
   4. Be sure to attend clinic follow-up appointments for monitoring of partial thromboplastin time (PTT) while taking Coumadin at home.
   5. Do not take over-the-counter (OTC) drugs containing aspirin.

G. Next-Generation NCLEX® Examination-Style Questions

Read the following situation and answer the questions below.

A 78-year-old woman is admitted to the hospital with viral pneumonia. Problems include inadequate oxygenation and inadequate nutrition. The nurse reviews her Nurse's Notes and Vital Signs.

Vital Signs:	
Temperature	103.5° F
Pulse	102 BPM
Blood Pressure	160/94 mm Hg
Respirations	28 BPM

Nurse's Notes:
0800: Client states she has "shortness of breath" and tires very easily. She complains of restlessness. Her chest pain is aggravated by coughing. Client states that she has a history of hypertension and congestive heart failure, for which she takes a diuretic and an ACE inhibitor. *S. Bailey, RN*

Complete the following sentence by choosing from the lists of options.

1. The assessment findings that indicate hypoxemia include _____ 1 [Select], _____ 2 [Select], and _____ 3 [Select].

Options for 1:	Options for 2:	Options for 3:
Temperature 103.5°F	Shortness of breath	Respiration 28
Pulse 102	Chest pain	History of congestive heart failure
Blood Pressure 160/94 mm Hg	Restlessness	Inadequate nutrition

2. For each body system listed below, select the potential nursing intervention(s) that would be appropriate for the care of the client at this time.
   Gastrointestinal _____ 1 [Select]

   Respiratory _____ 2 [Select]

   Pain _____ 3 [Select]

Options for 1:	Options for 2:	Options for 3:
Suggest small, frequent meals	Administer carbon dioxide (CO_2) therapy	Splint painful areas
Weigh the patient q4h	Elevate head of bed	Encourage oral fluids
Position the patient in left sims position	Use relaxation techniques	Administer muscle relaxants

Read the following situation and answer the questions below.

A 48-year-old male client presents to the Emergency Department with complaints of shortness of breath, chest pain, and calf pain and swelling to the right lower extremity. The nurse reviews the nurse's notes and vital signs.

Nurse's Notes:

0700: A 48-year-old male client presents to the Emergency Department with complaints of shortness of breath, chest pain 8/10 on a numeric pain scale, and calf pain and swelling to the right lower extremity. His wife reports that he had a right total hip replacement 1 week ago.

0715: Assessment complete. Wheezing and crackles on auscultation of lungs. New orders received for computed tomography pulmonary angiography (CTPA).

0720 Vital Signs:

Temperature	102°F
Blood Pressure	130/80 mm Hg
SPO2	93%

0800: Spoke with Dr. Jones. Dr. Jones states, "Client has a pulmonary embolism." Low-molecular-weight heparin is initiated as ordered.

---

1. Use an X for the nursing actions listed below that are indicated (appropriate or necessary) or contraindicated (could be harmful) for the patient's care at this time.

Nursing Action	Indicated	Contraindicated
Apply compression stockings as ordered		
Enforce prescribed activity limitations		
Place a pillow under her legs when in bed		
Monitor aPTT		
Encourage early ambulation after treatment has begun		
Encourage the client to report red or dark urine		
Administer O_2 via nasal cannula		

Chronic Lower Respiratory Tract Disorders

Go to http://evolve.elsevier.com/Linton/medsurg/ for additional activities and exercises.

NCLEX CATEGORIES

Safe and Effective Care Environment: Safety and Infection Control

Health Promotion and Maintenance

Psychosocial Integrity

Physiological Integrity: Pharmacological Therapies, Reduction of Risk Potential, Physiological Adaptation

PART I: MASTERING THE BASICS

A. Key Terms
Match the definition in the numbered column with the most appropriate term in the lettered column.

1. _____ One of many occupational diseases caused by inhalation of dusts from industrial substances

2. _____ Permanent dilation of a portion of the bronchi or bronchioles

3. _____ Clusters of cells and debris formed in tissues affected by an inflammatory process

4. _____ A condition characterized by episodes of bronchospasm and airway infection that causes wheezing and dyspnea; reactive airway disease

5. _____ A disorder characterized by loss of lung elasticity with trapping of air, retained carbon dioxide, and dyspnea

6. _____ Recurrent symptoms, sometimes called *attacks*

7. _____ Inflammation of the lung

8. _____ Right-sided heart failure secondary to pulmonary disease; enlargement of right ventricle

9. _____ Placement of a radiation source in the body to treat a malignancy

10. _____ Bronchial inflammation characterized by increased production of mucus and chronic cough

11. _____ Pneumoconiosis caused by occupational exposure to asbestos

A. Granuloma
B. Asthma
C. Brachytherapy
D. Pneumoconiosis
E. Asbestosis
F. Bronchiectasis
G. Pneumonitis
H. Bronchitis
I. Emphysema
J. Cor pulmonale
K. Exacerbations

B. COPD

Match the patient problem for the patient with chronic obstructive pulmonary disease (COPD) in the numbered column with the "related to" statement in the lettered column.

1. _____ Inadequate oxygenation
2. _____ Airway obstruction
3. _____ Anxiety
4. _____ Inadequate nutrition
5. _____ Potential for infection
6. _____ Decreased activity tolerance
7. _____ Decreased cardiac output

A. Decreased ciliary action, increased secretions, weak cough
B. Alveolar destruction, bronchospasm, air trapping
C. Anorexia, dyspnea
D. Right-sided heart failure
E. Increased secretions, weak cough
F. Inability to meet oxygen needs
G. Hypoxemia

8. Which conditions most frequently occur in conjunction with COPD? Select all that apply.
   1. Asthma
   2. Right-sided heart failure
   3. Pneumonia
   4. Chronic bronchitis
   5. Emphysema

9. Which are goals of medical treatment for COPD? Select all that apply.
   1. Attain symptom relief
   2. Slow disease progression
   3. Improve exercise tolerance
   4. Prevent and treat complications
   5. Radiotherapy and chemotherapy treatments

10. In the treatment of COPD, the initial flow of oxygen is usually 1–3 L/minute. Why are high levels of oxygen not administered to COPD patients?

C. Hypoxemia

1. Explain why the red blood cell count is typically elevated in patients with chronic hypoxemia.

D. Tuberculosis

1. Which diagnostic tests are done to confirm the diagnosis of tuberculosis? Select all that apply.
   1. Chest radiographs
   2. Solid or liquid media cultures
   3. Acid-fast bacilli smears of body fluids
   4. Tuberculin skin tests
   5. Auscultation of the lungs
   6. Pulmonary function tests

E. Pulmonary Disorders

Match the signs and symptoms in the numbered column with their respective conditions in the lettered column.

1. _____ Productive cough, exertional dyspnea, and wheezing
2. _____ Cough, night sweats, chest pain and tightness, fatigue, and anorexia
3. _____ Dyspnea on exertion; may display use of accessory muscles of respiration; barrel chest

A. Emphysema
B. Chronic bronchitis
C. Tuberculosis

4. Which are increased by cigarette smoking? Select all that apply.
   1. Tuberculosis
   2. Osteoporosis
   3. Renal disease
   4. Cataracts
   5. Reproductive complications

5. Which are examples of offending substances that may lead specifically to occupational lung diseases? Select all that apply.
   1. Bacteria
   2. Fungi
   3. Dust
   4. Chlorine
   5. Asbestos
   6. Coal dust
   7. Viruses

PART II: PUTTING IT ALL TOGETHER

F. Multiple Choice/Multiple Response

Choose the most appropriate answer or select all that apply.

1. What are the three major airway characteristics of a patient with asthma? Select all that apply.
    1. Inflammation
    2. Presence of mucus plugs
    3. Narrowing of bronchial airways
    4. Bronchial hyperresponsiveness
    5. Bronchodilation

2. What is one reason for the opening of the airways constricts in patients with asthma?
    1. Inflammatory process triggered
    2. Redness
    3. Loss of elasticity
    4. Pursed-lip breathing

3. A serious complication of bronchospasms is:
    1. hypoxemia.
    2. hypotension.
    3. drowsiness.
    4. bradycardia.

4. Which are the four key components of medical treatment for asthma? Select all that apply.
    1. Monitor over the long term to assess control and adjust therapy.
    2. Help patients learn self-management skills; education for partnership in care.
    3. Control of environmental factors.
    4. Provide appropriate medications.
    5. Eliminate risk factors.

5. The best position for patients with bronchial asthma is:
    1. supine.
    2. prone.
    3. side lying.
    4. Fowler.

6. Arterial blood gas findings that should be reported to the health care provider if they occur in patients with inadequate oxygenation include:
    1. PaO_2 decreases, pH increases.
    2. PaO_2 increases, pH increases.
    3. PaO_2 decreases, $PaCO_2$ increases.
    4. PaO_2 increases, $PaCO_2$ increases.

7. A nasal cannula is preferred over a face mask because the mask may increase the patient's feeling of:
    1. insecurity.
    2. safety.
    3. suffocation.
    4. self-esteem.

8. In patients with emphysema, which of the following causes patients to use accessory muscles for breathing? Select all that apply.
    1. Hyperinflated lungs
    2. Flattened diaphragm
    3. Pursed-lip breathing
    4. Hyperventilation
    5. Left-sided heart failure

9. The most serious complications of COPD are respiratory failure and:
    1. kidney failure.
    2. heart failure.
    3. brain hemorrhage.
    4. hypovolemic shock.

10. When a patient has increased mucus production and a chronic cough for 3 or more months over at least 2 years, then the patient is diagnosed with which disorder?
    1. Emphysema
    2. Pneumonia
    3. Adult respiratory distress syndrome
    4. Chronic bronchitis

11. Some patients with emphysema have normal skin color due to:
    1. normal arterial blood gases.
    2. unlabored respirations.
    3. barrel-chest formation.
    4. normal body temperature.

12. What is the most reliable diagnostic test for COPD?
    1. Chest radiograph
    2. Magnetic resonance imaging (MRI)
    3. Pulmonary function test
    4. Complete blood count (CBC)

13. Drugs that are prescribed to decrease airway resistance and the work of breathing for patients with COPD are called:
    1. vasoconstrictors.
    2. diuretics.
    3. calcium channel blockers.
    4. bronchodilators.

14. The preferred route of administration of bronchodilator drugs for patients with COPD is by:
    1. mouth.
    2. inhalation.
    3. intramuscular injection.
    4. intravenous injection.

15. During the physical examination of patients with COPD, the nurse observes the neck for:
    1. edema.
    2. distended veins.
    3. enlarged lymph nodes.
    4. cyanosis.

16. What is the recommended daily fluid intake to help thin secretions in patients with inadequate oxygenation?
    1. 600–800 mL
    2. 1000–1500 mL
    3. 2500–3000 mL
    4. 4000–5000 mL

17. Which contributes to increased feelings of restlessness and anxiety in the asthma patient?
    1. Decreased arterial oxygen
    2. Increased arterial carbon dioxide
    3. Increased heart rate
    4. Increased respiratory rate

18. During the physical examination of patients with COPD, the thorax is inspected for the classic:
    1. pink color.
    2. blue tinge.
    3. pulmonary edema.
    4. barrel-chest shape.

19. Which are signs and symptoms of airway obstruction in the patient with COPD? Select all that apply.
    1. Headache
    2. Tachycardia
    3. Abnormal breath sounds
    4. Dyspnea
    5. Dizziness

20. Why are patients with COPD encouraged to drink extra fluids each day?
    1. Decrease body temperature
    2. Increase circulation
    3. Liquefy secretions
    4. Prevent kidney stones

21. The work of breathing is increased with COPD, which in turn increases the patient's:
    1. caloric requirements.
    2. calcium requirements.
    3. sodium requirements.
    4. protein requirements.

22. The recommended diet for the patient who is dyspneic is a soft diet with:
    1. low salt.
    2. low protein.
    3. low calories.
    4. frequent, small meals.

23. If the COPD patient becomes excessively dyspneic or develops tachycardia during activity, the patient should:
    1. increase the activity slowly.
    2. pause until the patient recovers.
    3. sit down briefly and then resume activity.
    4. drink a full glass of water.

24. The nurse monitors the patient with COPD for which signs of heart failure? Select all that apply.
    1. Bradycardia
    2. Tachycardia
    3. Increasing dyspnea
    4. Dehydration
    5. Dependent edema

25. A persistent, productive cough with bloody sputum (hemoptysis) is a common symptom of:
    1. emphysema.
    2. cystic fibrosis.
    3. sinusitis.
    4. tuberculosis.

26. The most common preventive drug therapy for tuberculosis is:
    1. prednisone.
    2. isoniazid.
    3. gamma globulin.
    4. aminophylline.

27. The patient who is thought to have active tuberculosis is isolated at first. Which is *not* necessary related to the care of the patient?
    1. Good hand hygiene
    2. Wearing masks
    3. Wearing gowns
    4. Standard precautions

PART III: CHALLENGE YOURSELF!

G. Getting Ready for NCLEX
Choose the most appropriate answer or select all that apply.

1. Which problems develop when status asthmaticus is not treated? Select all that apply.
   1. Pneumothorax
   2. Acidosis
   3. Right-sided heart failure
   4. Renal failure
   5. Liver failure

2. Which complications occur when severe, persistent bronchospasm (status asthmaticus) is not corrected? Select all that apply.
   1. Constriction of bronchial smooth muscle
   2. Thickening of airway tissues
   3. Air trapping in the alveoli
   4. Hypoinflation of the lungs
   5. Decreased secretions

3. What is the treatment for a patient with a positive TB skin test, a negative chest radiograph, and who is at risk for tuberculosis?
   1. Treat prophylactically to prevent development of active tuberculosis.
   2. Repeat the chest radiograph in 6 months.
   3. No treatment is needed.
   4. Take isoniazid for 9–12 months.

4. Which are appropriate nursing interventions to help a patient with active tuberculosis who is experiencing social isolation due to medically imposed isolation? Select all that apply.
   1. Good hand hygiene by patient and health care providers.
   2. Wear particulate masks (disposable respirators) during contact with the patient.
   3. Wear gowns during all contact with the patient.
   4. Explain to the patient that isolation is temporary to protect others from infection.
   5. Encourage the patient to express feelings about the diagnosis and isolation.

5. Which foods must be avoided by patients who are taking isoniazid?
   1. Aged cheese
   2. Dairy products
   3. Grapefruit
   4. Bananas

6. The nurse is taking care of a patient with asthma. What are signs and symptoms of impending respiratory failure to monitor with this patient who is experiencing inadequate oxygenation? Select all that apply.
   1. Easy bruising
   2. Tachypnea
   3. Deep respirations
   4. Diaphoresis
   5. Bradycardia
   6. Loss of consciousness

H. Next-Generation NCLEX® Examination-Style Questions
A 73-year-old woman is admitted for increasing dyspnea. She has had chronic bronchitis and emphysema for 3 years. She has had frequent upper respiratory infections and was hospitalized with pneumonia twice. She is taking verapamil for hypertension. She uses a tiotropium (Spiriva) inhaler once a day. The review of symptoms notes fatigue, increasing dyspnea with exertion and at rest, orthopnea, and productive cough with yellow sputum. She has smoked one pack of cigarettes daily for 45 years. Physical examination: BP 140/94 mm Hg, pulse 100 bpm, respiration 28 breaths per minute, and temperature 100.6°F. She is seated with her hands on her knees to elevate her shoulders. She appears to be in mild distress. Pursed-lip breathing is noted. Accessory muscles of respiration are tense. The thorax is barrel-shaped. Abdominal muscles are used in respirations. No peripheral edema.

1. Highlight the signs and symptoms of COPD that this patient is exhibiting.
2. Complete the following sentence by choosing from the list of options below.

The priority problem for this patient

is _____ (1)

Options for 1:
Anxiety
Decreased activity tolerance
Risk for infection
Inadequate oxygenation
Decreased cardiac output

Read the following situation and answer the question below.

A 13-year-old male client admitted to the medical unit with dyspnea, chest tightness, productive cough, and audible expiratory wheezing was diagnosed with an acute asthma exacerbation. The nurse reviews the Past Medical History, Nurse's Notes, and Physician's Progress Note.

Past Medical History: Heart murmur Seasonal allergies. Physician's Progress Notes: Client has been treated with bronchodilators and inhaled glucocorticoids. Client ready for discharge. Nurse's Notes: 0800: Client resting in bed. His mother is at the bedside with her service dog. Vital signs:	

Blood pressure	110/62 mm Hg
Pulse	70 BPM
Respirations	16 BPM
SpO2	98%
Temp.	98.7°F

3. Based on the client information provided, what should the nurse include in the client's discharge planning? Select all that apply.
   1. "Your asthma can be triggered by playing soccer, you will need to keep a long-acting inhaled beta-adrenergic agonist inhaler to relieve symptoms during an asthma attack."
   2. "To reduce environmental triggers, you may need to keep the service dog confined to specific rooms."
   3. "During allergy season, stay indoors with the windows closed as much as possible."
   4. "If you need to take your reliever more than once per week, inform your health care provider."
   5. "If you have symptoms during exercise, use your prescribed inhaler as directed 2 hours before you exercise."
   6. "Drink 10–14 8-oz glasses of fluids daily."
   7. "It is best to use a metered dose inhaler when administering your inhalant medications."

Hematologic System Introduction

Go to http://evolve.elsevier.com/Linton/medsurg/ for additional activities and exercises.

NCLEX CATEGORIES

Safe and Effective Care Environment: Safety and Infection Control

Health Promotion and Maintenance

Psychosocial Integrity

Physiological Integrity: Pharmacological Therapies, Reduction of Risk Potential, Physiological Adaptation

PART I: MASTERING THE BASICS

A. Key Terms
Match the definition in the numbered column with the most appropriate term in the lettered column. Some definitions may be matched with more than one term.

1. _____ Person with type AB-positive blood who can receive transfusions with any type of blood because all the common antigens (A, B, and Rh) are present in the blood

2. _____ A purplish skin lesion resulting from blood leaking outside the blood vessels

3. _____ A reduction in the number of red blood cells or in the quantity of hemoglobin

4. _____ Small (1–3 mm) red or reddish-purple spots on the skin resulting from blood capillaries breaking and leaking small amounts of blood into the tissues

5. _____ A primary function of the hematologic system

6. _____ Person with type O-negative blood who can donate blood to anyone because none of the common antigens are present in the blood

7. _____ Changes in blood pressure and pulse as person moves from lying to sitting to standing positions

8. _____ Red or reddish-purple skin lesion 3 mm or more in size that results from blood leaking outside of the blood vessels

9. _____ Control of bleeding

A. Anemia
B. Oxygenation
C. Ecchymosis
D. Orthostatic vital sign changes
E. Petechiae
F. Purpura
G. Universal donor
H. Universal recipient
I. Hemostasis

B. Components of the Hematologic System
Match the descriptions in the numbered column with the appropriate component in the lettered column.

1. _____ Refers to a mixture of factors that transports gases between the lungs and tissues.

2. _____ Clear, straw-colored fluid that carries blood components through the circulatory system.

3. _____ Spongy center of bones where the stem cells are manufactured.

4. _____ Red blood cells (RBCs).

5. _____ Removes old RBCs from circulation.

6. _____ Forms a stable fibrin matrix over wounded area, protecting the injured site while healing.

7. _____ Manufactures hematopoietin, a hormone that is released in response to hypoxia.

8. _____ Platelets that activate the clotting factors.

9. _____ Manufactures clotting factors and clears old and damaged RBCs from circulation.

A. Bone marrow
B. Kidneys
C. Liver
D. Spleen
E. Blood
F. Erythrocytes
G. Thrombocytes
H. Clotting factors
I. Plasma

PART II: PUTTING IT ALL TOGETHER

C. Multiple Choice/Multiple Response

Choose the most appropriate answer or select all that apply.

1. For each unit of packed red blood cells (PRBCs) transfused, the patient's hemoglobin should increase approximately:
   1. 10 g/dL.
   2. 5 g/dL.
   3. 3 g/dL.
   4. 1 g/dL.

2. What is the primary function of the hematologic system?
   1. Circulation and regulation of blood pressure
   2. Oxygenation and hemostasis
   3. Transportation of nutrients and vitamins
   4. Hydration and fluid balance

3. Patients with low red blood cell counts may have:
   1. bradycardia.
   2. hypertension.
   3. bleeding problems.
   4. tachycardia.

4. The patient is receiving PRBCs because of low hematocrit and hemoglobin. Which of the following are symptoms of low hematocrit and hemoglobin? Select all that apply.
   1. Shortness of breath
   2. Bradycardia
   3. Decreased blood pressure
   4. Chest pain
   5. Fatigue
   6. Lightheadedness

5. Once blood is picked up from the blood bank, the transfusion should be started within:
   1. 5 minutes.
   2. 20 minutes.
   3. 30 minutes.
   4. 2 hours.

6. Platelets are generally administered when a patient's platelet count drops below:
   1. $10,000/mm^3$.
   2. $15,000/mm^3$.
   3. $20,000/mm^3$.
   4. $300,000/mm^3$.

7. If platelets are prescribed before a procedure such as a lumbar puncture or endoscopy to prevent postprocedure bleeding, the platelets should be administered:
   1. 1 week before the procedure.
   2. 1 day before the procedure.
   3. 6 hours before the procedure.
   4. immediately before the procedure.

8. Four types of blood transfusion reactions include hemolytic, circulatory overload, febrile, and:
   1. thrombocytopenic.
   2. anaphylactic.
   3. anemic.
   4. leukopenic.

9. Feverfew, garlic, and ginkgo are herbs that affect:
   1. wound healing.
   2. blood clotting.
   3. resistance to infection.
   4. kidney function.

10. What is the role of the spleen related to the hematologic system?
    1. Produces platelets
    2. Manufactures clotting factors
    3. Removes old red blood cells from circulation
    4. Synthesizes vitamins

11. A healthy adult has how many liters of blood circulating through the body?
    1. 3 liters
    2. 6 liters
    3. 12 liters
    4. 24 liters

12. What is the most common site for a bone marrow biopsy?
    1. Posterior iliac crest
    2. Sternum
    3. Femur
    4. Tibia

13. What is a term used to describe the series of events that occurs in the process of blood clotting?
    1. Anticoagulation
    2. Hemostasis
    3. Hemolysis
    4. Coagulation cascade

14. Which are antigens found on the cell membranes of red blood cells? Select all that apply.
    1. A antigens
    2. B antigens
    3. AB antigens
    4. O antigens
    5. Rhesus (Rh) antigens
    6. pH antigens

15. Which are types of blood transfusion reactions? Select all that apply.
    1. Hemolytic
    2. Anaphylactic
    3. Febrile
    4. Circulatory overload
    5. Anemic

16. Which functions of the liver are related to hematologic functions? Select all that apply.
    1. Manufactures red blood cells
    2. Manufactures clotting factors
    3. Clears old and damaged red blood cells from the circulation
    4. Stores glucose in the form of glycogen
    5. Aids in phagocytosis of bacteria

17. Match the drug action and the appropriate nursing intervention in the numbered column with the name of the drug(s) in the lettered column. Questions may have more than one answer, and answers may be used more than once.
    1. _____ Replaces iron
    2. _____ Stimulates the bone marrow to produce red blood cells
    3. _____ Intramuscular injection; must be given for the rest of the person's life if the patient has pernicious anemia
    4. _____ May be given by intravenous or subcutaneous injection; patient is usually treated three times per week until the hematocrit is 30–33

    A. Vitamin B_{12}
    B. Ferrous iron salts
    C. Epoetin alfa
    D. Iron dextran

PART III: CHALLENGE YOURSELF!

D. Getting Ready for NCLEX
Choose the most appropriate answer or select all that apply.

1. The nurse is assisting with a staff in-service program on hematologic disorders. The nurse includes information about bone marrow sites that produce the majority of red blood cells and platelets. Which are these bone marrow sites? Select all that apply.
   1. Humerus
   2. Sternum
   3. Pelvis
   4. Radius
   5. Clavicle

2. The nurse is taking care of a patient who has the potential for injury from a low red blood cell count. Which are appropriate nursing actions for this patient? Select all that apply.
   1. Allow for rest between periods of activity.
   2. Elevate the patient's head on pillows to reduce shortness of breath.
   3. Administer analgesics as prescribed.
   4. Decrease daily fluid intake.
   5. Increase food intake of iron.

3. The nurse is caring for a patient with anemia who has the potential for injury from bleeding. Which are nursing actions for this patient? Select all that apply.
   1. Avoid intramuscular injections.
   2. Use a soft-bristled toothbrush.
   3. Avoid foods high in vitamin D.
   4. Avoid the use of suppositories.
   5. Increase fiber in the diet.

4. The nurse is caring for a patient with iron deficiency anemia. Which foods are high in iron content? Select all that apply.
   1. Fish
   2. Dark green vegetables
   3. Red meats
   4. Beans
   5. Pasta
   6. Rice

5. The nurse is collecting data from a patient with a hematologic disorder. What characteristics may be indicative of an underlying hematologic disorder? Select all that apply.
   1. Kussmaul respirations
   2. Easy bruising
   3. Elevated temperature
   4. Chronic fatigue
   5. Periods of unusually long bleeding
   6. Hypertension

6. The patient with anemia has been prescribed ferrous iron salts. Which are nursing actions related to administration of this drug? Select all that apply.
   1. Have the patient take the drug with milk.
   2. Encourage the patient to take the drug with food.
   3. Tell the patient to drink through a straw if the ferrous sulfate is given in liquid form.
   4. Explain that stools may turn black.
   5. Avoid taking with foods containing tyramine.

7. The nurse is administering iron dextran to a patient with anemia. Which are appropriate nursing actions for the administration of this medication? Select all that apply.
   1. Monitor the patient for hypersensitivity reactions.
   2. Monitor the patient for signs of liver toxicity.
   3. Give intramuscular injections only in the lower outer quadrant of the buttock.
   4. Use the Z-track technique when giving an intramuscular injection.
   5. Inject the medication slowly.

8. The nurse is taking care of a patient with anemia who is experiencing orthostatic vital sign changes. Which should be increased in this patient's diet?
   1. Carbohydrates
   2. Fiber
   3. Fluids
   4. Vitamins

Hematologic Disorders

Go to http://evolve.elsevier.com/Linton/medsurg/ for additional activities and exercises.

NCLEX CATEGORIES

Safe and Effective Care Environment: Safety and Infection Control

Health Promotion and Maintenance

Psychosocial Integrity

Physiological Integrity: Pharmacological Therapies, Reduction of Risk Potential, Physiological Adaptation

PART I: MASTERING THE BASICS

A. Key Terms
Match the definition in the numbered column with the most appropriate term in the lettered column.

1. _____ Misshapen red blood cells become fragile and rupture easily

2. _____ Genetic disease in which a person lacks blood-clotting factors normally found in the plasma

3. _____ Hypercoagulable state with thrombosis and hemorrhage

4. _____ Occurs when a person does not absorb vitamin B_{12} from the stomach

5. _____ Destroys blood cells once they are released into circulation from the bone marrow

6. _____ Disorder in which too few platelets are circulating in the blood

7. _____ Increased RBC production that hampers circulation due to blood thickness

A. Disseminated intravascular coagulation
B. Hemolytic anemia
C. Hemophilia
D. Polycythemia vera
E. Pernicious anemia
F. Sickle cell anemia
G. Thrombocytopenia

B. Anemia and Coagulation Disorders
Match the descriptions in the numbered column with the appropriate type of anemia or coagulation disorder in the lettered column. Answers may be used more than once.

1. _____ Results from complete failure of bone marrow

2. _____ A genetic disease carried on a recessive gene

3. _____ Results from diet low in iron or inability of the body to absorb enough iron from GI tract

4. _____ Causes include cancer chemotherapy and radiation

5. _____ Secondary disorder to another pathologic process such as sepsis, shock, burns, or obstetric complications

6. _____ May be caused by drugs (such as streptomycin and chloramphenicol) and exposure to toxic chemicals and radiation

7. _____ Symptoms include weakness, sore tongue, and numbness of hands or feet

A. Thrombocytopenia
B. Disseminated intravascular coagulation (DIC)
C. Pernicious anemia
D. Sickle cell anemia
E. Iron-deficiency anemia
F. Aplastic anemia

PART II: PUTTING IT ALL TOGETHER

C. Multiple Choice/Multiple Response
Choose the most appropriate answer or select all that apply.

1. A condition in which there are too many blood cells is called:
   1. pernicious anemia.
   2. aplastic anemia.
   3. hemolytic anemia.
   4. polycythemia vera.

2. The treatment for autoimmune hemolytic anemia is:
   1. vitamin B_{12} injections.
   2. ferrous sulfate and high-iron diet.
   3. iron dextran and high-carbohydrate diet.
   4. corticosteroids and blood transfusions.

3. The treatment for aplastic anemia is:
   1. vitamin B_{12} injections.
   2. ferrous sulfate and high-iron diet.
   3. iron dextran and high-carbohydrate diet.
   4. transfusions, antibiotics, and immunosuppressants.

4. Treatment for sickle cell crisis includes:
   1. ferrous sulfate and high-iron diet.
   2. iron dextran and high-carbohydrate diet.
   3. aggressive intravenous hydration and IV opioids.
   4. corticosteroids and platelet transfusions.

5. Patients with aplastic or hemolytic anemia may have (Select all that apply):
   1. bradycardia.
   2. hypotension.
   3. bleeding problems.
   4. tachycardia.

6. The treatment for hemophilia is:
   1. plasma and cryoprecipitate transfusions.
   2. red blood cell transfusions and antibiotics.
   3. white blood cell transfusions and potassium.
   4. platelet and anticoagulant transfusions.

7. Symptoms of thrombocytopenia include:
   1. fatigue and pallor.
   2. petechiae and purpura.
   3. nausea and vomiting.
   4. tachycardia and palpitations.

8. Treatment for thrombocytopenia in cancer patients receiving chemotherapy or radiation therapy includes:
   1. red blood cell transfusions and iron.
   2. white blood cell transfusions and antibiotics.
   3. platelet transfusions.
   4. cryoprecipitate transfusions and anticonvulsants.

9. The condition in which a person has too few platelets circulating in the blood is called:
   1. leukemia.
   2. anemia.
   3. lymphoma.
   4. thrombocytopenia.

10. Which type of anemia may be caused by blood transfusions if lymphoctyes in the transfused blood make antibodies against the person receiving the blood?
    1. Vitamin B_{12} anemia
    2. Autoimmune hemolytic anemia
    3. Iron-deficiency anemia
    4. Aplastic anemia

11. Which are ways the body compensates when a person is anemic with chronic blood loss? Select all that apply.
    1. Increased heart rate
    2. Decreased respiratory rate
    3. Blood redistributed toward the skin
    4. Increased production of erythropoietin
    5. Blood redistributed to the heart and brain

12. Which are signs and symptoms of thrombocytopenia? Select all that apply.
    1. Petechiae
    2. Gingival bleeding
    3. Fever
    4. Orthostatic hypotension
    5. Epistaxis
    6. Purpura

13. Match the drug action and the appropriate nursing intervention in the numbered column with the name of the drug(s) in the lettered column. Questions may have more than one answer, and answers may be used more than once.
    1. _____ Replaces iron
    2. _____ Stimulates production of a type of hemoglobin resistant to sickling
    3. _____ Intramuscular injection; must be given every month if the patient has neurologic symptoms
    4. _____ Can reduce sickle cell crises

    A. Vitamin B$_{12}$
    B. Ferrous sulfate
    C. Hydroxyurea
    D. Iron dextran

14. Patients with red blood cell disorders usually have which problems? Select all that apply.
    1. Too few red blood cells
    2. Red blood cell distillation
    3. Overproduction of red blood cells
    4. Small or oversized red blood cells

15. What distinguishes aplastic anemia from all other anemic disorders?
    1. RBC count is normal.
    2. Bone marrow overproduces WBCs.
    3. Bone marrow only produces platelets.
    4. Bone marrow is also not producing WBCs.

16. A patient with sickle cell anemia informs the nurse that she is going skiing in Colorado. Why is this a concern for the nurse?
    1. Injuries could not heal properly due to improper blood flow.
    2. Increased danger of frostbite due to lack of RBCs.
    3. Decreased O$_2$ in higher altitudes could initiate a crisis.
    4. Lack of RBCs weakens individuals with sickle cell anemia.

17. In discussing a patient's diagnosis of aplastic anemia, he is told that the exact cause may never be identified or it could be related to what? Select all that apply.
    1. Exposure to toxic chemicals
    2. Genetics
    3. Radiation
    4. Certain drugs

18. What is an important consideration when teaching a patient with iron-deficiency anemia about supplements?
    1. Select only supplements recommended by health care provider.
    2. Doses that exceed recommended amounts can be toxic.
    3. Supplements should be taken with grapefruit juice.
    4. Eliminate the need for supplements by eating an iron-rich diet.

19. When a patient presents with fatigue and pallor, as well as weakness, a sore tongue, and numbness of the hands or feet, what RBC disorder is suspected?
    1. Pernicious anemia
    2. Aplastic anemia
    3. Hemolytic anemia
    4. Autoimmune anemia

20. What is usually the cause of hemolytic anemia in newborns?
    1. Passes from the mother
    2. Blood loss during delivery
    3. Rh– mother and Rh+ newborn
    4. Genetic mutation passed from one or both parents

PART III: CHALLENGE YOURSELF!

D. Getting Ready for NCLEX
Choose the most appropriate answer or select all that apply.

1. A patient is sent to a blood bank where 1 unit of blood is removed with a large-bore intravenous needle. What hematologic disorder is being treated?
   1. Sickle cell crisis
   2. Polycythemia vera
   3. Streptomycin
   4. Thrombocytopenia

2. The nurse is preparing a young African-American male patient recently diagnosed with sickle cell anemia to make the best choices to avoid stressors. Which teaching points the nurse should convey to the patient? Select all that apply.
   1. Drink 4–6 L of fluids, preferably water, each day.
   2. Genetic counseling is a good idea if children are planned.
   3. Identify and develop strategies to avoid stressors.
   4. Drinking alcohol is a suitable method for reducing stress.
   5. Strenuous exercise should not be attempted.
   6. Smoking is a common stressor and should be avoided.

3. A patient with iron-deficiency anemia asks the nurse to recommend foods that contain iron. Which foods should the nurse recommend? Select all that apply.
   1. Red wine
   2. Dried beans
   3. Dark green vegetables
   4. Red meat including liver
   5. Aged cheeses
   6. Fish and oysters
   7. Whole-grain breads and cereals
   8. Yogurt

4. What information should the nurse provide to the certified nursing assistants (CNAs) so that they can assist with the care of patients with blood disorders? Select all that apply.
   1. Instruct the CNAs to provide supplements as needed for patients with anemia.
   2. Instruct the CNAs to ensure patients with low RBC counts get adequate rest.
   3. Instruct the CNAs to ensure patients with sickle cell anemia do not smoke.
   4. Instruct the CNAs on how to prevent trauma and bleeding in patients who have low platelet counts.
   5. Instruct the CNAs on the importance of maintaining accurate oral fluid intake of patients in sickle cell crisis.
   6. Instruct the CNAs on ensuring that patients with iron-deficiency anemia are eating an iron-rich diet.

5. When teaching patients with hemophilia and their families about self-care, what are some of the key points the nurse should discuss? Select all that apply.
   1. Patients with hemophilia bleed from even the smallest incident, so it is important to monitor their environment as much as possible.
   2. It is unlikely that hemophilia will be passed on to children, so persons with hemophilia should not be concerned with possible genetic risks.
   3. If approved by the patients' health care provider, patients and families can be taught to administer the concentrate at home.
   4. Patients and their families should know emergency treatment of bleeding episodes.
   5. Patients with hemophilia should severely restrict all activities and avoid public areas.
   6. First-aid measures for a patient who begins bleeding include pressure, immobilization, and elevation.

E. Next-Generation NCLEX® Examination-Style Questions

Refer to the Nursing Care Plan, The Patient in Sickle Cell Crisis in the textbook, and answer the questions below.

A 19-year-old African-American woman was diagnosed with sickle cell anemia at age 12 years. The nurse reviews the health history and physical examination.

> Health History:
> A 19-year-old African-American woman was diagnosed with sickle cell anemia at age 12 years. She was in stable health until 3 days ago, when she complained of nausea and had diarrhea and vomiting. Since that time, she only drank soup and cola beverages. Her mother brought her to the emergency department, suspecting sickle cell crisis, when the patient complained of severe pain in her abdomen.
> Physical examination:
> BP 110/56 mm Hg, pulse 106 bpm, respiration 24 breaths per minute, oral temperature 102°F. Skin dry and warm to touch. Breath sounds clear. Abdomen soft but tender to light palpation. Bowel sounds hyperactive in all four quadrants. No bladder distention. Mild joint enlargement noted in both knees.

1. Which physician orders would the nurse anticipate being prescribed? Select All That Apply.
   1. Soft diet
   2. Complete bedrest
   3. Check the patient's blood pressure in lying, sitting, and standing positions
   4. IV infusion NS at 125 mL/hour
   5. Daily weights
   6. PCA Morphine
   7. Monitor intake and output
   8. Acetaminophen 650 mg q 4h prn

2. Which physician orders would the nurse anticipate being prescribed? Select All That Apply.
   1. Administer 2 units of fresh frozen plasma
   2. Administer 2 units of packed red blood cells
   3. 2 mg morphine IV Q4H PRN
   4. Shave left lower extremity for surgical prep
   5. Dangle lower extremities on side of bed Q2H
   6. Aspirin 81 mg daily
   7. Leave wound open to air

Read the situation below and answer the question.

A 32-year-old male client presents to the Emergency Department unconscious after a motor vehicle accident with a head contusion and severe bleeding to the left lower extremity. The first responders have been applying pressure to the site of injury, but have been unable to stop the bleeding. When his wife arrives, she informs the health care team that the client has a medical history of Hemophilia A. The nurse reviews the vital signs and lab values.

Vital Signs:	
Blood Pressure	90/50 mm Hg
Pulse	100 BPM
Respirations	22 breaths/min
Temperature	98.8°F
SPO2	96%

Lab values:	
Platelets	140,000 K/uL
Hemoglobin	6.8 g/dL
Hematocrit	30%

Immunologic System Introduction

Go to http://evolve.elsevier.com/Linton/medsurg/ for additional activities and exercises.

NCLEX CATEGORIES

Health Promotion and Maintenance

Physiological Integrity: Reduction of Risk Potential, Physiological Adaptation

PART I: MASTERING THE BASICS

A. Key Terms
Match the definition or description in the numbered column with the most appropriate term in the lettered column.

1. _____ Hormones secreted by cells to signal other cells

2. _____ Transplanted organ or tissue

3. _____ When monocytes enter tissue

4. _____ A complication of allogeneic bone marrow transplants in which T lymphocytes in the transplanted bone marrow identify the patient's tissue as foreign and try to destroy the patient's tissues

5. _____ Antigen-binding proteins

6. _____ A transplantation when the patient has an identical twin; therefore, the twin will be a perfect HLA match

7. _____ Type of transplant that is the best option for patients with a solid tumor that has not metastasized to the bone marrow; for example, patients with lymphoma

8. _____ A class of fatty acids that regulate vasodilation, temperature elevation, WBC activation, and other physiologic processes involved in immunity

9. _____ A transplantation that requires a donor whose human leukocyte antigens (HLAs) match those of the patient

A. Allogeneic bone marrow transplant
B. Allograft
C. Autologous bone marrow transplant
D. Cytokines
E. Eicosanoids
F. Graft-versus-host disease
G. Immunoglobulin
H. Macrophages
I. Syngeneic bone marrow transplant

B. The Immune System and Immunity
Match the organ in the numbered column with its function in the lettered column.

1. _____ Lymph nodes
2. _____ Bone marrow
3. _____ Spleen
4. _____ Thymus

A. Participate(s) in the maturation of T lymphocytes
B. Act(s) as filter to remove microorganisms from the lymph fluid before it returns to the blood
C. Filter(s) and destroy(s) microorganisms in the blood
D. Produce(s) white blood cells

5. Which are descriptions of innate immunity? Select all that apply.
   1. System consists of anatomic and physiologic barriers, inflammatory response, and action of phagocytic cells.
   2. Response initiated when IgM immunoglobulins on the surface of B lymphocytes detect a foreign antigen.
   3. System activated only when needed in response to a specific antigen; can be antibody-mediated or cell-mediated.
   4. Defense systems specific to a particular pathogen.
   5. Immunity aimed at invading microorganisms such as bacteria.
   6. Defense systems present at birth.

C. White Blood Cells

Match the type of white blood cell in the numbered column with its function in the lettered column.

1. _____ Basophils
2. _____ B lymphocytes
3. _____ Neutrophils
4. _____ Monocytes
5. _____ Eosinophils
6. _____ Mast cells
7. _____ T lymphocytes

A. Called *macrophages* when they enter tissue; powerful phagocytes.
B. Initiate inflammatory response; circulate in blood and release histamine.
C. Fight bacterial infections; most numerous type of white blood cell.
D. Combat parasitic infections; associated with allergies.
E. Manufacture immunoglobulins and stimulate the production of antibodies.
F. Store histamine; located in body tissues.
G. Secrete cytokines, facilitating body's immune system.

D. Lymphatic System

Using the figure below (Figure 31.2), label the parts of the lymphatic system.

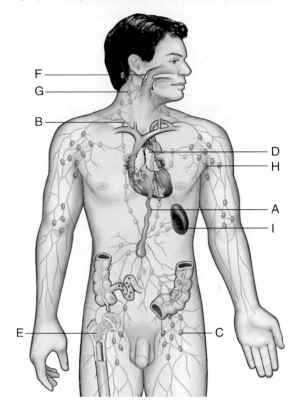

A. _____

B. _____

C. _____

D. _____

E. _____

F. _____

G. _____

H. _____

I. _____

PART II: PUTTING IT ALL TOGETHER

E. Multiple Choice/Multiple Response
Choose the most appropriate answer or select all that apply.

1. The body's defense network against infection is the:
   1. cardiovascular system.
   2. respiratory system.
   3. immune system.
   4. circulatory system.

2. Which anatomic and physiologic barrier is the body's first defense against pathogens?
   1. Inflammation
   2. Phagocytosis
   3. Antibodies and antigens
   4. Skin and mucous membranes

3. The most numerous white blood cells are the:
   1. neutrophils.
   2. basophils.
   3. lymphocytes.
   4. eosinophils.

4. Which are related to active acquired antibody immunity? Select all that apply.
   1. Occurs when a person synthesizes his or her own antibodies in response to a pathogen
   2. Occurs when a person receives a vaccination
   3. Permanent type of immunity
   4. Occurs when an antibody produced by a person is transferred to another person
   5. Immunity lasts only 1–2 months after antibodies have been received
   6. Occurs when a person has an infection and manufactures his or her own antibodies

5. Which leukocyte initiates an inflammatory response that brings all the other leukocytes to the site of infection?
   1. Eicosanoids
   2. Eosinophils
   3. Basophils
   4. Cytokines

6. When there is a breakdown of tolerance, what types of diseases occur?
   1. Autoimmune
   2. Viral
   3. Bacterial
   4. Cancers

7. Which are examples of autoimmune disorders? Select all that apply.
   1. Rheumatoid arthritis
   2. Systemic lupus erythematosus (SLE)
   3. Graves' disease
   4. Leukemia
   5. Type 1 diabetes mellitus

8. The process of the immune system to recognize its own proteins and not attack itself is called:
   1. tolerance.
   2. phagocytosis.
   3. immunity.
   4. inflammation.

9. A common blood test that measures various blood components including total number of WBCs is:
   1. complete blood count (CBC).
   2. Western blot test.
   3. antinuclear antibody test.
   4. T cell counts.

10. Which diagnostic procedure is done to detect and identify microorganisms in blood?
    1. Western blot
    2. Viral load
    3. CBC
    4. Blood culture

11. Colony-stimulating factors (CSFs) are examples of which hormone?
    1. Eicosanoids
    2. Basophils
    3. Cytokines
    4. Lymphocytes

12. What minimizes the chance of the recipient's immune system attacking the transplanted organ?
    1. Administration of steroids
    2. Tissue matching of donor to recipient
    3. Administration of antibiotics
    4. Administration of platelets

13. Which are major complications of bone marrow and peripheral blood stem cell transplants? Select all that apply.
    1. Hemorrhage
    2. Infection
    3. Shock
    4. Thrombocytopenia
    5. Graft-versus-host disease

14. Which are allergens used in skin testing for hyposensitivities or hypersensitivities? Select all that apply.
    1. Animal dander
    2. Pollen
    3. Organ transplant cells; transplanted graft rejection
    4. Blood transfusion cells; mismatched blood transfusion
    5. Dust

15. Which are anatomic and physiologic barriers that help remove pathogens from the body? Select all that apply.
    1. Skin
    2. Sweat glands
    3. Inflammation
    4. Gastrointestinal (GI) and genitourinary (GU) mucosae
    5. Phagocytosis
    6. Respiratory and gastrointestinal secretions
    7. Cardiac cells

16. Which describe peripheral blood stem cell transplants? Select all that apply.
    1. The most common type of transplant
    2. Procedure in which a patient's own bone marrow is harvested after chemotherapy and radiation therapy
    3. Following harvesting of stem cells through apheresis, the patient is treated with chemotherapy and radiation therapy
    4. Procedure in which CSFs are administered to the patient to stimulate the bone marrow to produce white blood cells
    5. Procedure that reduces the duration of neutropenia

PART III: CHALLENGE YOURSELF!

F. Getting Ready for NCLEX

Choose the most appropriate answer or select all that apply.

1. Which are nursing actions indicated for a patient who has potential for injury from infection who is on compromised host precautions? Select all that apply.
    1. All staff and visitors entering the patient's room must wash their hands before touching the patient for any reason.
    2. Masks are required for all staff and visitors.
    3. Serve only cooked or canned foods to the patient.
    4. The patient should wear a clean mask while in his or her room.
    5. Scheduling of patient appointments: Plan follow-up appointment at clinic in 1 week.
    6. The patient should have a private room.

2. When completing a nursing assessment, what symptoms might indicate that a patient has an immunologic disorder? Select all that apply.
    1. Bruises easily
    2. Weight loss
    3. Frequent or persistent infections
    4. Excessive thirst
    5. Bleeds for a long time when cut
    6. Chronic fatigue

3. A 65-year-old patient may have inadequate immune response under stress, infection, or after cancer treatment. Why is this true of an older patient?
    1. Lymph nodes are smaller and fewer.
    2. Bone marrow is less productive with age.
    3. Lymphatic tissue shrinks.
    4. Tolerance breaks down.

4. A nurse is caring for a patient who has had an organ transplant and is taking immunosuppressant drugs. What conditions are a risk for this patient? Select all that apply.
    1. Anemia
    2. Neutropenia
    3. Leukocytopenia
    4. Thrombocytopenia

5. A patient develops rejection 24 hours after an organ or tissue transplantation. How is rejection treated?
   1. Increased use of immunosuppressant drugs
   2. Stem cell transplantation
   3. Removal of the transplanted tissue or organ
   4. Administer chemotherapy drugs

6. What major complications should a nurse be aware of for a patient who has had a bone marrow transplant? Select all that apply.
   1. Infection
   2. Edema
   3. Thrombocytopenia
   4. Renal insufficiency
   5. Myalgia
   6. Hepatic veno-occlusive disease
   7. Graft-versus-host disease

Immunologic Disorders

chapter
32

Go to http://evolve.elsevier.com/Linton/medsurg/ for additional activities and exercises.

NCLEX CATEGORIES

Safe and Effective Care Environment: Safety and Infection Control

Physiological Integrity: Pharmacological Therapies, Physiological Adaptation

PART I: MASTERING THE BASICS

A. Key Terms
Match the definition or description in the numbered column with the most appropriate term in the lettered column.

1. _____ The total number of neutrophils is abnormally low (an absolute neutrophil count of fewer than 1500 cells/μL), putting the patient at increased risk of infection.

2. _____ Disease that is now viewed less as a fatal illness than as a manageable chronic condition.

3. _____ Medication regimen or a combination of drugs that is recommended when the viral load reaches certain levels.

4. _____ Retrovirus that causes AIDS.

5. _____ Diseases that occur when immune system inappropriately identifies its own proteins as foreign and mounts a response to destroy them.

A. Acquired immunodeficiency syndrome (AIDS)
B. Antiretroviral therapy (ART)
C. Autoimmune disorder
D. Human immunodeficiency virus (HIV)
E. Neutropenia

B. Cancers with HIV Infection
List four types of cancers that may occur in 40% of patients with HIV infection.

1. _____

2. _____

3. _____

4. _____

5. Explain why patients with HIV infection are at increased risk for cancer.

C. Transmission of HIV

1. How is HIV transmitted? Select all that apply.
   1. Saliva
   2. Breast milk
   3. Semen
   4. Urine
   5. Blood
   6. Vaginal fluids
   7. Tears
   8. Sweat

PART II: PUTTING IT ALL TOGETHER

D. Multiple Choice/Multiple Response
Choose the most appropriate answer or select all that apply.

1. What is the leading cause of death in people with AIDS?
   1. Kaposi sarcoma
   2. Malnutrition
   3. Infection
   4. Encephalopathy

2. About how long after infection does the body produce enough antibodies to be detected by standard HIV testing?
   1. 2–3 days
   2. 1 week
   3. 12 weeks
   4. 6 months

3. Which substances remain at high levels throughout the course of HIV infection? Select all that apply.
   1. HIV antibodies
   2. CD8 cells
   3. CD4 cells
   4. Red blood cells

4. Antiretroviral medications are given to patients with HIV infection to: **(Select all that apply.)**
   1. reduce the viral load.
   2. prevent and treat infections.
   3. cure the HIV infection.
   4. treat malignancies.

5. Which test for HIV infection can be used at home?
   1. Nucleic acid test
   2. CBC test
   3. OraQuick test
   4. Antigen test

6. Approximately how many HIV infections were newly diagnosed in 2018?
   1. 20,000
   2. 40,000
   3. 100,000
   4. 540,000

7. Which drug is used to treat opportunistic fungal infections in people with HIV infection?
   1. AZT
   2. Retrovir
   3. Amphotericin B
   4. Bactrim

8. What is the usual combination of drugs for HIV patients who are started on the medication regimen highly active antiretroviral therapy (**HAART**)?
   1. Antimicrobials and protease inhibitor
   2. Nucleoside reverse transcriptase inhibitors (NRTIs) and protease inhibitor
   3. NRTIs, nonnucleoside reverse transcriptase inhibitors (NNRTIs), and protease inhibitors
   4. Antimycotics and NNRTIs

9. What is the most serious problem with HAART therapy?
   1. Resistance
   2. Hypolipidemia
   3. Renal failure
   4. Infection

10. What type of cells does HIV over time destroy faster than the body can replace?
    1. CD4+ T cells
    2. T4 cells
    3. B cells
    4. Eosinophils

11. HIV is passed from person to person primarily through:
    1. air droplet contact.
    2. hand-to-mouth contact.
    3. exposure to body fluids.
    4. mouth-to-mouth contact.

12. A patient with HIV has developed some GI infections causing diarrhea, nausea, vomiting, and poor appetite. What is the priority nursing intervention for this patient?
    1. Provide periods of rest during the day.
    2. Ensure adequate intake of nutrients and fluids.
    3. Report fluid and electrolyte imbalances.
    4. Monitor for signs of infection.

13. What are two other nursing interventions for an HIV patient who is experiencing nausea, vomiting, diarrhea, and a poor appetite?
    1. Discuss ways to conserve energy and promote restful sleep.
    2. Talk to nurse practitioner about prescribing antinausea medication, an appetite stimulant, and an antidiarrheal.
    3. Encourage patient to ask questions and talk about feelings.
    4. Teach the importance of regular dental care.
    5. Provide a diet high in protein and calories.

14. A type of skin cancer that has dramatically increased as a result of AIDS is:
    1. basal cell carcinoma.
    2. melanoma.
    3. Kaposi sarcoma
    4. venereal warts.

15. The risk of transmission of HIV increases with:
    1. donating blood.
    2. unprotected sex.
    3. hugging and kissing.
    4. using public restrooms.

16. The patient with AIDS is at high risk for opportunistic infections because of:
    1. altered skin integrity.
    2. increased HIV antibodies.
    3. decreased CD4 cells.
    4. fatigue.

17. Patients with AIDS may have confusion due to:
    1. anxiety.
    2. dementia.
    3. anemia.
    4. brain damage.

18. Which tissue can be infected by HIV?
    1. Pancreas
    2. Stomach
    3. Kidney
    4. Lymph nodes

19. Which are common signs and symptoms of HIV infection? Select all that apply.
    1. Heart palpitations
    2. Abdominal pain
    3. Fever
    4. Night sweats
    5. Swollen lymph nodes

20. Which are major complications of HIV infection? Select all that apply.
    1. Hemorrhage
    2. Opportunistic infections
    3. Weight loss
    4. Edema
    5. Dementia
    6. Malnutrition

21. Which factors contribute to the wasting syndrome experienced by patients with HIV infection? Select all that apply.
    1. Liver disorder
    2. Kidney failure
    3. Malabsorption of nutrients
    4. Reduced food intake
    5. Extreme fatigue

22. A patient with leukemia can have a high WBC count crowding out platelets and RBCs, leaving the patient at risk for what? Select all that apply.
    1. Infection
    2. Anemia
    3. Bleeding
    4. Sepsis

23. When a patient has a abnormally low number of total neutrophils and has an increased potential for infection, what condition occurs?
    1. Leukemia
    2. Neutropenia
    3. HIV
    4. Herpes simplex

24. A patient with systemic lupus erythematosus (SLE) may experience pain related to:
    1. skin rash.
    2. low RBC count.
    3. proteinuria.
    4. inflammation of joints and muscles.

25. A 20-year-old African-American woman comes to the community clinic complaining of fatigue, fever, anorexia, joint pain, and muscle pain. She has a butterfly rash on her face. These are common signs and symptoms of:
    1. Hodgkin's disease.
    2. leukemia.
    3. systemic lupus erythematosus (SLE).
    4. multiple myeloma.

26. The reason pus may not be seen even though infection is present in a patient with leukemia is that patients with leukemia do not have normal:
    1. platelets.
    2. red blood cells.
    3. white blood cells.
    4. cytokines.

27. Exaggerated immune responses that are uncomfortable and potentially harmful are:
    1. hypersensitivity reactions.
    2. bacterial lung infections.
    3. tachycardic reactions.
    4. peripheral neuropathy reactions.

28. Which of the following are the causes of neutropenia? Select all that apply.
    1. Decreased bone marrow production
    2. Chemotherapy
    3. Hypersensitivity reactions
    4. Radiation therapy
    5. Autoimmune disorders

E. HIV Drug Therapy

Match the description in the numbered column with the correct drug(s) used to treat patients with HIV infection in the lettered column. There may be two or more answers to each question.

1. _____ Used in patients with HIV to slow the progression of the virus by interfering with HIV replication inside the CD4 cell.

2. _____ Prevents HIV from entering CD4 T cells.

3. _____ Used in patients with HIV to slow the replication and progression of HIV by blocking an enzyme so that the infected cell cannot produce any more HIV proteins.

A. Nucleoside reverse transcriptase inhibitors (NRTIs) (AZT, Retrovir)
B. Protease inhibitors (Invirase, Norvir)
C. Nonnucleoside reverse transcriptase inhibitors (NNRTIs) (Viramune)
D. Fusion inhibitors (Enfuvirtide or Fuzeon)

PART III: CHALLENGE YOURSELF!

F. Getting Ready for NCLEX

Choose the most appropriate answer or select all that apply.

1. A patient has an appointment at the clinic to follow-up about the combination drug therapy she is receiving for her HIV infection. Which of the following are the common side effects of HAART therapy for this patient? Select all that apply.
   1. Decreased triglycerides
   2. Increased cholesterol
   3. Nausea and vomiting
   4. Peripheral neuropathy
   5. Kidney toxicity

2. The nurse is making a home health visit to see a patient with HIV. Which are nutrition teaching points for this patient?
   1. Thoroughly cook meats and poultry.
   2. Thaw frozen foods at room temperature.
   3. Eat small, frequent meals high in lactose.
   4. Eat meals low in calories.

3. A patient with HIV returns to the community health clinic for a follow-up visit because he is receiving combination drug therapy. He states he does not always take his medications every morning. What is one of the major reasons for noncompliance among patients receiving HAART therapy?
   1. Muscle weakness
   2. Nightmares
   3. Gastrointestinal upset
   4. Hypersensitivity reactions

4. The nurse is teaching a class at the community clinic on HIV transmission. The nurse emphasizes that the best way to prevent transmission of HIV is to:
   1. use condoms during all sexual contact.
   2. wash hands thoroughly following contact with HIV-positive people.
   3. practice safe sexual habits.
   4. get plenty of rest and eat a nutritious diet.

5. A patient tells the nurse that she has just been diagnosed with HIV infection and that she is "scared that she will die." Which are therapeutic communication techniques that the nurse can use to show support for this patient with HIV infection? Select all that apply.
   1. Be reassuring.
   2. Be positive.
   3. Be accepting.
   4. Be sensitive.
   5. Be courteous.

A 58-year-old woman has acute leukemia. She has been initially treated with high doses of chemotherapy in the hospital.

Choose the most appropriate answer or select all that apply.

6. The nurse is checking the patient's vital signs every 2–4 hours while she is receiving chemotherapy in the hospital. Which change in her vital signs may indicate sepsis?
   1. Tachycardia
   2. Dyspnea
   3. Hypertension
   4. Decreased temperature

7. The patient's hematocrit has dropped to 28 g/dL and her hemoglobin has dropped to 8 g/dL. These laboratory results indicate that she has developed:
   1. anemia.
   2. thrombocytopenia.
   3. leukopenia.
   4. sepsis.

8. Which problem presents the greatest risk to this patient with leukemia?
   1. Hemorrhage
   2. Anemia
   3. Infection
   4. Fatigue

G. Nursing Care Plan
Refer to Nursing Care Plan, The Patient with HIV Infection, in the book and answer questions 1–3.

A 25-year-old divorced mother of two children works as an accountant and lives with her parents. She was diagnosed with HIV infection during her pregnancy with her daughter, who is now 3 years old and shows no signs of HIV infection. The mother reports that she tires easily, but she is able to work 6 hours a day and care for her children. She is taking three medications (Crixivan, Zerit, and Videx) and is seen monthly by a nurse practitioner in a community clinic. She reports bouts of depression and anxiety about her future. Her most recent blood studies show a decline in the number of T helper (CD4) cells. She has been treated for two upper respiratory infections and does not sleep well. She reports a 10-pound weight loss in the past 3 months, as well as a poor appetite and frequent diarrhea.

1. Which nursing interventions for this patient could be assigned to unlicensed assistive personnel? Select all that apply.
   1. Advise patient of the kinds of side effects and adverse effects that she might experience.
   2. Explain the importance of continuing the drugs under medical supervision.
   3. Discuss ways to conserve energy.
   4. Assist patient with ambulation.
   5. Weigh weekly.
   6. Assist with oral hygiene.

2. This patient is now beginning to develop signs of wasting syndrome. Which are nutrition considerations that the nurse should teach this patient? Select all that apply.
   1. Do not buy expired foods.
   2. Wash hands thoroughly when placing foods into the pan for cooking.
   3. Wash all fruits and vegetables before eating.
   4. Thaw frozen foods at room temperature before cooking.
   5. Your diet should be low-calorie and low-carbohydrate.
   6. Weigh yourself weekly and report patterns of weight loss or weight gain to your health care provider.

3. This patient has also developed a thrush infection in her mouth. Which instruction should you give this patient about mouth care?
   1. Instruct her to use a soft toothbrush.
   2. Encourage her to ask questions and talk about her feelings.
   3. Discuss ways to conserve energy and promote restful sleep.
   4. Advise her to talk to her health care provider to see about getting antinausea medication.

H. Next-Generation NCLEX® Examination-Style Questions

Read each situation and answer the questions that follow.

A 49-year-old male client with a history of HIV infection presents to the medical unit with a diagnosis of Herpes Zoster Virus and oral candidiasis. He has been prescribed nystatin and acyclovir by mouth. The nurse reviews the physical assessment and vital signs.

Physical Assessment:
Client has a stripe of blisters that wraps around the left side of his torso. The client appears visibly upset and complains of pain 8/10 on a numeric scale to his left side.

Vital signs:

Blood Pressure	110/60 mm Hg
Pulse	90 BPM
Respirations	20 breaths/min
Temperature	99.9°F

---

1. Which of the following instructions should be included In the client's teaching plan?
    1. Maintain good hygiene without drying out the skin.
    2. Avoid deodorant astringent soap.
    3. Use cold water; leave the skin moist.
    4. Apply lotion after bathing.
    5. Scratch the area if itching occurs.
    6. Use a separate cloth for affected areas.
    7. Avoid contact with people who have never had chickenpox.

A 35-year-old male client with a history of HIV infection presents to his primary care provider (PCP). The nurse reviews the physical assessment and physician's progress notes.

Physical Assessment:
A 35-year-old male client with a history of HIV infection presents with fatigue, severe diarrhea, and reports a 7 lb weight loss over 1 month. He appears visibly concerned. He has no fever. Skin is intact. Lungs are clear on auscultation. Abdomen is soft with bowel sounds present in all four quadrants.

Physician's Progress Notes:
Client's most recent blood studies show a decline in the number of T helper (CD4) cells. The CD4 cell count today is 450 cells/mm^3. He has been treated twice within the last 6 months for oral candidiasis. Recommend the addition of Carnation Instant Breakfast to his daily diet to increase calorie intake, weekly weigh Ins, and loperamide to manage the diarrhea.
S. Lance, MD

Complete the following sentence by choosing from the list of options in the menus below.

2. The priority patient problems are _____ 1 (Select) and _____ 2 (Select) .

Options for 1:	Options for 2:
impaired oral tissue integrity	fluid volume deficit
inadequate nutrition	potential for infection
risk for impaired skin integrity	ineffective management of therapeutic regimen
inadequate coping	anxiety

Cardiovascular System Introduction

Go to http://evolve.elsevier.com/Linton/medsurg/ for additional activities and exercises.

NCLEX CATEGORIES

Physiological Integrity: Pharmacological Therapies, Reduction of Risk Potential, Physiological Adaptation

PART I: MASTERING THE BASICS

A. Key Terms

Match the definition in the numbered column with the most appropriate term in the lettered column. Some terms may not be used.

1. _____ A heart rate of 60 bpm or less

2. _____ Occurs during ventricular relaxation as they are being refilled with blood coming from the atria

3. _____ A disturbance of the rhythm of the heart caused by a problem in the conduction system

4. _____ The sound produced by turbulent blood flow across the valves

5. _____ Fainting

6. _____ Characterized by a heart rate in excess of 100 bpm

7. _____ Describes the thickness of the blood

8. _____ Occurs when the ventricles contract and blood is ejected into the pulmonary artery

9. _____ The amount of pressure the ventricles must overcome to eject the blood volume

10. _____ The amount of blood remaining in a ventricle at the end of diastole or the pressure generated at the end of diastole

11. _____ Monitoring of patients who have central venous catheters, pulmonary artery catheters, or arterial lines

12. _____ The ability of cardiac muscle fibers to shorten and produce a muscle contraction

A. Afterload
B. Bradycardia
C. Contractility
D. Diastole
E. Dysrhythmia
F. Hemodynamic
G. Murmur
H. Perfusion
I. Preload
J. Syncope
K. Systole
L. Tachycardia
M. Viscosity
N. Vasoconstriction

B. Vascular System

Match the definition or description in the numbered column with the most appropriate term in the lettered column. Some terms may be used more than once, and some may not be used.

1. _____ Vessels that return blood to the heart

2. _____ Cusps that are attached by chordae tendineae to the papillary muscles that line the floor of the ventricles

3. _____ These vessels accommodate the collection of lymph fluid from the peripheral tissues and the transportation of the fluid to the venous circulatory system

4. _____ Vessels that carry blood away from the heart

5. _____ Transfer of oxygen and nutrients between the blood and the tissue cells occurs here

6. _____ They keep blood flowing in one direction by opening and closing passively in response to changes in pressure and volume

A. Veins
B. Valves
C. Leaflets
D. Capillaries
E. Lymph vessels
F. Arteries

C. Heart Circulation

In Figure 33.2 from the book, label the parts (A–I) of the heart.

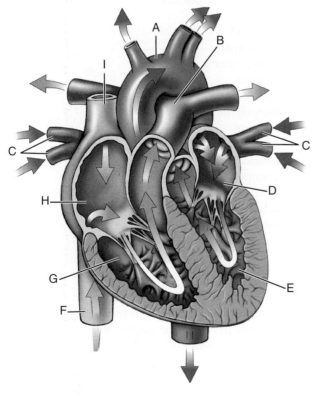

A. _____

B. _____

C. _____

D. _____

E. _____

F. _____

G. _____

H. _____

I. _____

D. Cardiac Function

Match the definition or description in the numbered column with the most appropriate term in the lettered column.

1. _____ The delivery of an electrical shock to the heart in an effort to restore normal cardiac conduction and contraction

2. _____ Place where electrical impulse is initiated in the heart (also called the *pacemaker* of the heart)

3. _____ Contraction phase of the cardiac cycle

4. _____ The amount of blood (measured in liters) ejected by each ventricle per minute

5. _____ For the heart to pump blood through the chambers, nerves must stimulate muscle contractions in an orderly fashion. This pattern is called _____.

6. _____ The terminal ends of the right and left branches of the bundle of His are called the _____.

7. _____ The delivery of a synchronized shock to terminate atrial or ventricular tachydysrhythmias (rapid, abnormal heart rhythms)

A. Cardiac output
B. Systole
C. Conduction
D. SA node
E. Defibrillation
F. Cardioversion
G. Purkinje fibers

E. Diagnostic Tests and Procedures
Match the definition or description in the numbered column with the appropriate diagnostic test or procedure in the lettered column. Some answers may be used more than once.

1. _____ An ambulatory ECG that provides continuous monitoring

2. _____ A transducer used to pick up sound waves and convert them to electrical impulses

3. _____ A high-resolution, three-dimensional image of the heart; cardiac tissue is imaged without lung or bone interference

4. _____ An exercise tolerance test that is a recording of an individual's cardiovascular response during a measured exercise challenge

5. _____ Study of the electrical activity of the heart

6. _____ A procedure in which a catheter is advanced into the heart chambers or coronary arteries under fluoroscopy

7. _____ Electrodes placed on the surface of the skin pick up the electrical impulses of the heart

8. _____ The patient ambulates on a treadmill or a stationary bicycle while connected to a monitor

9. _____ Noninvasive measurement of oxygen saturation

10. _____ Use of catheters with multiple electrodes inserted through the femoral vein to record the heart's electrical activity

11. _____ Fast form of imaging technology that allows for high-quality images of the heart as it contracts and relaxes

A. Stress test
B. Cardiac catheterization
C. Electrocardiogram (ECG)
D. Echocardiogram
E. Electrophysiology study (EPS)
F. Magnetic resonance imaging (MRI)
G. Holter monitor
H. Pulse oximetry
I. Ultrafast computed tomography (electron-beam CT)

F. Drug Therapy

1. Which type of drug is used to treat Raynaud disease?
   1. Alpha-adrenergic blockers
   2. Thrombolytic agents
   3. Anticoagulants
   4. Platelet aggregation inhibitors

2. List two primary anticoagulants and their antidotes.
   1. Oral drug and antidote: _____

   2. Parenteral drug and antidote: _____

Match the drug classification in the numbered column with its use and action in the lettered column.

3. _____ Diuretics
4. _____ Antianginals
5. _____ Antiplatelets
6. _____ Cardiac glycosides
7. _____ Thrombolytics

A. Increase cardiac output
B. Dissolve clots
C. Prevent strokes
D. Decrease fluid retention
E. Relieve pain

G. Heart Chambers
Match the characteristic in the numbered column with the appropriate heart chamber in the lettered column. Some terms may be used more than once.

1. _____ Contains the highest pressure in the heart
2. _____ Receives blood through the tricuspid valve
3. _____ Cone-shaped, has the thickest muscle mass of the four chambers
4. _____ Receives blood saturated with oxygen from the four pulmonary veins
5. _____ Receives blood from the inferior and superior vena cava

A. Right atrium (RA)
B. Right ventricle (RV)
C. Left atrium (LA)
D. Left ventricle (LV)

H. Tissue Layers of Veins and Arteries

Using Figure 33.6 from the book and the word bank below, label the structures of the artery, vein, and capillary using the following numbers. Structures may be used more than once.

1. Tunica adventitia
2. Endothelium
3. Tunica media
4. Elastic tissue
5. Tunica intima
6. Connective tissue
7. Valve

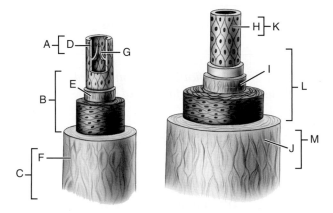

A. _____

B. _____

C. _____

D. _____

E. _____

F. _____

G. _____

H. _____

I. _____

J. _____

K. _____

L. _____

M. _____

PART II: PUTTING IT ALL TOGETHER

I. Multiple Choice/Multiple Response

Choose the most appropriate answer or select all that apply.

1. The pressure is highest in which heart chamber?
   1. Right atrium
   2. Left atrium
   3. Right ventricle
   4. Left ventricle

2. Which are age-related changes in the heart? Select all that apply.
   1. Decreased density of heart muscle connective tissue
   2. Decreased elasticity of myocardium
   3. Increased cardiac contractility
   4. Valves may thicken and stiffen
   5. Cardiac output decreases
   6. Increased number of pacemaker cells in the SA node
   7. Increased number of nerve fibers in ventricles
   8. Cardiac response to stress is slower

3. The first branches of the systemic circulation are the:
   1. subclavian arteries.
   2. coronary arteries.
   3. carotid arteries.
   4. brachial arteries.

4. Which are factors that increase preload? Select all that apply.
   1. Dehydration
   2. Hemorrhage
   3. Increased venous return to the heart
   4. Overhydration
   5. Venous vasodilation

5. Which of these factors increase afterload?
   1. Vasodilation
   2. Hypertension
   3. Vasoconstriction
   4. Aortic stenosis
   5. Overhydration

6. The ventricles contract when the electrical impulse reaches the:
   1. SA node.
   2. AV node.
   3. Purkinje fibers.
   4. bundle of His.

7. Stroke volume, the amount of blood ejected with each ventricular contraction, depends on myocardial:
   1. contractility.
   2. excitability.
   3. conductivity.
   4. automaticity.

8. Which are ways to increase oxygen supply to the myocardium? Select all that apply.
   1. Administer supplemental oxygen.
   2. Increase the rate of myocardial contraction.
   3. Coronary artery vasodilation.
   4. Increase antiplatelet activity.
   5. Increase exercise activity.

9. Which is more likely to occur in older adults as the cardiovascular system adapts more slowly to changes in position?
   1. Tachycardia
   2. Bradycardia
   3. Postural hypotension
   4. Headache

10. A noninvasive measure of cardiac output is:
    1. cardiac catheterization.
    2. blood pressure.
    3. angioplasty.
    4. blood gas measurement.

11. A normal ECG finding is documented as a normal:
    1. tachycardia.
    2. sinus rhythm.
    3. bradycardia.
    4. ventricular gallop.

12. The patient is taking a stress test. Which symptoms require that the stress test be stopped immediately? Select all that apply.
    1. Angina
    2. Dysrhythmias
    3. Diaphoresis
    4. Slower respirations
    5. Falling blood pressure

13. The normal cardiac output is:
    1. 1–3 L/minute.
    2. 4–8 L/minute.
    3. 10–13 L/minute.
    4. 15–20 L/hour.

14. Patients with MI often exhibit:
    1. respiratory acidosis.
    2. respiratory alkalosis.
    3. elevated cholesterol levels.
    4. decreased white blood cell count.

15. What type of diet is generally recommended for cardiac patients?
    1. Low-fat, high-calcium
    2. Low-fat, high-fiber
    3. Low-sodium, low-protein
    4. High-sodium, low-potassium

16. If fluid retention accompanies the cardiac problem, the health care provider may prescribe restriction of:
    1. potassium.
    2. sodium.
    3. fat.
    4. calcium.

17. The purpose of temporary and permanent pacemakers is to improve cardiac output and tissue perfusion by restoring regular:
    1. blood volume.
    2. blood pressure.
    3. impulse conduction.
    4. rhythm.

18. The delivery of a synchronized shock to terminate atrial or ventricular tachyarrhythmias is called:
    1. a pacemaker.
    2. cardiac catheterization.
    3. angioplasty.
    4. cardioversion.

19. During open-heart surgery, the patient's core temperature is reduced to decrease the body's need for:
    1. oxygen.
    2. sodium.
    3. potassium.
    4. ATP.

20. Heparin is given intravenously for immediate response for:
    1. pulmonary embolism.
    2. thrombophlebitis.
    3. varicose vein disease.
    4. ventricular tachycardia.

21. The internal cardiac defibrillator is used to treat patients with life-threatening recurrent:
    1. hypertension.
    2. aortic stenosis.
    3. ventricular fibrillation.
    4. endocarditis.

22. A low-molecular-weight heparin (LMWH), Lovenox, is prescribed for a patient with unstable angina. Which is an advantage of using LMWHs over other anticoagulants?
    1. They are administered SubQ once or twice a day.
    2. The anticoagulant effect is more predictable.
    3. They require very frequent monitor checks for aPTT.
    4. They will dissolve clots.

23. Which heart sound is normal in children and young adults but is pathologic if it is heard after the age of 30?
    1. S_1
    2. S_2
    3. S_3, ventricular gallop
    4. S_4, atrial gallop

24. Questran, lopid, and niacin are drugs classified as:
    1. cardiac glycosides.
    2. nitrates.
    3. lipid-lowering drugs.
    4. antiplatelets.

25. Any interruption of the blood flow to the distal regions of the body, as occurs in peripheral vascular disease (PVD), results in:
    1. kidney failure.
    2. cardiac shock.
    3. dyspnea.
    4. hypoxia.

26. The nervous system that acts on the smooth muscles of vessels, resulting in dilation and constriction of the artery walls, is:
    1. autonomic.
    2. somatic.
    3. central.
    4. cranial.

27. In the evaluation of edema, when the thumb is depressed in the area for 5 seconds and the depression of the thumb remains in the edematous area, the edema is said to be:
    1. 1+.
    2. 2+.
    3. 3+.
    4. pitting.

28. Nurses should teach patients with PVD to stop smoking because smoking causes:
    1. intermittent claudication.
    2. skin ulceration.
    3. vasoconstriction.
    4. vasodilation.

29. Which works as a vasodilator that promotes arterial flow to the peripheral tissues?
    1. TED hose
    2. Intermittent pneumatic compression
    3. Heat
    4. Cold

30. Thrombolytic therapy is employed to:
    1. shorten the clotting time.
    2. increase clot formation.
    3. prevent the formation of new clots.
    4. dissolve an existing clot.

31. The use of vasodilators results in increased blood flow by relaxing the vascular smooth muscle and causing:
    1. increased clotting time.
    2. decreased elasticity in vessels.
    3. reduced resistance in vessels.
    4. increased narrowing in vessels.

32. The placement of an antiembolism hose on patients with peripheral vascular disease (PVD) is done to improve:
    1. infection.
    2. blood flow.
    3. hemorrhage.
    4. ulceration.

33. Intermittent pneumatic compression is used for patients:
    1. with paresthesia.
    2. with intermittent claudication.
    3. confined to bed following surgery.
    4. on moderate exercise programs.

34. Which medications intensify anticoagulant effects?
    1. Antacids
    2. Barbiturates
    3. Oral contraceptives
    4. NSAIDs

35. Which herbal remedy decreases the effectiveness of warfarin?
    1. Garlic
    2. Ginger root
    3. St. John's wort
    4. Ginkgo

36. For patients with PVD, prolonged standing puts strain on the:
    1. venous system.
    2. varicosities.
    3. aneurysms.
    4. aortic dissection.

PART III: CHALLENGE YOURSELF!

J. Getting Ready for NCLEX
Choose the most appropriate answer.

1. The nurse is checking on a patient with PVD. The patient is complaining of pain during Buerger-Allen exercises. It is a priority for the nurse to:
    1. encourage the exercises to be done gradually.
    2. stop the exercises immediately.
    3. ambulate the patient to promote venous return.
    4. administer muscle relaxants as prescribed.

2. The clinic nurse is taking care of a patient with PVD. What is a priority in caring for this patient?
    1. Pain management
    2. Stress management
    3. Regular exercise
    4. A low-sodium diet

3. The nurse is preparing a patient with PVD for discharge from the hospital. The nurse teaches the patient that when intermittent claudication occurs, the patient should:
    1. stop smoking.
    2. avoid constrictive clothing.
    3. use antiembolism hose.
    4. stop exercise.

4. A patient with PVD is being treated with a vasodilator. Patients taking vasodilators for PVD must be monitored for:
    1. hypotension.
    2. hemorrhage.
    3. increased vascular resistance.
    4. hypocalcemia.

5. The nurse is planning to administer the prescribed warfarin for a patient with a cardiac disorder. Warfarin dosage is adjusted according to the patient's:
    1. hemoglobin.
    2. prothrombin time.
    3. partial thromboplastin time.
    4. hematocrit.

Hypertension

Go to http://evolve.elsevier.com/Linton/medsurg/ for additional activities and exercises.

NCLEX CATEGORIES

Physiological Integrity: Pharmacological Therapies, Reduction of Risk Potential, Physiological Adaptation

PART I: MASTERING THE BASICS

A. Key Terms
Match the definition in the numbered column with the most appropriate term in the lettered column.

1. _____ Sudden drop in systolic blood pressure when changing from a lying or sitting position to a standing position
2. _____ Nosebleed
3. _____ Persistent elevation of arterial blood pressure of 140/90 mm Hg or greater
4. _____ Fainting
5. _____ Enlargement
6. _____ Abnormal amounts of lipids or lipoproteins in the blood

A. Dyslipidemia
B. Epistaxis
C. Hypertension
D. Hypertrophy
E. Orthostatic hypotension
F. Syncope

B. Risk Factors

1. What are significant risk factors for primary (essential) hypertension? Select all that apply.
   1. Varicose veins
   2. Dyslipidemia
   3. Tobacco use
   4. Obesity
   5. Thrombophlebitis
   6. Atherosclerosis
   7. Family history

2. How does stress contribute to hypertension?
   1. Increases secretion of catecholamine
   2. Constricts blood vessels and delays the release of epinephrine and norepinephrine
   3. Increases lipids and lipoproteins in the blood, leading to atherosclerosis
   4. Decreases the elasticity of the arteries and arterioles, causing increased peripheral vascular resistance (PVR)

C. Drug Therapy
Match the names of the medications in the numbered column with the correct classification of drugs in the lettered column.

1. _____ Prazosin (Minipress), doxazosin (Cardura)
2. _____ Hydrochlorothiazide (HCTZ), furosemide (Lasix)
3. _____ Losartan potassium (Cozaar), valsartan (Diovan)
4. _____ Clonidine (Catapres), methyldopa (Aldomet)
5. _____ Propranolol (Inderal), atenolol (Tenormin)
6. _____ Hydralazine (Apresoline)
7. _____ Captopril (Capoten) and enalapril (Vasotec)
8. _____ Verapamil (Calan) and diltiazem (Cardizem)

A. Calcium channel blockers
B. Beta blockers
C. Direct vasodilators
D. Angiotensin II receptor antagonists
E. Diuretics
F. Alpha-adrenergic receptor blockers
G. Centrally acting drugs (alpha-2 agonists)
H. ACE inhibitors

Match the actions of the medications in the numbered column with the correct classification of drugs in the lettered column. Some classifications may be used more than once.

9. _____ Block the effects of norepinephrine, causing vasodilation
10. _____ Decrease fluid retention by decreasing the production of aldosterone
11. _____ Reduce blood pressure by blocking the beta effects of catecholamines
12. _____ Act on the central nervous system (CNS) to block vasoconstriction
13. _____ Prevents vasoconstriction from angiotensin and prevents the release of aldosterone

14. _____ Reduce blood volume through the promotion of renal excretion of sodium and water
15. _____ Block the movement of calcium into cardiac and vascular smooth muscle cells, reducing heart rate, decreasing the force of cardiac contraction, and dilating peripheral blood vessels
16. _____ Relax vascular smooth muscle, causing vasodilation
17. _____ Prevent the conversion of angiotensin I to angiotensin II, a potent vasoconstrictor, decreasing peripheral resistance

A. Centrally acting drugs (alpha-2 agonists)
B. Calcium channel blockers
C. Alpha-adrenergic receptor blockers
D. ACE inhibitors
E. Direct vasodilators
F. Beta-adrenergic receptor blockers
G. Diuretics
H. Angiotensin II receptor antagonists

D. Complications

1. *Using Figure 34.2 from the book, list four body structures (A–D) damaged by long-term blood pressure elevation in the figure below.*

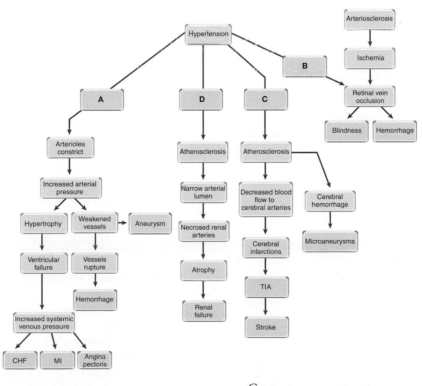

A. _____

B. _____

C. _____

D. _____

2. As blood pressure rises, what are complications that may occur? Select all that apply.
   1. Heart failure
   2. Heart attack
   3. Blindness
   4. Kidney disease
   5. Hypoglycemia
   6. Stroke

E. Blood Pressure

Refer to Table 34.2 in the book to answer the following questions.

1. What is the average systolic blood pressure reduction range for a person who walks briskly 30 minutes/day, most days of the week?

2. What is the average systolic blood pressure reduction range for a person who adopts the DASH eating plan?

3. What is the average systolic blood pressure reduction range for a person who maintains body weight with a body mass index between 18.5 and 24.9 kg/m²?

PART II: PUTTING IT ALL TOGETHER

F. Multiple Choice/Multiple Response

Choose the most appropriate answer or select all that apply.

1. What are the characteristics of hypertensive Risk Group C?
   1. Diabetes
   2. Target organ damage
   3. Clinical cardiovascular disease
   4. Any or all of the above conditions, with or without other risk factors

2. The cause of primary (essential) hypertension is:
   1. kidney disease.
   2. drugs.
   3. pregnancy.
   4. unknown.

3. Hypertension is usually a higher risk for which age group?
   1. Age 30 for men and age 50 for women
   2. Older than age 55 for men and older than age 65 for women
   3. Age 20 for men and age 29 for women
   4. Age 40–49 for men and women

4. A blood pressure of 135/87 mm Hg is considered to be:
   1. stage 1 hypertension.
   2. normal.
   3. prehypertension.
   4. stage 2 hypertension.

5. In which risk group is a hypertensive patient who smokes half a pack of cigarettes a day and who has no heart disease or heart damage classified?
   1. Risk A
   2. Risk B
   3. Risk C
   4. Risk D

6. Isolated systolic blood pressure elevations of 160 mm Hg in older adults are most often due to:
   1. decreased cardiac output.
   2. atherosclerosis.
   3. increased peripheral vascular resistance.
   4. increased pulse pressure.

7. The diameter of blood vessels is regulated primarily by:
   1. the heart muscles.
   2. adrenal gland hormones.
   3. the vasomotor center.
   4. thyroid gland hormones.

8. Patients with systolic pressures between 120 and 139 mm Hg and with diastolic pressures between 80 and 89 mm Hg are said to:
   1. have normal blood pressure.
   2. be in risk group B.
   3. have prehypertension.
   4. have stage I hypertension.

9. Beta blockers are contraindicated in patients with:
   1. hypertension.
   2. edema.
   3. osteoporosis.
   4. asthma.

10. Which group of patients responds better to diuretics as treatment for hypertension?
    1. Caucasians
    2. African Americans
    3. Asians
    4. Hispanics

11. Older patients taking antihypertensives are more susceptible to orthostatic hypotension, increasing their potential for:
    1. confusion.
    2. myocardial infarction.
    3. falls.
    4. congestive heart failure.

12. When body position is changed from supine to standing, the systolic pressure normally:
    1. rises about 5 mm Hg.
    2. rises about 10 mm Hg.
    3. falls about 5 mm Hg.
    4. falls about 10 mm Hg.

13. People with increased blood pressure should not take over-the-counter:
    1. analgesics.
    2. cold remedies.
    3. antacids.
    4. laxatives.

14. A common side effect of many antihypertensives is:
    1. GI distress.
    2. sexual dysfunction.
    3. respiratory depression.
    4. rebound hypertension.

15. Without appropriate treatment, the patient in hypertensive crisis may develop:
    1. cerebrovascular accident.
    2. hyperglycemia.
    3. respiratory acidosis.
    4. adrenal insufficiency.

16. What is the medical treatment blood pressure goal for patients with diabetes or renal disease?
    1. Lower than 110/70 mm Hg
    2. 120/80 mm Hg
    3. Less than 130/80 mm Hg
    4. 140/90 mm Hg

17. How does a blood pressure cuff which is too small affect the blood pressure reading?
    1. False high reading
    2. False low reading
    3. Systolic reading too high
    4. Diastolic reading too low

18. Patients taking antihypertensive medications are encouraged to rise slowly from a lying or sitting position to prevent:
    1. syncope.
    2. orthostatic hypotension.
    3. hypertensive crisis.
    4. confusion.

19. What is the percentage of people with hypertension who have primary or essential hypertension?
    1. 10%–15%
    2. 25%–30%
    3. 45%–50%
    4. 90%–95%

20. What is the effect of epinephrine on blood vessels? Select all that apply.
    1. Dilates blood vessels
    2. Increases blood pressure
    3. Pulse pressure widens
    4. Increases the force of cardiac contraction
    5. Constricts blood vessels

21. Which statement is true about blood pressure?
    1. When body position is altered from supine to standing, the diastolic blood pressure decreases.
    2. In response to increased peripheral vascular resistance, the systolic pressure decreases.
    3. When there is narrowing of the arteries and arterioles, peripheral vascular resistance increases.
    4. When body position is altered from supine to standing, the systolic pressure normally increases.

22. Which factor does not contribute to hypertension?
    1. Cardiac stimulation
    2. Retention of fluid
    3. Vasodilation
    4. Sympathetic nervous system stimulation

23. Which stimulants may contribute to hypertension? Select all that apply.
    1. Caffeine
    2. Nicotine
    3. Alcohol
    4. Amphetamines
    5. Diuretics

24. Which are symptoms of hypertensive crisis? Select all that apply.
    1. Nausea
    2. Restlessness
    3. Drowsiness
    4. Blurred vision
    5. Bradycardia

25. Which are lifestyle modifications related to exercise that are benefits for patients with high blood pressure? Select all that apply.
    1. Reduces water in the body, decreasing the circulating blood volume
    2. Decreases blood glucose and cholesterol levels, increasing the sense of well-being
    3. Eliminates vasoconstriction caused by nicotine
    4. Reduces stress and lowers blood pressure
    5. Improves cardiac efficiency by increasing the cardiac output and decreasing peripheral vascular resistance
    6. Reduces blood pressure by reducing the workload of the heart

26. What are the leading causes of death in people with hypertension? Select all that apply.
    1. CVA
    2. Renal failure
    3. Cardiac failure
    4. Pneumonia

27. What are long-term effects of hypertension on the eyes? Select all that apply.
    1. Retinal hemorrhages
    2. Pupil dilation
    3. Papilledema
    4. Narrowing of retinal arterioles
    5. Conjunctival infections

28. What are long-term effects of hypertension on the heart? Select all that apply.
    1. Angina
    2. Myocardial infarction
    3. Vasodilation
    4. Coronary artery disease
    5. Decreased cardiac contractility

29. Which is a long-term effect of hypertension on the brain?
    1. Dehydration
    2. Transient ischemic attacks
    3. Decreased blood flow
    4. Aneurysm

G. Matching

Match the side effect or caution in the numbered column with the correct classification of drugs in the lettered column. Some classifications may be used more than once.

1. _____ Palpitations, dizziness, headache, drowsiness
2. _____ Hypoglycemia
3. _____ Hyponatremia and hypokalemia
4. _____ Flushing, dizziness, headache
5. _____ Skin rash, cough
6. _____ Use cautiously in patients with asthma and diabetes
7. _____ Fluid volume deficit
8. _____ Dry mouth, weakness

A. Centrally acting drugs
B. Beta blockers
C. Calcium channel blockers
D. Alpha-adrenergic receptor blockers
E. Diuretics
F. ACE inhibitors

Use Table 34.1 from the book to match the blood pressure categories in the numbered columns with the labels in the lettered columns.

9. _____ What is the category for a person with blood pressure of 150/95 mm Hg?
10. _____ What is the category for a person with blood pressure of 122/84 mm Hg?
11. _____ What is the category for a person with blood pressure of 118/78 mm Hg?
12. _____ What is the category for a person with blood pressure of 180/110 mm Hg?

A. Prehypertension
B. Normal
C. Stage 1 hypertension
D. Stage 2 hypertension

PART III: CHALLENGE YOURSELF!

H. Getting Ready for NCLEX

Choose the most appropriate answer or select all that apply.

1. The nurse is speaking about the DASH diet with a group of patients who have hypertension. Which food groups are emphasized in the DASH diet? Select all that apply.
    1. Vegetables
    2. Fruits
    3. Nuts and seeds
    4. Whole milk
    5. Meats

2. The nurse is taking care of a patient in hypertensive crisis. Which blood tests are likely to be prescribed for this patient? Select all that apply.
    1. Arterial blood gases (ABGs)
    2. Complete blood count (CBC)
    3. Electrolytes
    4. Blood urea nitrogen (BUN)
    5. Creatinine
    6. Prothrombin time

3. A nurse is taking care of a patient with hypertension in the hospital. Which are the teaching points about orthostatic hypotension that the nurse will explain to this patient? Select all that apply.
    1. Eat a low-sodium diet.
    2. Avoid prolonged standing.
    3. Avoid cholesterol in diet.
    4. Avoid hot baths and showers.
    5. Rise slowly.

4. The nurse is teaching a staff development program about primary and secondary hypertension. What are causes of secondary hypertension that the nurse should include in this program? Select all that apply.
    1. Renal disease
    2. Sedentary lifestyle
    3. Tobacco use
    4. Narrowing of the aorta
    5. Increased intracranial pressure

5. An older patient taking furosemide (Lasix) for hypertension complains of muscle weakness, confusion, and irritability. Which patient teaching is correct for this patient?
    1. Decrease sodium in the diet.
    2. Increase potassium in the diet.
    3. Increase fluid intake.
    4. Decrease vitamin K intake.

6. A patient with diabetes is taking a beta blocker for hypertension. Which is the only sign of hypoglycemia that may be present in this patient?
    1. Diaphoresis
    2. Fatigue
    3. Hunger
    4. Excessive thirst

7. The nurse is taking care of a 75-year-old patient in a nursing home who is taking a beta blocker for hypertension. The nurse recognizes that older patients taking beta blockers are at greater risk than younger people for:
    1. bradycardia.
    2. hypoglycemia.
    3. bronchoconstriction.
    4. GI upset.

8. If a patient's diastolic pressure is 120 mm Hg, the nurse should:
    1. try a larger blood pressure cuff.
    2. reassess it in 30 minutes.
    3. notify the health care provider.
    4. encourage the patient to stay on bedrest.

9. The nurse is assisting with discharge teaching of a patient with hypertension who is leaving the hospital. The health care provider has prescribed lisinopril for the patient to take at home. The nurse explains that the patient must take this medication as prescribed because if antihypertensive drugs are stopped abruptly, what may occur?
    1. Hypotensive crisis
    2. Orthostatic hypotension
    3. Rebound hypertension
    4. Bradycardia

I. Next-Generation NCLEX® Examination-Style Questions

Read the situations below and answer the questions that follow.

A 66-year-old female client presents to her primary care provider with complaints of severe headaches on arising, light-headedness, and occasional epistaxis. The nurse reviews the health history and vital signs.

Health History:

A 66-year-old female client presents to her primary care provider with complaints of severe headaches on arising, light-headedness, and occasional epistaxis. She has a history of diabetes mellitus type II, dyslipidemia, and a 10-year smoking history. Her family history reveals that her father was diagnosed with hypertension at age 45. She works as a lawyer and spends many hours at her computer. She states that she has been feeling unmotivated to workout due to the stress of her job.

Vital Signs:

Blood Pressure	172/90 mm Hg
Pulse	89 beats/minute
Respirations	18 breaths/minute
Temperature	98.8°F

---

1. Highlight the risk factors that place the client at risk for primary (essential) HTN.

A 35-year-old African American male client presents to the Emergency Department with severe headache, blurred vision, and nausea. He states that his symptoms began abruptly approximately one hour prior to arrival. The nurse reviews the health history and vital signs.

He has a medical history that includes hypertension, 15-year smoking history, and BMI 30 kg/m². He states that he recently stopped taking his hydrochlorothiazide (HCTZ) because he did not like the way it made him feel. Vital signs: 200/140 mm Hg, pulse 104, respirations 22, temperature 97.9°F.

Health History:

Hypertension, 15-year smoking history, and BMI 30 kg/m². He states that he recently stopped taking his hydrochlorothiazide (HCTZ) because he did not like the way it made him feel.

Vital signs:

Blood Pressure	200/140 mm Hg
Pulse	104 beats/minute
Respirations	22 breaths/minute
Temperature	97.9°F

---

2. Which physician orders would the nurse anticipate being prescribed? Select all that apply.

   1. Insert peripheral IV STAT
   2. Thiazide diuretics
   3. Monitor fluid intake and output
   4. Seizure precautions
   5. NPO
   6. Insert straight catheter
   7. Total parenteral nutrition
   8. Head CT

Cardiac Disorders

chapter

35

Go to http://evolve.elsevier.com/Linton/medsurg/ for additional activities and exercises.

NCLEX CATEGORIES

Physiological Integrity: Basic Care and Comfort, Reduction of Risk Potential, Physiological Adaptation

PART I: MASTERING THE BASICS

A. Key Terms
Match the definition or description in the numbered column with the most appropriate term in the lettered column. Some terms may not be used.

1. _____ An inflammatory disease that begins with endothelial injury and progresses to the complicated lesion seen in advanced stages of the disease process

2. _____ The inability of the valve to close completely, allowing the blood to flow backward when a valve does not close (also called *insufficiency*)

3. _____ The death of myocardial tissue due to prolonged lack of blood and O_2 supply

4. _____ Inflammation of the pericardial sac

A. Pericarditis
B. Atherosclerosis
C. Myocardial infarction
D. Regurgitation
E. Syncope
F. Thromboembolism

B. Complications of Coronary Artery Disease
Match the description of complications of coronary artery disease (CAD) in the numbered column with the most appropriate term in the lettered column. Some terms may not be used.

1. _____ Disturbances in heart rhythm

2. _____ When an injured ventricle is unable to meet the body's circulatory demands

3. _____ The most frequent cause of death after an acute myocardial infarction (AMI); marked by hypotension and decreasing alertness

4. _____ A fatal complication in which weakened areas of the ventricular wall bulge and burst

A. Ventricular aneurysm/rupture
B. Mitral stenosis
C. Dysrhythmias
D. Hemorrhage
E. Cardiogenic shock
F. Thromboembolism
G. Heart failure

C. Mitral Stenosis
Complete the statement in the numbered column with the most appropriate term in the lettered column. Some terms may not be used.

1. _____ The leading cause of mitral stenosis

2. _____ The chamber of the heart that dilates to accommodate the amount of blood not ejected in patients with mitral stenosis

3. _____ When collecting data for the assessment of the patient with mitral stenosis, the nurse takes the vital signs and auscultates for _____.

A. Heart murmur
B. Rheumatic heart disease
C. Left ventricle
D. Left atrium
E. Right ventricle

D. Heart Failure

For the following signs and symptoms of heart failure (HF), indicate whether they are indicative of (A) right-sided or (B) left-sided failure.

1. _____ Dependent edema
2. _____ Decreasing BP readings
3. _____ Increased central venous pressure
4. _____ Anxious, pale, and tachycardic
5. _____ Jugular venous distention
6. _____ Abdominal engorgement
7. _____ Crackles, wheezes, dyspnea, and cough
8. _____ Restless and confused
9. _____ Decreased urinary output

E. Matching

Match the drug used for cardiac disorders in the numbered column with its classification in the lettered column. Some terms may not be used.

1. _____ Nitroglycerin
2. _____ Aspirin, dipyridamole (Persantine), and clopidogrel (Plavix)
3. _____ Heparin and warfarin (Coumadin)
4. _____ Furosemide (Lasix) and hydrochlorothiazide (Esidrix, HCTZ, and Oretic)
5. _____ Streptokinase, sotalol hydrochloride (Betapace), and tissue plasminogen activator
6. _____ Digoxin (Lanoxin) and digitoxin
7. _____ Dabigatran (Pradaxa) and rivaroxaban (Xarelto)

A. Anticholinergics
B. Antianginals
C. Analgesics
D. Antiplatelet agents
E. Antidysrhythmics
F. Diuretics
G. Fibrinolytics (thrombolytics)
H. Anticoagulants
I. Cardiac glycosides
J. ACE inhibitors
K. Anticoagulants classified as direct thrombin inhibitors

Match the use(s) of AMI drug therapy in the numbered column with the specific drug in the lettered column. Some drugs may be used more than once, and some may not be used.

8. _____ Used for chest pain
9. _____ Administered through an IV or into the coronary arteries to dissolve thrombi
10. _____ Following the administration of antithrombolytics, this drug is administered to prevent further clot formation
11. _____ Increases myocardial contractility and decreases the heart rate

A. Furosemide (Lasix)
B. Streptokinase
C. Digoxin
D. Morphine sulfate
E. Atropine sulfate
F. Lidocaine
G. Heparin

Match the actions of drugs used to treat HF in the numbered column with the drug or drug classification in the lettered column. Some answers may be used more than once, and some answers may not be used.

12. _____ Improve(s) pump function by increasing contractility and decreasing heart rate
13. _____ Decrease(s) circulating fluid volume and decrease(s) preload
14. _____ Decrease(s) anxiety, dilate(s) the vasculature, and reduce(s) myocardial oxygen consumption in the acute stage

A. Heparin
B. Morphine
C. Diuretics
D. Streptokinase
E. Cardiac glycosides or inotropic agents

PART II: PUTTING IT ALL TOGETHER

F. Multiple Choice/Multiple Response

Choose the most appropriate answer or select all that apply.

1. If the valves of the heart do not close properly, the patient is said to have:
    1. infarction.
    2. mitral regurgitation.
    3. necrosis.
    4. tachycardia.

2. When the demand for O_2 by the myocardial cells exceeds the supply of O_2 delivered, the patient has a condition called:
    1. heartburn.
    2. dyspnea.
    3. pleurisy.
    4. angina.

3. Which drug is administered to dilate coronary arteries and increase blood flow to the damaged area of a patient with AMI?
    1. Nitroglycerin
    2. Furosemide
    3. Dipyridamole (Persantine)
    4. Streptokinase

4. Which vein is often used as grafts in coronary artery bypass surgery?
    1. Subclavian
    2. Femoral
    3. Inferior vena cava
    4. Saphenous

5. What is the reason for placing patients with HF in a semi-Fowler or high-Fowler position?
    1. Decrease cardiac workload
    2. Decrease aspiration
    3. Lessen fatigue
    4. Breathe easier by reducing pressure of organs on the diaphragm

6. The most common adverse effects of diuretic therapy for patients with HF are:
    1. hypertension and tachycardia.
    2. fluid and electrolyte imbalances.
    3. headache and oliguria.
    4. confusion and weakness.

7. A common finding in patients with right-sided HF is:
    1. increased urinary output.
    2. dependent edema.
    3. weight loss.
    4. cough.

8. The most common site for organisms to accumulate in patients with infective endocarditis is the:
    1. mitral valve.
    2. tricuspid valve.
    3. aortic valve.
    4. pulmonary valve.

9. The main drugs used for endocarditis are:
    1. cardiac glycosides.
    2. diuretics.
    3. calcium channel blockers.
    4. antimicrobials.

10. The hallmark symptom of pericarditis is:
    1. chest pain.
    2. headache.
    3. hypertension.
    4. indigestion

11. A procedure in which a peripherally inserted catheter is passed into an occluded artery and a balloon is inflated to dilate the artery is:
    1. percutaneous transluminal angioplasty (PTCA).
    2. coronary atherectomy.
    3. intracoronary stent placement.
    4. laser angioplasty.

12. Lifelong medications that must be given to patients with heart transplants include:
    1. antihistamines.
    2. analgesics.
    3. antimicrobials.
    4. immunosuppressives.

13. The two major valve problems of the heart are stenosis and:
    1. inflammation.
    2. insufficiency
    3. emboli.
    4. hemorrhage.

14. Before each dose of digoxin, the apical pulse is counted for 1 full minute; the drug is withheld, and the health care provider notified if the pulse is below:
    1. 60 bpm.
    2. 70 bpm.
    3. 72 bpm.
    4. 80 bpm.

15. The first medication given to patients with chest pain is:
    1. morphine.
    2. aspirin.
    3. Demerol.
    4. nitroglycerin.

16. The pain of heart problems may radiate or may be referred to other areas. Which are areas to which pain may radiate? Select all that apply.
    1. Down either arm
    2. Just below the sternum
    3. Umbilicus
    4. Jaw
    5. Lower abdomen

17. What are reasons that PTCA may be a preferred treatment over bypass surgery? Select all that apply.
    1. Done under local anesthesia instead of general anesthesia
    2. Less invasive than bypass surgery
    3. Faster recovery time
    4. Tiny holes are drilled in the myocardium using a laser
    5. Higher-resolution image of heart activity

18. Which drugs are used to treat chronic stable angina? Select all that apply.
    1. Antidysrhythmics
    2. Nitrates
    3. Beta-adrenergic blockers
    4. Antiplatelets
    5. Calcium channel blockers
    6. Diuretics

PART III: CHALLENGE YOURSELF!

G. Getting Ready for NCLEX
Choose the most appropriate answer or select all that apply.

1. The nurse is taking care of a patient with stable angina. Which are words that this patient may use to describe anginal pain? Select all that apply.
   1. Burning
   2. Squeezing
   3. Aching
   4. Dull
   5. Viselike
   6. Smothering

2. A patient who has been diagnosed with mitral stenosis comes to the community clinic. Which findings would the nurse expect to observe in this patient? Select all that apply.
   1. Bradycardia
   2. Tachypnea
   3. Increasing pulse pressure
   4. Jugular vein distention
   5. Wheezing lung sounds
   6. Rumbling, low-pitched murmur sounds

3. The nurse is collecting data from a cardiac patient about his diet. Which areas of intake should the nurse especially document in the patient record? Select all that apply.
   1. Calcium
   2. Vitamin D
   3. Salt
   4. Protein
   5. Fat
   6. Iron

4. The nurse is assisting with the presentation of a community health program about risk factors for atherosclerosis. Which are modifiable risk factors for atherosclerosis that should be a part of the presentation? Select all that apply.
   1. Tobacco use
   2. High blood pressure
   3. Sedentary lifestyle
   4. Age
   5. Heredity
   6. Obesity

H. Nursing Care Plan

Refer to Nursing Care Plan, The Patient with Heart Failure, in the book and answer questions 1–6.

A 73-year-old Chinese-American woman is admitted through the Emergency Department. She lives by herself with no immediate family in the area. She began having dyspnea and orthopnea that became progressively worse over the past 3 days. She had a myocardial infarction 1 year ago and a 10-year history of hypertension treated with diet and verapamil. She complains of fatigue, restlessness, nervousness, irritability, insomnia, anorexia, and a productive cough with pink sputum.

Physical exam: BP, 168/96 mm Hg. Pulse 104 bpm with slight irregularity. Respiration, 24 breaths per minute. Weight, 152 lbs (7-lb increase in 1 week). Alert, anxious, pale skin, and diaphoretic. An S_3 is present. Jugular vein distention is noted. Crackles in the lower lobes of both lungs. Distended abdomen. 3+ pitting edema in both feet and ankles.

She is being admitted to the telemetry unit for treatment, where she will have continuous ECG monitoring and be placed on O_2.

1. Which abnormal findings were found on physical examination for this patient related to HF?

    1. _____

    2. _____

    3. _____

    4. _____

    5. _____

    6. _____

    7. _____

    8. _____

    9. _____

    10. _____

    11. _____

2. What is the primary patient problem to be addressed?

3. Why is this patient more susceptible to adverse drug effects?

4. If she is started on digoxin, what are early signs of digoxin toxicity that the nurse would be watching for?

5. Why is it important for her to remain on bedrest?

6. Which tasks can be assigned to unlicensed assistive personnel?

I. Next-Generation NCLEX® Examination-Style Questions

A 56-year-old male client with a history of stable angina presents to the Emergency Department with complaints of chest pain. The nurse reviews the health history.

Health History:
A 56-year-old male client with a history of stable angina. Experienced an episode of chest pain while exercising and took his nitroglycerin. He states that after 5 minutes the chest pain was not relieved by rest or with nitroglycerin. The client is now experiencing shortness of breath, diaphoresis, and nausea.

1. Which physician orders would the nurse anticipate being prescribed? Select all that apply.

1. Soft diet
2. Cardiac catheterization
3. Complete bedrest
4. 81 mg aspirin daily
5. Nitroglycerin
6. Metoprolol
7. Simvastatin
8. Low molecular weight heparin

The nurse reviews the physical assessment, labs, and vital signs of a 50-year-old female admitted with left- sided heart.

Physical Assessment:
A client presents with crackles, wheezes, shortness of breath, and cough. Her husband reports that she has been restless and confused at times. S3 and S4 heard upon auscultation of heart.

Labs:

Sodium	125 mEq/L
BUN	24 mg/dL
B-type natriuretic peptide (BNP)	500 pg/mL

Vital Signs:

	0700	0800
Blood Pressure	108/62 mm Hg	90/50 mm Hg
Pulse	108 beats/minute	110 beats/minute
Respiration	18 breaths/minute	18 breaths/minute
Temp	98.8°F	98.8°F
SPO2	93% Room air	90% Room air

2. **Complete the following sentence by choosing from the list of options below.**

The priority patient problem is _____ (1), related to _____ (2).

Options for 1	Options for 2
Inadequate pulmonary oxygenation	Mechanical failure
Inadequate cardiac circulation	Decreased pulmonary perfusion
Increased extracellular fluid volume	Difficulty breathing
Anxiety	Ineffective cardiac pumping

Vascular Disorders

chapter
36

Go to http://evolve.elsevier.com/Linton/medsurg/ for additional activities and exercises.

NCLEX CATEGORIES

Physiological Integrity: Reduction of Risk Potential, Physiological Adaptation

PART I: MASTERING THE BASICS

A. Key Terms
Match the definition in the numbered column with the most appropriate term in the lettered column.

1. _____ Deficient blood flow due to obstruction or constriction of blood vessels

2. _____ Inflammation of a vein

3. _____ Development or presence of a thrombus

4. _____ A balloon-like bulge in an artery

A. Thrombosis
B. Phlebitis
C. Ischemia
D. Aneurysm

5. Which are factors contributing to varicosities? Select all that apply.
   1. Hereditary weakness
   2. Aging
   3. Pregnancy
   4. Prolonged standing
   5. Orthostatic hypotension

6. What are common sites for varicosities? Select all that apply.
   1. Esophageal veins
   2. Renal veins
   3. Coronary veins
   4. Peripheral veins
   5. Hemorrhoidal veins

PART II: PUTTING IT ALL TOGETHER

B. Multiple Choice/Multiple Response
Choose the most appropriate answer or select all that apply.

1. Thrombolytic therapy is employed to:
   1. shorten the clotting time.
   2. increase clot formation.
   3. prevent the formation of new clots.
   4. dissolve an existing clot.

2. A serious risk with a diagnosis of deep vein thrombosis is the development of:
   1. hemorrhage.
   2. pneumonia.
   3. pulmonary embolus.
   4. infection.

3. Which of the following are the classifications of drugs that are used in the general management of PVD to improve peripheral circulation? Select all that apply.
   1. Antimicrobials
   2. Diuretics
   3. Anticoagulants
   4. Thrombolytics
   5. Vasoconstrictors

4. During repair of an abdominal aneurysm, the aorta is clamped for a period of time. This poses a risk of:
   1. dyspnea.
   2. renal failure.
   3. pneumonia.
   4. incontinence.

5. Varicose veins develop as a result of incompetent:
   1. elasticity.
   2. smooth muscle.
   3. thickness.
   4. valves.

6. Chronic venous insufficiency may develop from:
   1. varicose veins.
   2. plaque formations.
   3. thrombophlebitis.
   4. aortic dissection.

7. Signs of chronic venous insufficiency include stasis dermatitis of lower legs and:
   1. redness.
   2. infection.
   3. edema.
   4. cyanosis.

8. The nurse is taking care of a patient with Raynaud disease. This patient is experiencing inadequate peripheral tissue oxygenation related to:
   1. vascular occlusion.
   2. atherosclerosis.
   3. vasoconstriction.
   4. open wound.

9. Chronically cold hands and numbness are symptoms of:
   1. Buerger disease.
   2. Raynaud disease.
   3. atherosclerosis.
   4. deep vein thrombosis.

10. An alternative therapy for vasospastic episodes of Raynaud disease is:
    1. guided imagery.
    2. meditation.
    3. biofeedback.
    4. yoga.

11. What factors (called *Virchow's triad*) contribute to venous thrombus formation? Select all that apply.
    1. Stasis of the blood
    2. Damage to the vessel walls
    3. Hypertension
    4. Hypercoagulability
    5. Vasodilation

12. What are symptoms of a deep vein thrombosis in the lower leg? Select all that apply.
    1. Area is edematous.
    2. Area is cool.
    3. Area is dry.
    4. Area is tender to touch.
    5. Area is red.

13. What is the most serious complication of deep vein thrombosis?
    1. Hemorrhage
    2. Venous stasis
    3. Pulmonary embolism
    4. Hypovolemic shock

14. Which are complications of aneurysms? Select all that apply.
    1. Emboli
    2. Infection
    3. Rupture
    4. Thrombus forms, obstructing blood flow
    5. Pressure on surrounding structures
    6. Liver failure

15. Which are primary diagnostic examinations used in the detection of venous thrombi? Select all that apply.
    1. Doppler ultrasonography
    2. Duplex ultrasonography
    3. Exercise treadmill test
    4. Venography
    5. Magnetic resonance imaging (MRI)

16. Which are characteristics of venous insufficiency in the legs? Select all that apply.
    1. Capillary refill greater than 3 seconds
    2. Lower leg edema
    3. Pale skin color when elevated
    4. Varicose veins may be visible
    5. Dark reddish color in dependent position
    6. Bronze-brown pigmentation
    7. Cool skin
    8. Intermittent claudication or rest pain
    9. Dull ache, heaviness in calf or thigh
    10. Absent peripheral pulses

17. Thromboangiitis obliterans, also called *Buerger disease*, is an inflammatory thrombotic disorder of the lower and upper extremities. Which statements about the disorder are true? Select all that apply.
    1. Uncommon in the United States
    2. Cold hands and numbness are common symptoms
    3. Only smokers are affected
    4. Very common in Korea, India, and Japan
    5. Stress effects the process of the disease

PART III: CHALLENGE YOURSELF!

C. Getting Ready for NCLEX
Choose the most appropriate answer or select all that apply.

1. The nurse is teaching a program at a community health clinic on the risk factors for the development of deep vein thrombosis. Which are risk factors the nurse should include in the program? Select all that apply.
   1. Prescribed bedrest
   2. Obesity
   3. Malnourishment
   4. Use of oral contraceptives
   5. Use of anticoagulants
   6. Prescribed cast or traction for fractures

2. The nurse is checking on a patient who has deep vein thrombosis in the acute phase. Which are treatments for this patient? Select all that apply.
   1. Frequent ambulation initially
   2. Elevate extremity
   3. Apply warm compresses
   4. Anticoagulant therapy
   5. Antiembolism hose

3. The nurse in a community health clinic is reviewing the records of patients who are receiving anticoagulants. The nurse makes a list of patients with conditions in which anticoagulants are contraindicated. In the list below, when are anticoagulants contraindicated? Select all that apply.
   1. Venous thrombosis
   2. Active bleeding
   3. Recent major surgery
   4. Patients on bedrest
   5. Uncontrolled hypertension

4. The nurse is taking care of a patient with thrombosis. The nurse instructs the patient not to massage or rub the site because of the possible development of:
   1. severe infection.
   2. hemorrhage.
   3. skin breakdown.
   4. pulmonary emboli.

5. A patient complains of persistent, aching pain in his left foot after lying quietly in bed. This type of rest pain is a symptom of:
   1. peripheral arterial disease (PAD).
   2. PVD.
   3. deep vein thrombosis.
   4. Raynaud disease.

6. A patient has Raynaud disease. What is related to the inadequate peripheral tissue oxygenation problem for this patient?
   1. Compromised circulation
   2. Vascular occlusion
   3. Graft thrombosis
   4. Vasoconstriction

D. Nursing Care Plan
Refer to Nursing Care Plan, The Patient with a Venous Stasis Ulcer, in the book and answer questions 1–5.

A 75-year-old man is being seen in the community clinic for an ulcer on the medial malleolus of the right ankle. He describes a "heavy burning sensation" in the lower legs. He worked for many years as a toll-booth attendant, often in a standing position. He reports having had hypertension in the past but takes no medication for it now.

Physical examination: Blood pressure 194/102 mm Hg; pulse 64 bpm; respirations 16. Alert and oriented. Walks with slight limp. 2+ edema both ankles. Varicosities noted in both legs. Stasis dermatitis in ankles and calves. Ulcer present. Ankles and feet are cooler than calves. Pedal pulses faint but palpable, slightly stronger in left foot.

1. Which eight findings on the physical examination are abnormal?

    1. _____
    2. _____
    3. _____
    4. _____
    5. _____
    6. _____
    7. _____
    8. _____

2. How does this patient describe his pain?

3. What is a risk factor for PVD for this patient?

4. What are steps this patient can take to lessen his pain?

5. Which tasks can be assigned to unlicensed assistive personnel? Select all that apply.
    1. Check vital signs.
    2. Instruct the patient in measures to improve circulation.
    3. Assess condition of ulcer, peripheral pulses, skin color and warmth, pain, and edema.
    4. Teach hygienic techniques of handwashing and wound care.
    5. Teach signs and symptoms of infection that should be reported to health care provider.
    6. Teach pain-relief measures.
    7. Explain the use of analgesics.
    8. Assist the patient with ambulation.
    9. Document the condition of the ulcer during each clinic visit.
    10. Weigh the patient.

E. Next-Generation NCLEX® Examination-Style Questions

A 56-year-old male client presents to his primary care provider (PCP) office. The nurse reviews the physician's progress notes, physical assessment, and vital signs.

Physician's Progress Notes:

A 56-year-old male client presents with complaints of aching, cramping, and weakness in his right lower extremity. He states that the symptoms occur with walking and is relieved by rest. He rates the pain 5/10 on a numeric scale when ambulating, but states he is not having any pain at this time.

Physical Assessment:

Right lower extremity is pale in color with muscle atrophy noted. Toenails are thickened to the right lower extremity and there is minimal hair growth to the leg.

Vital Signs:

Blood Pressure	150/90 mm Hg
Pulse	88 BPM
Respirations	20 breaths/minute
Temperature	98.9°F

---

1. Based on the client information provided, what would be the nurse's first action?
   1. Apply a nicotine patch
   2. Administer analgesics for pain
   3. Administer an antihypertensive
   4. Apply an ice pack to the right lower extremity
   5. Educate the patient on the need for an endarterectomy
   6. Elevate the right lower extremity
   7. Administer tPA

A 30-year-old female client who is pregnant with her first child presents to her obstetrics appointment. The nurse reviews the physician's progress notes.

Physician's Progress Notes:

A 30-year-old pregnant female reports dull aching sensations to her bilateral lower extremities when walking, muscle cramps at night, and bilateral ankle edema. Purple colored veins to the back of the client's bilateral lower extremities. Probable varicose veins. *K. Long, MD*

---

2. Based on the client information provided, what should be included in the client's teaching plan? Select all that apply.
   1. Exercise regularly to promote circulation.
   2. Avoid prolonged standing, sitting, and crossing your legs.
   3. Wear restrictive clothing to reduce pain.
   4. Elevate extremities whenever possible.
   5. Wear support hose.
   6. Apply ice to bilateral lower extremities.
   7. Begin bedrest immediately.

Digestive System Introduction

Go to http://evolve.elsevier.com/Linton/medsurg/ for additional activities and exercises.

NCLEX CATEGORIES

Safe and Effective Care Environment: Safety and Infection Control

Health Promotion and Maintenance

Physiological Integrity: Basic Care and Comfort, Pharmacological Therapies, Reduction of Risk Potential, Physiological Adaptation

PART I: MASTERING THE BASICS

A. Key Terms
Match the definition in the numbered column with the most appropriate term in the lettered column.

1. _____ Regurgitation and passage of fluids into the respiratory tract.

2. _____ Characterized by the digestive disturbances of nausea, vomiting, dyspepsia, heartburn, fat intolerance, change in stool frequency, or characteristics.

3. _____ One of the processes by which the liver maintains blood glucose. Fats and protein are broken down in response to low blood glucose levels and the molecules are used to make new glucose.

4. _____ This term refers to the liver.

5. _____ After a meal, excess glucose molecules are taken up by the liver, combined, and then stored as glycogen.

6. _____ Direct inspection of hollow interior organs through a lighted tube.

7. _____ Intense, rapid-acting laxative.

8. _____ Fluid accumulation in the peritoneal cavity that causes the abdomen to be distended.

9. _____ When the glucose level in the blood falls, glycogenesis is reversed by this process and the glucose molecules are returned to the blood.

10. _____ Liver enlargement.

11. _____ A golden-yellow skin color associated with liver dysfunction or bile obstruction.

12. _____ Stretch marks.

13. _____ The sclera may turn yellow with liver disease.

A. Ascites
B. Aspiration
C. Cathartic
D. Dysphagia
E. Endoscope
F. Gluconeogenesis
G. Glycogenesis
H. Glycogenolysis
I. Hepatic
J. Hepatomegaly
K. Icterus
L. Jaundice
M. Striae

B. Drug Therapy

Match the drugs in the numbered column with their actions in the lettered column.

1. _____ Anticholinergic agents
2. _____ Antivirals
3. _____ Antiemetics
4. _____ Antacids
5. _____ Mucosal barriers (cytoprotective)
6. _____ Antidiarrheals
7. _____ Antibacterials
8. _____ Antifungals
9. _____ Proton pump inhibitors

A. Treat ulcerative colitis and *H. pylori*
B. Neutralize gastric acid
C. Cling to the surface of the ulcer and protect it so that healing can take place
D. Treat yeast infections
E. Prevent and treat nausea
F. Decrease intestinal motility so that liquid portion of feces is reabsorbed
G. Reduce gastrointestinal motility and secretions; block acetylcholine
H. Used to treat adults with chronic hepatitis C
I. Inhibit gastric acid secretion and used in peptic ulcer disease and GERD

C. GI Tubes

Answer questions 1–4 with the terms in the lettered column. Some questions will have more than one answer. Some answer choices may not be used.

1. _____ Which nasogastric tubes are used for gastric decompression (GI suction)?
2. _____ Which nasoenteric tubes are used for intestinal decompression?
3. _____ Which esophageal-gastric balloon tube is used to control bleeding in the esophagus, usually in patients with severe complications of liver disease?
4. _____ Which feeding tube is placed in the stomach through an opening (stoma) in the abdominal wall?

A. Miller-Abbott tube
B. Sengstaken-Blakemore tube
C. Levin tube
D. Salem sump tube
E. Cantor tube
F. Dobhoff
G. Gastrostomy (PEG)

D. Digestive Tract

In Figure 37.1 from the book, label the parts (A–L) of the digestive tract.

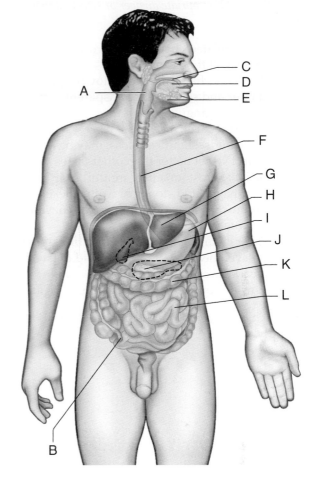

A. _____

B. _____

C. _____

D. _____

E. _____

F. _____

G. _____

H. _____

I. _____

J. _____

K. _____

L. _____

PART II: PUTTING IT ALL TOGETHER

E. Multiple Choice/Multiple Response
Choose the most appropriate answer or select all that apply.

1. Some age-related changes to the digestive tract are: (Select all that apply.)
   1. Teeth: mechanically worn down; appear darker and somewhat transparent with receding gingiva
   2. Jaw: osteoarthritis
   3. Taste buds: significant loss; may be able to detect sweet better than other tastes
   4. Saliva: xerostomia (dry mouth)
   5. Esophagus and stomach: walls thicken
   6. Hydrochloric acid and digestive enzymes: production decreases
   7. Liver changes include reduced blood flow, delayed healing after injury, and delayed clearance of some drugs
   8. Lower esophageal sphincter: more rigid

2. Which herbs can harm the liver? Select all that apply.
   1. Comfrey
   2. Borage
   3. Ginger root
   4. Garlic
   5. Coltsfoot
   6. Chaparral
   7. Germander

3. After insertion of a gastric tube, feedings are not started until:
   1. the patient requests food.
   2. adequate oxygen levels are achieved on blood gases.
   3. placement of tube is certain.
   4. oral fluids are tolerated.

4. What is the peritoneum?
   1. A two-layer membrane that lines the abdominal cavity and covers the surfaces of the abdominal organs
   2. Organ that secretes fluid containing specialized enzymes into the digestive tract
   3. A gland that produces saliva
   4. The sphincter that keeps food in the stomach until it is properly mixed

5. What is the semiliquid mass that food becomes when churned in the stomach and mixed with gastric secretions?
   1. Peristalsis
   2. Chyme
   3. Amylase
   4. Glycerol

6. TPN feeding tubes should be clearly labeled and a TPN catheter should never be used:
   1. for administering medication.
   2. directly feeding into a large vein.
   3. when a patient's head is elevated.
   4. at a slow rate.

7. What are the three major functions of the digestive tract?
   1. Digestion, absorption, and elimination
   2. Metabolism, glucose regulation, and nutrient absorption
   3. Ingestion, digestion, and elimination
   4. Ingestion, absorption, and elimination

8. Where in the digestive tract does chemical digestion and absorption of nutrients occur?
   1. Through the stomach after the food is converted into chyme
   2. In the large intestine while water is being absorbed from the chyme
   3. Through the villi in the small intestine
   4. Through the rectum right before wastes leave the body

9. Patients with liver disorder have an increased risk for:
   1. decreased production of bile.
   2. inability to absorb fat-soluble vitamins.
   3. toxic effects of drugs.
   4. infections.

10. The function of the pancreas includes: (Select all that apply.)
    1. converting bile into urobilinogen and then into stercobilin.
    2. exocrine function (metabolism).
    3. breaking down fats and protein (gluconeogenesis).
    4. endocrine function (regulation of blood glucose).

11. What is the most serious complication of gastric endoscopy?
    1. Shock
    2. Pulmonary embolism
    3. Infection
    4. Perforation of digestive tract

12. Which statements are true about capsule endoscopy? Select all that apply.
    1. Transmits video images of the entire digestive tract
    2. May detect obscure GI bleeding
    3. Detects inflammation caused by NSAIDs and radiotherapy
    4. Measures HCl and pepsin secreted in the stomach
    5. Patients fast overnight before swallowing the capsule
    6. Detects small bowel tumors

PART III: CHALLENGE YOURSELF!

F. Getting Ready for NCLEX
Choose the most appropriate answer or select all that apply.

1. After a patient has a liver biopsy, a pressure dressing is placed on the puncture wound. How often should the nurse check the wound?
   1. Every 15 minutes for the first hour, every 30 minutes for the next hour, and then hourly or according to agency protocol
   2. Once per shift
   3. Every hour
   4. Every 15 minutes until there is no sign of bleeding

2. The nurse is taking care of a patient who needs TPN. The nurse knows radiography is the most reliable method for determining placement of the tube. However, as this is not practical before each feeding, what is most accurate way to assess tube placement at the bedside?
   1. Listening over the stomach area with a stethoscope while injecting air through the tube
   2. Placing the end of the tube in water to see if bubbles appear
   3. Testing the patient's ability to speak and observing respiratory patterns
   4. Observation of aspirated material and assessment of pH

3. What should the nurse observe when verifying correct tube placement before beginning TPN?
   1. There are bubbles in the water when placing the end of the tube in water.
   2. There are sounds of air moving in the stomach area.
   3. Stomach contents are green, clear, colorless, or brown and pH is less than 5.
   4. Stomach contents are green, clear, colorless, or brown and pH is 6 or higher.

4. A patient has just had a liver biopsy and is showing signs of tachycardia, restlessness, and hypotension. What condition could these signs indicate to the nurse?
   1. Pulmonary embolism
   2. Hemorrhage
   3. Pneumothorax
   4. Perforation of the liver

5. How long does it typically take for food to reach the sigmoid colon?
   1. 6 hours
   2. 4 hours
   3. 12–24 hours
   4. 2.5 hours

6. A nurse is caring for a patient who has had a liver biopsy. The patient complains of dyspnea. What condition could this indicate to the nurse?
   1. Pulmonary embolism
   2. Hemorrhage
   3. Pneumothorax
   4. Perforation of the liver

7. Which diagnostic test detects abnormalities in the large intestine?
   1. Barium swallow
   2. Barium enema
   3. Cholangiography
   4. Small bowel series

Upper Digestive Tract Disorders

chapter

38

Go to http://evolve.elsevier.com/Linton/medsurg/ for additional activities and exercises.

NCLEX CATEGORIES

Safe and Effective Care Environment: Safety and Infection Control

Health Promotion and Maintenance

Physiological Integrity: Basic Care and Comfort, Pharmacological Therapies, Reduction of Risk Potential

PART I: MASTERING THE BASICS

A. Key Terms

Match the definition in the numbered column with the most appropriate term in the lettered column.

1. _____ The forceful expulsion of stomach contents through the mouth
2. _____ Inflammation of the oral mucosa
3. _____ Inflammation of the peritoneum
4. _____ The gentle ejection of food or fluid without nausea or retching
5. _____ Lack of appetite
6. _____ Inflammation of the gums

A. Anorexia
B. Emesis
C. Gingivitis
D. Peritonitis
E. Regurgitation
F. Stomatitis

B. Esophageal Disorders

Match or complete the statements in the numbered column with the most appropriate term in the lettered column. Some terms may be used more than once, and some terms may not be used.

1. _____ Inflammation of the esophagus caused by acidic gastric fluids

2. _____ A feeling of burning and tightness rising from the lower sternum to the throat
3. _____ Hiatal hernia is thought to be caused by weakness in the _____
4. _____ The opening in the diaphragm through which the esophagus passes is the esophageal _____
5. _____ Detects structural abnormalities
6. _____ Procedure that measures the pressures in the stomach and the esophagus
7. _____ The protrusion of the lower esophagus and stomach upward through the diaphragm into the chest
8. _____ A surgical procedure that strengthens the lower esophageal sphincter by suturing the fundus of the stomach around the esophagus and anchoring it below the diaphragm

A. Hiatus
B. Pyloric sphincter
C. Hiatal hernia
D. Esophagoscopy
E. Gastrectomy
F. Esophagitis
G. Heartburn
H. Palpation
I. Stomatitis
J. Heartburn
K. Fundoplication
L. Esophageal manometry
M. Lower esophageal sphincter

Match or complete the statements in the numbered column with the most appropriate term in the lettered column.

9. _____ Removal of all or part of the esophagus and replacement of the resected part with a Dacron graft

10. _____ Replacement of the diseased part of the esophagus with a segment of colon

11. _____ Resection of the diseased part of the esophagus and attachment of the remaining esophagus to the stomach

A. Esophagectomy
B. Esophagogastrostomy
C. Esophagoenterostomy

C. Drug Therapy
Give three examples of types of antisecretory drugs that can be used to treat patients with ulcers, hiatal hernia, and GERD.

1. _____

2. _____

3. _____

D. Common Types of Stomatitis
Match the statements in the numbered column with the most appropriate term in the lettered column.

1. _____ Canker sores

2. _____ Cold sores

3. _____ Thrush

A. Candidiasis
B. Herpes simplex I
C. Aphthous

PART II: PUTTING IT ALL TOGETHER

E. Multiple Choice/Multiple Response
Choose the most appropriate answer or select all that apply.

1. What are the two types of malignant tumors that occur in the mouth?
   1. Erythroleukoplakia and erythroplakia
   2. Leukoplakia and nasopharyngeal cancer
   3. Squamous cell and basal cell carcinoma
   4. Osteoma and fibroma

2. Which herb is effective in calming an upset stomach, reducing flatulence, and preventing motion sickness?
   1. Ginkgo
   2. Ginseng
   3. Ginger root
   4. Garlic

3. What are the signs of a patient being in the last stage of dumping syndrome? Select all that apply.
   1. Occurs 1–3 hours after the episode started
   2. The patient may perspire
   3. Increase in eructation
   4. Patient may feel weak, shaky, anxious, or hungry

4. The patient who is experiencing severe or prolonged vomiting has the potential for:
   1. fluid volume deficit.
   2. inadequate circulation.
   3. hemorrhage.
   4. infection.

5. Sudden, sharp pain starting in the midepigastric region and spreading across the entire abdomen in patients with peptic ulcer may indicate:
   1. infection.
   2. perforation.
   3. dyspnea.
   4. kidney failure.

6. The most prominent symptom of pyloric obstruction is persistent:
   1. eructation.
   2. heartburn.
   3. vomiting.
   4. hemorrhage.

7. What is the cause of most peptic ulcers?
   1. *H. pylori*
   2. *E. coli*
   3. Stress
   4. Infection

8. What are two symptoms of peritonitis?
   1. Shock
   2. Pulmonary embolism
   3. Rigid, tender abdomen
   4. Drawing knees toward chest

9. What is the most serious complication of peptic ulcer?
   1. Infection
   2. Hemorrhage
   3. Shock
   4. Intractable pain

10. Why is the head of the bed elevated 30° at times for patients who have had esophageal stents placed after esophageal cancer surgery?
    1. Prevent hemorrhage
    2. Prevent dumping syndrome
    3. Prevent regurgitation of stomach contents
    4. Prevent hypotension

11. What color will blood in feces be since it has passed through the digestive tract?
    1. Black or maroon
    2. Bright red
    3. Greenish
    4. Pink

12. What are some factors that may increase the risk of gastric cancer? Select all that apply.
    1. *H. pylori* infection
    2. Pernicious anemia
    3. Inflammation caused by NSAIDs
    4. Type A blood
    5. Family history of stomach cancer
    6. Smoking and diet high in starch, salt, pickled foods, salted meats, and nitrates

13. Which describe the first stage of dumping syndrome? Select all that apply.
    1. Occurs 1–3 hours after eating.
    2. Patient experiences abdominal fullness and nausea within 10–20 minutes after eating.
    3. Patient feels flushed and faint.
    4. Symptoms in this stage are probably caused by distention of the small intestine by the consumed food and fluids.
    5. Patient's heart races and patient breaks into a sweat as a result of pooling of blood in the abdominal organs.
    6. Symptoms in this stage are a result of hypoglycemia caused by an exaggerated rise in insulin secretion in response to the rapid delivery of carbohydrates into the intestine.

14. Which patient is most likely to experience decreased cardiac output related to hypovolemia secondary to dumping syndrome?
    1. Patient with abdominal hernia
    2. Patient with anorexia
    3. Patient who has had gastric surgery
    4. Patient with peritonitis

PART III: CHALLENGE YOURSELF!

F. Getting Ready for NCLEX
Choose the most appropriate answer or select all that apply.

1. The nurse is taking care of a patient who is vomiting and is unconscious. The patient has difficulty swallowing and has the potential for aspiration. What is the correct position for this patient?
   1. Lying flat in bed
   2. With head of bed elevated at least 90°
   3. Side-lying
   4. With head of bed slightly elevated; for example, at 30°

2. A patient with hiatal hernia is getting ready to be discharged. The nurse reinforces teaching about how to prevent nighttime reflux. The best sleeping position for this patient is:
   1. side-lying.
   2. with head of bed at 90° angle.
   3. flat.
   4. with head of bed elevated 6–12 inches.

3. What is a complication that some patients experience after completing gastric surgery?
   1. Dumping syndrome
   2. Orthostatic hypotension
   3. Diuresis
   4. Diarrhea

4. Which aspects of care should the nurse teach the patient who experiences dumping syndrome? Select all that apply.
   1. Follow a diet low in fat and protein.
   2. Drink fluids between meals, not with them.
   3. Lie down for about 30 minutes after meals.
   4. Follow a low-carbohydrate diet.
   5. Sleep with head of bed elevated.

G. Nursing Care Plan

Read the following situation and answer questions 1-9. For more information, refer to Nursing Care Plan, The Patient with a Peptic Ulcer in your textbook.

A 47-year-old male patient has recently been diagnosed with duodenal ulcers. He has a history of burning pain 2–3 hours after meals. The pain is located just beneath the sternum and is relieved by antacid agents. He sometimes has nausea but not vomiting. He noticed that his stools have been darker than usual this week. He describes his health as good, but he is being treated for hypertension. He states that he rarely drinks alcoholic beverages, but smokes 1½ packs of cigarettes daily.

Physical examination: BP, 136/82 mm Hg; pulse, 76 bpm; respiration, 16/minute; temperature 97.6°F measured orally. Alert and oriented. Abdomen soft. Bowel sounds present in all four quadrants.

1. What is the primary problem the nurse should address?

2. What are this patient's risk factors for duodenal ulcers?

3. What findings indicate the presence of duodenal ulcers?

4. What diet is this patient on?

5. What are signs and symptoms of bleeding the nurse would be monitoring with this patient? Select all that apply.
   1. Clay-colored stools
   2. Bradycardia
   3. Pallor
   4. Hypotension
   5. Cyanosis

6. If hemorrhage occurs in this patient, what will the nurse do?

7. What is the main symptom of perforation for which the nurse would monitor?

8. What is the main sign of pyloric obstruction for which the nurse would monitor in this patient?

9. What are the basic types of medications for peptic ulcer disease? Select all that apply.
   1. Proton pump inhibitors
   2. H_2 antagonists
   3. Antacids
   4. Anticoagulants
   5. Mucosal barrier agents

H. Next-Generation NCLEX® Examination-Style Questions

A 35-year-old female client is admitted with complaints of tongue irritation and pain in the tongue. The nurse reviews the health history. Upon further inspection, the nurse notes small lip and buccal ulcerations. The client reports a 15-year tobacco history. She states that she drinks 2–3 beers per week. She has been a lifeguard for 10 years and states that she prefers to snack on chips and cookies during the day, rather than eat lunch due to her work schedule.

Health History:
A 35-year-old female client presents with tongue irritation and pain in the tongue. Client has small lip and buccal ulcerations. The client reports a 15-year tobacco history. She states that she drinks 2–3 beers per week. She has been a lifeguard for 10 years and states that she prefers to snack on chips and cookies during the day, rather than eat lunch due to her work schedule.

1. Highlight the risk factors that increase the risk of oral cancers.

A 45-year-old male client presents to his primary care provider with difficulty swallowing. The nurse reviews the physician's progress notes.

Physician's Progress Notes:
A 45-year-old male client presents with difficulty swallowing. He states that he is unable to swallow meats for the past 2 weeks and tries to limit his meals to soft foods and liquids. He states that he sometimes feels like he is choking when eating, so he tries to eat only once per day. He rates his pain 6/10 on a numeric scale when swallowing and states that it radiates to his right ear. Magnetic resonance imaging (MRI) scan reveals esophageal cancer.

2. Complete the following sentence by choosing from the list of options in the menu below.

The priority problems for this client include _____ (1) and _____ (2) .

Priority Problems:
Acute pain
Anxiety
Potential for injury
Inadequate nutrition
Inability to manage self-care

Lower Digestive Tract Disorders

chapter

39

Go to http://evolve.elsevier.com/Linton/medsurg/ for additional activities and exercises.

NCLEX CATEGORIES

Safe and Effective Care Environment:
Coordinated Care, Safety, and Infection Control

Health Promotion and Maintenance

Psychosocial Integrity

Physiological Integrity: Basic Care and Comfort, Pharmacological Therapies, Reduction of Risk Potential, Physiological Adaptation

PART I: MASTERING THE BASICS

A. Key Terms
Match the statement in the numbered column with the most appropriate term in the lettered column.

1. _____ A condition in which the bowel becomes twisted due to intestinal obstruction
2. _____ The presence of excessive fat in the stool due to malabsorption
3. _____ A worm classified as a parasite

A. Helminths
B. Steatorrhea
C. Volvulus

B. Abdominal Hernia Disorders
Complete the statements in the numbered column with the most appropriate term in the lettered column.

1. _____ The repair of the muscle defect in abdominal hernia by suturing
2. _____ A pad placed over the hernia to provide support for weak muscles; for patients who cannot tolerate the stress of surgical hernia repair
3. _____ The bulging portion of the large intestine pushing through weak muscle in the abdominal wall
4. _____ Weak location where hernias occur, in addition to the lower inguinal areas of the abdomen

A. Umbilicus
B. Hernia
C. Truss
D. Herniorrhaphy

C. Intestinal Disorders
Match the statements in the numbered column with the most appropriate term in the lettered column. Some answers may be used more than once or not at all.

1. _____ A genetic abnormality characterized by severe changes in the intestinal mucosa and impaired absorption of most nutrients
2. _____ Caused by an infectious agent and results in the malabsorption of fats, folic acid, and vitamin B_{12}
3. _____ Located in the sacrococcygeal area; appears to result from an infolding of skin causing a sinus that is easily infected because of its closeness to the anus

4. _____   The medical specialty that treats obesity

5. _____   An inflammatory bowel disease in which the inflammation typically begins in the rectum and gradually extends up the bowel toward the cecum

6. _____   A condition in which the large intestine loses the ability to contract effectively enough to propel the fecal mass toward the rectum

7. _____   A laceration between the anal canal and the perianal skin related to constipation, diarrhea, Crohn disease, tuberculosis, leukemia, trauma, or childbirth

8. _____   A complication of diverticulitis in which an abnormal opening develops between the colon and the bladder

9. _____   An inflammatory bowel disease also known as _regional enteritis_; can affect any part of the GI tract

A. Crohn disease
B. Ulcerative colitis
C. Anal fissure
D. Fistula
E. Abdominal pain
F. Bariatric
G. Celiac disease
H. Tropical sprue
I. Megacolon
J. Pilonidal cyst

PART II: PUTTING IT ALL TOGETHER

D. Multiple Choice/Multiple Response

Choose the most appropriate answer or select all that apply.

1. What type of bowel sounds should a nurse expect to hear when auscultating a patient with an intestinal obstruction?
   1. Rapid, high-pitched, tinkling sounds
   2. Clicks and gurgles 5–30 times/minute
   3. Steady, consistent gurgling sounds
   4. No sounds for 1 full minute

2. In addition to monitoring vital signs, what should a nurse watch for that may indicate decreased cardiac output when a patient is being treated for peritonitis? Select all that apply.
   1. Increasing pulse
   2. Restlessness
   3. Kidney failure
   4. Pyloric obstruction
   5. Pallor
   6. Decreasing blood pressure

3. A major complication of appendicitis is:
   1. diarrhea.
   2. constipation.
   3. fluid volume deficit.
   4. peritonitis.

4. The classic symptom of appendicitis is pain at:
   1. McBurney's point.
   2. the xiphoid process.
   3. right hypochondriac region.
   4. inguinal node.

5. When appendicitis is suspected, the patient is allowed:
   1. clear liquids.
   2. full liquids.
   3. nothing by mouth.
   4. soft foods.

6. In addition to a fluid volume deficit, patients with peritonitis may go into shock because of:
   1. edema.
   2. convulsions.
   3. septicemia.
   4. paralysis.

7. Following abdominoperineal resection, a procedure that cleans, soothes, and increases circulation to the perineum is:
   1. use of a TENS unit.
   2. Kegel exercises.
   3. the sitz bath.
   4. débridement.

8. Which natural substance can help control diarrhea?
   1. Garlic
   2. Rice water
   3. Kava kava
   4. _Ephedra sinica_

9. Which type of laxative may not be effective for several days?
    1. Bulk-producing laxative
    2. Intestinal stimulant
    3. Osmotic suppository
    4. Stool softener

10. One of the nutritional goals of therapy for patients with diarrhea is to replace:
    1. potassium.
    2. sodium.
    3. calcium.
    4. fluids.

11. Which is a sign of intestinal rupture in a patient with intestinal obstruction?
    1. Sudden vomiting of blood
    2. Sudden sharp pain
    3. Sudden increased temperature and chills
    4. Sudden diarrhea

12. Which factors may cause constipation in older adults? Select all that apply.
    1. Long-term laxative and enema use
    2. Inactivity
    3. Hyperthyroidism
    4. Drug therapy

13. What are the local complications of inflammatory bowel disease? Select all that apply.
    1. Hemorrhage
    2. Perforation of the bowel
    3. Gastritis
    4. Fistulas
    5. Obstructions
    6. Stomach and peptic ulcers
    7. Abscesses in the anus or rectum

14. Which disorders may result in the patient experiencing a fluid volume deficit? Select all that apply.
    1. Abdominal hernia
    2. Diarrhea
    3. Inflammatory bowel disease
    4. Nausea and vomiting
    5. Gastritis
    6. Peptic ulcer
    7. Stomach cancer

15. A patient has just been admitted to the hospital with appendicitis. What is the primary concern to be addressed for this patient?
    1. Pain related to abdominal cramping and rectal irritation
    2. Potential infection (peritonitis) related to rupture
    3. Fluid volume deficit
    4. Anxiety related to the threat of serious illness

16. Which patient has the greatest potential for injury related to wound dehiscence?
    1. Patient with diverticulosis
    2. Patient with hiatal hernia
    3. Patient with intestinal obstruction
    4. Patient with abdominal hernia repair

17. What is the diet recommended for outpatient acute diarrhea?
    1. Clear liquids
    2. Nothing by mouth
    3. Soft diet
    4. Bland diet

18. A male patient has had an abdominal hernia repair. What is a common complication of this procedure?
    1. Fever
    2. Vomiting
    3. Scrotal swelling
    4. Bradycardia

19. The Roux-en-Y gastric bypass (RNYGBP) and sleeve gastroplasty are restrictive procedures used to treat:
    1. peptic ulcer.
    2. extreme obesity.
    3. stomach cancer.
    4. hiatal hernia.

20. The most common bariatric surgeries are RNYGBP, sleeve gastroplasty, duodenal switch, and gastric banding. What is an alternative to these surgeries?
    1. vBloc Maestro System
    2. Comprehensive daily coaching
    3. Stomach stapling
    4. Obalon Balloon System

PART III: CHALLENGE YOURSELF!

E. Getting Ready for NCLEX

Choose the most appropriate answer or select all that apply.

1. Pain is severe for several postoperative days following abdominoperineal resection. At first, the patient will probably be most comfortable in which position?
   1. Supine
   2. Side-lying
   3. Prone
   4. Fowler

2. The nurse is teaching a patient with moderate inflammatory bowel disease about diet. Which type of diet is appropriate for this patient?
   1. Low-residue diet
   2. High-fiber diet
   3. Low-potassium diet
   4. Low-salt diet

3. The nurse is taking care of a patient with diverticulosis. Which side effect of opiates (such as morphine) result in opiates not being given to this patient?
   1. Respiratory depression
   2. Constipation
   3. Hypersensitivity
   4. Diarrhea

4. A patient has been admitted to the hospital for an abdominal hernia repair and is experiencing signs and symptoms of strangulation. Which are signs and symptoms of strangulation? Select all that apply.
   1. Nausea
   2. Vomiting
   3. Coffee-ground emesis
   4. Pain
   5. Black, tarry stools
   6. Fever
   7. Tachycardia

5. The nurse is teaching a class at a community health clinic on colon cancer. Which are three classical signs of colorectal cancer? Select all that apply.
   1. Blood in stools
   2. Change in bowel habits (diarrhea or constipation)
   3. Steatorrhea
   4. Pencil-like stools
   5. Clay-colored stools
   6. Weight gain
   7. Feeling of fullness or pressure in the abdomen or rectum

6. What patient teaching is necessary after bariatric surgery to support the patient in managing dietary changes? Select all that apply.
   1. Diet should be high in protein and low in fat, carbohydrates, and roughage.
   2. Divide daily food into 4–6 small meals.
   3. Take *Ephedra sinica* supplements as prescribed.
   4. Do not drink liquids with meals.
   5. Excessive fat and sugar may cause diarrhea.
   6. Take dietary supplements as prescribed.

7. Which are risks for the bariatric surgical patient related to limited mobility after surgery? Select all that apply.
   1. Pulmonary emboli
   2. Infection
   3. Hemorrhage
   4. Deep vein thrombosis

F. Next-Generation NCLEX® Examination-Style Questions

A 22-year-old male client admitted with a ruptured appendix presents to the Emergency Department. The nurse reviews the physical assessment and vital signs.

Physical Assessment:
Client complains of pain 8/10 on a numeric scale to umbilicus and right upper quadrant of the abdomen. He states he has been having frequent episodes of nausea and vomiting. Upon palpation of abdomen rebound tenderness and abdominal rigidity and distention observed.

1. Based on the client information provided, which physician orders would the nurse anticipate being prescribed? Select all that apply.
   1. Insert NG tube
   2. 0.9% Normal saline 125 mL/h
   3. Piperacillin/tazobactam (Zosyn) 3.375 g IV q6hr
   4. Morphine 1 mg Q4 hours
   5. Obtain surgical consent
   6. Clear liquid diet
   7. Total parenteral Q24 hours

A 53-year-old female client presents to the Emergency Department with complaints of loose, liquid stools, cramps, abdominal pain rated 6/10 on a numeric pain scale. The nurse reviews the health history and vital signs.

Health History:
Client states that she recently returned from an international trip and began having her symptoms 24 hours ago. She states that she has had six loose stools since returning from her trip and has not eaten solid foods due to fear of diarrhea.

Vital Signs:

Blood Pressure	94/60 mm Hg
Pulse	100 beats/minute
Respirations	20 breaths/minute
Temperature	98.6°F

2. **Complete the following sentence by choosing from the list of options in the menus below.**

   The client is at highest risk for developing

   _____ 1 (Select) related to _____

   2 (Select).

Options for 1	Options for 2
Inadequate nutrition	Fluid loss from diarrhea
Acute pain	Failure to absorb nutrients
Deficient fluid volume	Irritation of diarrhea stool
Potential for disrupted tissue integrity	Abdominal cramping

Liver, Gallbladder, and Pancreatic Disorders

Go to http://evolve.elsevier.com/Linton/medsurg/ for additional activities and exercises.

NCLEX CATEGORIES

Physiological Integrity: Reduction of Risk Potential, Physiological Adaptation

PART I: MASTERING THE BASICS

A. Key Terms
Match the definition in the numbered column with the most appropriate term in the lettered column.

1. _____   Chronic, progressive liver disease
2. _____   The standard care for cholelithiasis; can be performed via laparoscopy or through a right subcostal incision
3. _____   Inflammation of the liver
4. _____   Belching
5. _____   Inflammation of the gallbladder
6. _____   Presence of gallstones in the gallbladder
7. _____   Obstruction in the common bile duct

A. Cholecystectomy
B. Cholecystitis
C. Choledocholithiasis
D. Cholelithiasis
E. Cirrhosis
F. Eructation
G. Hepatitis

B. Types of Hepatitis
Match the statements in the numbered column with the most appropriate term in the lettered column. Some terms may not be used.

1. _____   Caused by a virus known as the *delta agent*, which is a defective ribonucleic acid (RNA) virus that can survive only in the company of HBV. It is transmitted percutaneously (through the skin or mucous membranes) with or following an HBV infection.

2. _____   Similar to hepatitis A and is most commonly transmitted via water or food contaminated with infected fecal matter. It is rare in the United States, except among people who have traveled in developing countries where the virus is more common.

3. _____   Called *infectious hepatitis* and *epidemic hepatitis*. It is caused by a virus that is transmitted from one person to another by way of water, food, or medical equipment that has been contaminated with infected fecal matter. It is the most common type of viral hepatitis.

4. _____   Transmitted by contact with contaminated blood or medical equipment or by contact with infected body fluids. Commonly asymptomatic and undiagnosed.

5. _____   Caused by a virus found in all body fluids of infected persons; modes of transmission include intimate contact with carriers, as well as contact with contaminated blood or medical equipment.

A. Hepatitis A
B. Hepatitis B
C. Hepatitis C
D. Hepatitis D
E. Hepatitis E

C. Phases of Hepatitis

Match the symptoms in the numbered column with the most appropriate term in the lettered column. Some letters may be used more than once.

1. _____ Characterized by jaundice, light- or clay-colored stools, and dark urine. Lasts 2–4 weeks

2. _____ Symptoms include fatigue, malaise, and liver enlargement lasting for weeks-months

3. _____ Common findings are malaise, severe headache, right upper quadrant abdominal pain, anorexia, nausea, vomiting, fever, arthralgia (joint pain), rash, enlarged lymph nodes, urticaria, and enlargement and tenderness of the liver

4. _____ The accumulation of bile salts under the skin may cause pruritus during this phase

5. _____ This phase lasts 1–6 months and is when the patient is most infectious

A. Acute Hepatitis
B. Convalescence

D. Alcohol-Induced Liver Disease

List the three types of liver disease related to alcohol consumption.

1. _____

2. _____

3. _____

E. Cirrhosis

Using Figure 40.1 below, list the seven body systems where clinical manifestations of cirrhosis occur (A–G).

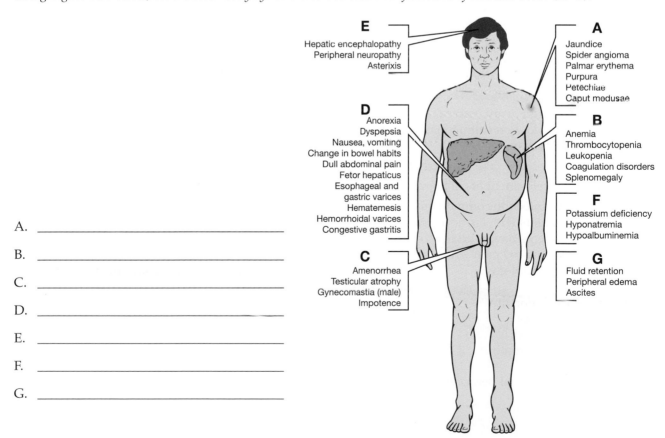

A. _____

B. _____

C. _____

D. _____

E. _____

F. _____

G. _____

Match the definition or description in the numbered column with the most appropriate term in the lettered column. Some terms may be used more than once.

1. _____ Develops as a result of obstruction of bile flow

2. _____ Results from severe right-sided heart failure

3. _____ A complication of hepatitis in which massive liver cell necrosis occurs

4. _____ Liver enlarges, becomes "knobby," and shrinks later; this cirrhosis is not reversible

A. Alcoholic cirrhosis
B. Biliary cirrhosis
C. Cardiac cirrhosis
D. Postnecrotic cirrhosis

Match the effects of cirrhosis complications in the numbered column with the most appropriate complication of cirrhosis in the lettered column. Some terms may be used more than once, and some may not be used.

5. _____ Results in leaking of lymph fluid and albumin-rich fluid from the diseased liver

6. _____ Renal failure following diuretic therapy, paracentesis, or GI hemorrhage

7. _____ Caused by excessive ammonia in the blood, resulting in cognitive disturbances

8. _____ May cause fatal hemorrhage

9. _____ Development of collateral vessels

10. _____ An infection common among patients with cirrhosis; some patients have jaundice, fever, and abdominal pain while others have no symptoms

A. Hepatic encephalopathy
B. Esophageal varices
C. Portal hypertension
D. Hepatorenal syndrome
E. Ascites
F. Spontaneous bacterial peritonitis

PART II: PUTTING IT ALL TOGETHER

F. Multiple Choice/Multiple Response
Choose the most appropriate answer or select all that apply.

1. Patients with liver disease are at increased risk for drug:
   1. incompatibilities.
   2. toxicities (hepatotoxic).
   3. idiosyncrasies.
   4. synthesis.

2. Clay-colored stools are characteristic of:
   1. acute stage of hepatitis.
   2. pancreatitis.
   3. gastritis.
   4. Crohn disease.

3. Which is a symptom common in cirrhosis that is characterized by tingling or numbness in the extremities thought to be caused by vitamin B deficiencies?
   1. Peripheral neuropathy
   2. Hepatic encephalopathy
   3. Portal hypertension
   4. Ascites

4. Patients with hepatitis may have skin breakdown due to:
   1. jaundice.
   2. pruritus and scratching.
   3. nausea and vomiting.
   4. fluid volume deficit.

5. Which drugs may be prescribed for pruritus in patients with hepatitis if conservative methods are not effective?
   1. Antihistamines
   2. Antiemetics
   3. Antibiotics
   4. Analgesics

6. To reduce the risk of heath care-associated infections, health care workers who work with hospitalized patients should receive:
   1. hepatitis B vaccinations.
   2. herpes zoster vaccine.
   3. influenza virus vaccine.
   4. immune globulin.

7. The medical management of ascites aims to promote reabsorption and elimination of the fluid by means of salt restriction and:
   1. antihistamines.
   2. analgesics.
   3. diuretics.
   4. antibiotics.

8. Potential complications of peritoneal-venous shunts used to allow ascitic fluid to drain from the abdomen and return to the bloodstream are tubing obstruction and:
   1. jaundice.
   2. peripheral neuropathy.
   3. pruritus.
   4. hepatic encephalopathy.

9. The patient with cirrhosis is at greater risk for injury or hemorrhage due to impaired:
   1. coagulation.
   2. immunity.
   3. bile production.
   4. breathing patterns.

10. Esophageal balloons are now uncommon. What methods are used to treat acute bleeding episodes for patients with esophageal varices? Select all that apply.
    1. Drug therapy
    2. Sclerotherapy
    3. Cholecystectomy
    4. Endoscopic ligation

11. When the patient's bile duct responds to obstruction from gallstones with spasms in an effort to move the stone, the intense spasmodic pain would be documented as:
    1. ascites pain.
    2. cholelithiasis.
    3. biliary colic.
    4. biliary obstruction.

12. A common symptom of cholecystitis is right-upper quadrant pain that radiates to the:
    1. sternum.
    2. shoulder.
    3. umbilicus.
    4. jaw.

13. When the cholecystectomy patient first returns from surgery, the drainage from the T-tube may be bloody, but it should soon become:
    1. dark amber.
    2. clay-colored.
    3. bright red.
    4. greenish brown.

14. Patients with obstructed bile flow may have a deficiency of vitamin:
    1. A.
    2. C.
    3. D.
    4. K.

15. A patient had an endoscopic sphincterotomy and developed pancreatitis as a complication, caused by accidental entry of the endoscope into the pancreatic duct. Early signs of pancreatitis in this patient would be:
    1. jaundice and confusion.
    2. nausea and vomiting.
    3. ascites and hypertension.
    4. pain and fever.

16. A gland that has both endocrine and exocrine functions is the:
    1. pancreas.
    2. adrenal gland.
    3. thyroid gland.
    4. sebaceous gland.

17. Vitamin K is needed for the production of:
    1. bile.
    2. calcium.
    3. prothrombin.
    4. thyroxine.

18. Specific blood studies used to assess pancreatic function include serum:
    1. bilirubin.
    2. amylase.
    3. prothrombin.
    4. albumin.

19. The most prominent symptom of pancreatitis is:
    1. jaundice.
    2. abdominal pain.
    3. hypertension.
    4. diarrhea.

20. Which is recommended for patients with acute pancreatitis to remove the stimulus for the secretion of pancreatic fluid?
    1. Nothing by mouth
    2. Low-fat diet
    3. Clear-liquid diet
    4. Low-sodium diet

21. Which drugs do patients with chronic pancreatitis need to take to digest food?
    1. Analgesics
    2. Anticholinergics
    3. Antiemetics
    4. Pancreatic enzymes

22. An early sign of shock that may occur in patients with pancreatitis includes:
    1. restlessness.
    2. bradycardia.
    3. hypotension.
    4. easy bruising.

23. The bile channels in the liver are compressed in patients with hepatitis, resulting in elevated:
    1. serum creatinine.
    2. BUN.
    3. serum bilirubin.
    4. hemoglobin.

24. Which cultural group has the highest rate of death from cirrhosis of the liver?
    1. American Indians and Alaska natives
    2. African Americans and Asians
    3. Caucasians
    4. Hispanics

25. The medical treatment of hepatic encephalopathy is directed toward:
    1. raising hemoglobin.
    2. reducing ammonia formation.
    3. decreasing urea.
    4. increasing prothrombin time.

26. Which is a common laboratory finding consistent with hepatitis?
    1. Decreased levels of serum enzymes (AST, ALT, GGT)
    2. Prolonged prothrombin time
    3. High albumin
    4. High gamma globulin

27. Which group of drugs is now being used in the treatment of patients with chronic hepatitis C?
    1. Antimicrobials
    2. Antivirals
    3. Anticoagulants
    4. Anticholinergics

PART III: CHALLENGE YOURSELF!

G. Getting Ready for NCLEX
Choose the most appropriate answer or select all that apply.

1. A patient has just had a liver biopsy. Which are the nursing interventions for this procedure? Select all that apply.
   1. Tell the patient to avoid strenuous activities and heavy lifting for 1–2 weeks and to report fever to the health care provider.
   2. Monitor vital signs and breath sounds.
   3. Keep the patient on the right side for 1–2 hours to maintain pressure on the puncture site.
   4. Place the patient in the semi-Fowler position after the biopsy.

2. What are primary complications the nurse should watch for in a patient with a liver biopsy when monitoring vital signs and breath sounds? Select all that apply.
   1. Hemorrhage
   2. Pneumothorax
   3. Hypertensive crisis
   4. Increased intracranial pressure
   5. Infection

3. The nurse is taking care of a patient with cirrhosis. The nurse recognizes which results of blood tests and procedures are consistent with cirrhosis? Select all that apply.
   1. Elevated serum and urine bilirubin
   2. Decreased serum enzymes
   3. Increased total serum protein
   4. Decreased cholesterol
   5. Prolonged prothrombin time

4. The nurse observes that the patient with cirrhosis is developing hepatic encephalopathy. What neurologic symptoms are caused by a failing liver and excessive ammonia in the blood? Select all that apply.
   1. Cognitive disturbances
   2. Declining level of consciousness
   3. Changes in neuromuscular function
   4. Numbness and tingling in the extremities
   5. Edema in the extremities

5. The nurse is taking care of a patient with hepatitis. The nurse teaches the patient that rest is necessary to allow the liver to heal by:
   1. producing more white blood cells to fight infection.
   2. producing more platelets to assist in clotting.
   3. regenerating new cells to replace damaged cells.
   4. regenerating new blood vessels to replace damaged ones.

6. The nurse should be alert for signs of fluid retention in patients with hepatitis. In addition to increasing abdominal girth and rising blood pressure, the nurse would expect to observe:
   1. dry mucous membranes.
   2. tachycardia.
   3. edema.
   4. concentrated urine.

7. A female patient comes to the community clinic and is diagnosed with hepatitis. This patient may be self-conscious about her appearance because of:
   1. skin rash.
   2. redness.
   3. ulcerations.
   4. jaundice.

8. The nurse is taking care of a patient with cirrhosis who has ascites. The best position to help this patient breathe more easily is:
   1. side-lying.
   2. prone.
   3. supine.
   4. with the head of the bed elevated.

9. The nurse is taking care of a patient with cholecystitis who is experiencing attacks of biliary colic. What type of diet is recommended for this patient to decrease attacks of biliary colic?
   1. Low protein
   2. Low fat
   3. Low carbohydrate
   4. Low salt

10. A patient with pancreatitis is on NPO to restrict oral intake and reduce pancreatic fluid secretion. What kind of diet is provided when oral intake is resumed?
    1. Increased protein
    2. Small frequent meals in a pleasant environment to manage anorexia
    3. A diet high in calories, carbohydrates, and vitamins
    4. Bland, high carbohydrate, and low fat

11. The nurse is teaching the patient about bile duct obstruction. Which are signs of bile duct obstruction that the nurse should emphasize? Select all that apply.
    1. Blood in the stool
    2. Dark urine
    3. Jaundice
    4. Steatorrhea
    5. Ascites

12. As a liver transplant is the only cure for a patient with end-stage liver disease, it is important that the nurse recognizes and monitors the signs of rejection, which include: (Select all that apply.)
    1. fever (sometimes the only sign of rejection).
    2. anorexia and depression.
    3. hemorrhage.
    4. vague abdominal pain.
    5. muscle and joint pain.

H. Nursing Care Plan

Refer to Nursing Care Plan, The Patient with Pancreatitis, in the textbook and answer questions 1–6.

A 57-year-old woman is admitted to the hospital with repeated attacks of severe pain in the upper-left quadrant that radiates to her back. She reports having vomited repeatedly over the past 24 hours. When the pain is severe, she reports feeling flushed, faint, and short of breath. She states that she had a gallbladder attack several months ago that resolved without surgery.

Physical examination: BP 144/84 mm Hg. Pulse 92 bpm. Respiration 24 breaths per minute. Temperature (oral) 100.2°F. Patient appears to be in acute distress, but she is alert and oriented. Abdomen is tender and distended, with hypoactive bowel sounds in all four quadrants.

1. What is the primary problem the nurse should address for this patient?

2. What is a risk factor for this patient?

3. What data was collected about this patient, indicating the presence of pancreatitis?

4. What are causes of pancreatitis? Select all that apply.
   1. Biliary tract disorders
   2. Alcoholism
   3. Peptic ulcer disease
   4. Hyperthyroidism
   5. Smoking

5. Which are common complications of pancreatitis? Select all that apply.
   1. Pseudocyst
   2. Abscess
   3. Hypercalcemia
   4. Renal complications
   5. Confusion

6. After oral intake is resumed, what are the nutritional interventions for patients with pancreatitis to avoid stimulating the pancreas and promote healing? Select all that apply.
   1. Full liquid
   2. Bland
   3. Low carbohydrate
   4. High fat
   5. Small meals

I. Next-Generation NCLEX® Examination-Style Questions

A 54-year-old male client presents to the Emergency Department. The nurse reviews the physician's progress notes and client's medical history.

Physician's Progress Notes:
A 54-year-old male presents with complaints of dull heaviness in the right upper quadrant of the abdomen, loss of appetite, nausea, vomiting, and complaints of tingling in his right lower extremity. The client states that his emesis often is bright red in color. He stated that he last vomited this morning. Findings associated with alcoholic cirrhosis and esophageal varices.

Medical History:
Client's wife states that the client has been drinking 1 bottle of liquor per week and 3 beers per day over the past 20 years.

---

1. **Using the assessment findings from the choices below, fill in each blank in the following sentence.**

   The assessment finding that requires immediate follow-up is _____.

Assessment findings:
Complaints of dull heaviness in the right upper quadrant of the abdomen
Complaints of loss of appetite
Complaints of bright red emesis
Complaints of tingling in the right lower extremity
Reports 20-year drinking history

A 50-year-old woman is admitted to the hospital. The nurse reviews the health history and physical assessment.

> Health History:
> A 50-year-old woman presents with nausea, chills, and right upper quadrant pain that radiates to the shoulder rated 7/10 on a numeric pain scale. She states that the pain typically occurs after meals. The client states that she was diagnosed with gallstones 6 months ago but did not undergo treatment. Results of transabdominal ultrasonography indicate cholelithiasis. Physician recommends a laparoscopic cholecystectomy.
>
> Physical Assessment:
> BP 140/80 mm Hg. Pulse 90 beats/minute. Respirations 22 breaths/minute. Temperature (oral) 101.2°F. Abdomen is tender and distended, with hypoactive bowel sounds in all four quadrants.

2. Which of the following patient teaching instructions will the patient need post-operatively? Select all that apply.
   1. Avoid protein for several weeks.
   2. Remove the dressings and bathe or shower normally the next day.
   3. Notify the physician if redness, drainage, or pus from the incision is noted.
   4. Report severe abdominal pain.
   5. Eat a low-carbohydrate diet for 4–6 weeks.
   6. Avoid heavy lifting for 4–6 weeks.
   7. Sexual intercourse can be resumed when you feel well enough.

Urologic System Introduction

Go to http://evolve.elsevier.com/Linton/medsurg/ for additional activities and exercises.

NCLEX CATEGORIES

Physiological Integrity: Reduction of Risk Potential, Physiological Adaptation

PART I: MASTERING THE BASICS

A. Key Terms
Match the description in the numbered column with the most appropriate term in the lettered column.

1. _____ Noninvasive procedure to break up calculi

2. _____ The absence of urine output

3. _____ Painful urination

4. _____ Involuntary loss of urine with laughing or sneezing

5. _____ Removal of the bladder

6. _____ The concentration of a urine sample to determine the ability of the kidneys to excrete or conserve electrolytes and water

7. _____ The presence of blood in the urine

8. _____ The inability to hold urine when feeling the need to void

9. _____ A large urine output

10. _____ Medications that are harmful to the kidneys

11. _____ A low output of urine

A. Cystectomy
B. Anuria
C. Dysuria
D. Hematuria
E. Lithotripsy
F. Nephrotoxic
G. Oliguria
H. Osmolality
I. Polyuria
J. Stress incontinence
K. Urge incontinence

B. Anatomy and Physiology
In Figure 41.1 from the book below, label the parts (A–G) of the urinary system.

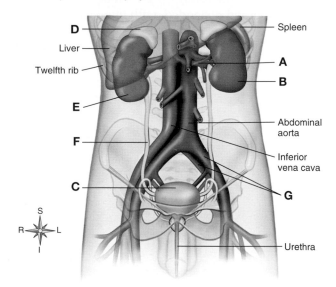

A. _____

B. _____

C. _____

D. _____

E. _____

F. _____

G. _____

Match the description or definition in the numbered column with the most appropriate term in the lettered column. Some terms may be used more than once.

1. _____ Causes reabsorption of water in the renal tubules, decreasing urine volume

2. _____ Released in response to inadequate renal blood flow or low arterial pressure

3. _____ The hormone secreted in the kidneys that stimulates the bone marrow to produce red blood cells

4. _____ The hormone that is released from the pituitary gland and affects the amount of water reabsorbed in the distal tubules and the collecting ducts

A. Erythropoietin
B. Renin
C. Antidiuretic hormone

C. Diagnostic Procedures

Match the statements in the numbered column with the most appropriate term in the lettered column. Some letters may be used twice.

1. _____ A general indicator of the kidneys' ability to excrete urea; values are raised by high-protein diets, gastrointestinal bleeding, dehydration, and some drugs

2. _____ The best laboratory test of overall kidney function

3. _____ Measures the rate of urine flow during voiding

4. _____ Outlines the contour of the bladder and shows reflux of urine

5. _____ Dye is injected IV, radiographs of kidney, ureters, and bladder are taken; used to assess kidney function

6. _____ Examination of voided urine (or from catheter) specimen for pH, blood, glucose, and protein

7. _____ Clean-catch or midstream urine specimen is collected to determine which antibiotics will be effective against the specific organisms found in the culture

8. _____ Collection of urine for 12 or 24 hours, which gives an estimate of the glomerular filtration rate

9. _____ A blood test that is indicative of the kidney's ability to excrete wastes

10. _____ A blood test that may show elevated sodium and potassium levels and decreased calcium levels, which indicate renal failure

A. Blood urea nitrogen (BUN)
B. Creatinine clearance
C. Cystogram
D. Intravenous pyelogram
E. Urodynamic study
F. Serum creatinine
G. Urinalysis
H. Serum electrolytes
I. Urine sensitivity

D. Age-Related Changes

1. Which are true statements about age-related changes in the urinary system? Select all that apply.
   1. The function of kidneys remains normal.
   2. The renal blood flow increases.
   3. The glomerular filtration rate declines.
   4. The antidiuretic hormone's effect on tubules is that the tubules are more responsive.
   5. The kidney's ability to concentrate and dilute urine decreases.
   6. The incidence of nocturia decreases.
   7. Waste removal is slowed.
   8. Incomplete bladder emptying leads to risk of bladder infection.

E. Urine Characteristics

Match the description in the numbered column with the appropriate term in the lettered column. Answers may be used more than once.

1. _____ Bleeding from lower urinary tract
2. _____ Small amounts of blood or bacterial infection
3. _____ Excessive fluid intake
4. _____ Chronic renal failure
5. _____ Normal
6. _____ Bleeding from kidneys
7. _____ Diabetes mellitus

A. Straw- or amber-colored
B. Bright red
C. Dark red or tea-colored
D. Cloudy or hazy appearance
E. Colorless

PART II: PUTTING IT ALL TOGETHER

F. Multiple Choice/Multiple Response

Choose the most appropriate answer or select all that apply.

1. Glomerular filtrate and blood plasma are essentially the same, except that the filtrate does not have:
   1. water.
   2. sodium.
   3. potassium.
   4. proteins.

2. As the blood passes through the glomerulus, which element is too large to pass through the semipermeable membrane?
   1. Serum sodium
   2. Serum potassium
   3. Plasma protein
   4. Glucose

3. The normal pH of urine is:
   1. 1.0–3.0.
   2. 4.6–8.0.
   3. 8.5–10.0.
   4. 10.5–3.0.

4. Two substances that are present in blood but not normally present in urine are:
   1. sodium and chloride.
   2. glucose and protein.
   3. calcium and magnesium.
   4. potassium and bicarbonate.

5. Glomerular damage may be indicated by the presence of what in the urine?
   1. Sodium
   2. Chloride
   3. Protein
   4. Potassium

6. The presence of how much urine in the bladder usually causes the urge to urinate?
   1. 100–150 mL
   2. 250–300 mL
   3. 500–600 mL
   4. 800–1000 mL

7. If blood volume decreases, which enzyme is secreted into the blood by the kidneys to regulate blood pressure?
   1. Aldosterone
   2. Renin
   3. Antidiuretic hormone
   4. Parathormone

8. Decreased oxygen in renal blood triggers the secretion of:
   1. aldosterone.
   2. antidiuretic hormone.
   3. epinephrine.
   4. erythropoietin.

9. A common age-related problem in males related to the urinary system is:
   1. urethral obstruction.
   2. incontinence.
   3. relaxed pelvic musculature.
   4. lack of testosterone.

10. If patients with urinary disorders have an odor of urine on their breath, this may indicate:
    1. urinary tract infection.
    2. renal failure.
    3. cardiac failure.
    4. diabetes mellitus.

11. What is the most serious complication of a renal biopsy?
    1. Blood clot
    2. Pneumonia
    3. Infection
    4. Hemorrhage

12. Following cystoscopy, at first the urine will be:
    1. colorless.
    2. pink-tinged.
    3. tea-colored.
    4. orange.

13. Following cystoscopy, urine should lighten to its usual color within:
    1. 4–6 hours.
    2. 8–10 hours.
    3. 24–48 hours.
    4. 60–72 hours.

14. Following cystoscopy, belladonna and opium suppositories may be prescribed by the health care provider to reduce:
    1. bladder spasms.
    2. hematuria.
    3. infection.
    4. back pain.

15. Bladder perforation is rare following cystoscopy, but it may be indicated by severe:
    1. hematuria.
    2. abdominal pain.
    3. tachycardia.
    4. hypotension.

16. Which procedure is contraindicated in patients with known renal insufficiency or diabetes mellitus?
    1. Intravenous pyelogram (IVP)
    2. Flat plate
    3. Renal scan
    4. Ultrasonography

PART III: CHALLENGE YOURSELF!

G. Getting Ready for NCLEX

Choose the most appropriate answer or select all that apply.

1. A nurse needs to complete an assessment of a patient's urinary function and problems. What should be included in the assessment? Select all that apply.
   1. Reason for seeking medical attention
   2. Preparation for a cystogram
   3. Present health including urination patterns
   4. IV fluids started
   5. Past health history
   6. Family health history
   7. Patient education about low-calcium diet
   8. Review of all body systems
   9. Functional assessment
   10. Administer antibiotics
   11. Physical exam

2. A patient is scheduled for a urine sensitivity culture. Which preparations would the nurse be responsible for? Select all that apply.
   1. Make sure it is the first voided urine of the day.
   2. Bladder palpation to encourage urination.
   3. Teach midstream, clean-catch technique.
   4. Cleanse genitalia.
   5. Collect initial stream of urine in a sterile cup.
   6. Begin antibiotic therapy before collecting urine.
   7. If collecting a specimen by catheterization, discard a small amount of urine before collecting the rest of the specimen.

3. A patient is having an intravenous pyelogram. How long before the test should a patient be placed on nothing by mouth (NPO)?
   1. 24 hours
   2. 8–10 hours
   3. 2 hours
   4. NPO is not necessary before an intravenous pyelogram.

4. What are common therapeutic measures for patients with urologic disorders that the nurse should be familiar with? Select all that apply.
   1. Catheterization
   2. Nephrostomy tube
   3. Standard precautions
   4. Urinary stent
   5. Urinalysis
   6. Pre- and postoperative care following urologic surgery
   7. Inhalation therapy
   8. Drug therapy

5. To measure residual volume, the patient must be catheterized immediately after voiding. Which is an abnormal finding?
   1. 5 mL
   2. 10 mL
   3. 25 mL
   4. 75 mL

6. A 75-year-old female patient has been seen by her health care provider for multiple urinary tract infections in the last year. What is an age-related factor that the nurse should be aware of that may contribute to these infections?
   1. Decline in renal blood flow and glomerular filtration
   2. Incomplete bladder emptying
   3. Nocturia is common
   4. Lack of estrogen after menopause

7. A 45-year-old male patient has been unable to urinate for 6 hours. What is the term the nurse would use to document this symptom?
   1. Dysuria
   2. Hematuria
   3. Oliguria
   4. Anuria

8. When collecting a urine specimen, the nurse notices dark red urine. What condition may this indicate?
   1. Bleeding from the kidney
   2. Bleeding from lower urinary tract
   3. Dehydration
   4. Excessive red meat in the patient's diet

9. A patient has been prescribed Lasix to increase urine output. What intervention should the nurse teach the patient?
   1. To administer at bedtime to avoid the sedative effect
   2. Encourage sodium-rich foods
   3. How to prevent orthostatic hypotension by changing position slowly and avoidance of prolonged standing
   4. Warn the patient to not discontinue the drug suddenly

Urologic Disorders

Go to http://evolve.elsevier.com/Linton/medsurg/ for additional activities and exercises.

NCLEX CATEGORIES

Health Promotion and Maintenance

Physiological Integrity: Pharmacological Therapies, Reduction of Risk Potential, Physiological Adaptation

PART I: MASTERING THE BASICS

A. Key Terms
Match the description in the numbered column with the most appropriate term in the lettered column.

1. _____ Incision of organ or duct to remove calculi

2. _____ The passage of molecules through a semipermeable membrane into a special solution called *dialysate solution*

3. _____ When calcium is lost from bones and is replaced with fibrous tissue

4. _____ The term used when whitish crystals composed of urea and other salts precipitate on the skin

5. _____ The formation of calculi (stones) in the urinary tract; often called *kidney stones*

6. _____ Most are precipitations of calcium salts (calcium oxalate or calciumphosphate), uric acid, magnesium ammonium phosphate (struvite), or cystine

7. _____ Process by which blood is removed from the body and circulated through an artificial kidney

A. Calculus (*plural:* calculi)
B. Dialysis
C. Hemodialysis
D. Lithotomy
E. Osteitis fibrosa
F. Uremic frost
G. Urolithiasis

B. Urinary Tract Inflammations and Infections
Match the statements in the numbered column with the most appropriate term in the lettered column.

1. _____ Inflammation of the urethra

2. _____ Inflammatory disease of the bladder that usually is chronic

3. _____ Inflammation of the urinary bladder

4. _____ Inflammation of the renal pelvis

5. _____ The most common infection associated with health care and caused by viruses, yeasts, and fungi

A. Pyelonephritis
B. Urinary tract infection (UTI)
C. Urethritis
D. Interstitial cystitis
E. Cystitis

C. Renal Disorders
Match the statements in the numbered column with the most appropriate term in the lettered column.

1. _____ Formation of stones in the urinary tract; often called *kidney stones*

2. _____ The term used for the symptoms that develop when chronic kidney disease advances to the point of end-stage renal disease and the kidneys are unable to maintain fluid and electrolyte or acid-base balance

3. _____ Injury that is penetrating or blunt

4. _____ Increased nitrogenous waste products in the blood

5. _____ As kidney function fails, potassium is retained, resulting in this condition, the most life-threatening effect of renal failure

6. _____ An immunologic disease characterized by inflammation of the capillary loops in the glomeruli

7. _____ Malignancies of the kidney or urinary tract

8. _____ Kidney failure that has a sudden onset and may be reversible

9. _____ A hereditary disorder characterized by grapelike cysts in place of normal kidney tissue

10. _____ Any condition that decreases the kidney's ability to function normally, usually with a slow onset (months to years) and is characterized by progressive, irreversible damage

11. _____ Characterized by progressive destruction of the nephrons of both kidneys that results in elevated urine albumin and decreased GFR for 3 or more months

12. _____ When diseased kidney tissue cannot activate vitamin D, and therefore calcium levels are depleted

A. Polycystic kidney disease
B. Glomerulonephritis
C. Renal calculi
D. Kidney failure
E. Azotemia
F. Chronic kidney disease
G. Uremia
H. Urologic trauma
I. Renal or bladder cancer
J. Hyperkalemia
K. Hypocalcemia
L. Acute kidney injury (AKI)

D. Drug Therapy

For the following drugs, indicate whether it is used to treat (A) oliguria or (B) hyperkalemia.

1. _____ Glucose and insulin

2. _____ Furosemide (Lasix)

3. _____ Calcium gluconate

4. _____ Sodium polystyrene sulfonate (Kayexalate)

E. Stages of AKI

Match the statements in the numbered column with the most appropriate term in the lettered column.

1. _____ As renal tissue recovers, serum electrolytes, BUN, and creatinine return to normal, and the glomerular filtration rate returns to 70%–80% of normal.

2. _____ The urine output during this phase decreases to 400 mL/day or less. The serum values for BUN, creatinine, potassium, and phosphorus increase. Serum calcium and bicarbonate decrease. The phase continues between 8 and 14 days.

3. _____ This phase is short, with a duration between hours and days. It is characterized by increasing BUN and serum creatinine with normal to decreased urine output. The primary treatment goal during this stage is reversal of failing renal function to prevent further damage.

4. _____ This phase begins when the cause of AKI is corrected. Urine output exceeds 400 mL/day and may rise above 4 L/day. Despite the production of large quantities of urine, few waste products are excreted, and wastes accumulate in the blood. Toward the end of the phase, the kidneys begin to excrete BUN, creatinine, potassium, and phosphorus and retain calcium and bicarbonate.

A. Initial (onset) phase
B. Oliguric (anuric) phase
C. Diuretic phase
D. Recovery phase

PART II: PUTTING IT ALL TOGETHER

F. Multiple Choice/Multiple Response
Choose the most appropriate answer or select all that apply.

1. When a patient is diagnosed with glomerulonephritis, glomerular permeability increases, allowing what substance to leak into the urine?
   1. Water
   2. Sodium
   3. Potassium
   4. Proteins

2. As urine output decreases due to glomerulonephritis, what color does the urine become?
   1. Straw-colored
   2. Tea-colored
   3. Rosy pink
   4. Dark yellow

3. Which foster development of renal calculi? Select all that apply.
   1. Concentrated urine
   2. Low dietary calcium intake
   3. Altered urine pH
   4. Low intake of vitamin D
   5. Antibiotic use
   6. Sedentary lifestyle

4. If a patient cannot pass a renal calculus spontaneously, what are the possible procedures used to destroy or remove it? Select all that apply.
   1. Percutaneous nephrolithotomy
   2. Dialysis
   3. Lithotripsy
   4. Laproscopic stone removal

5. Long-term management to prevent recurrence of renal calculi includes: (Select all that apply.)
   1. high fluid intake.
   2. limited activity.
   3. dietary restrictions (e.g. animal protein, purines).
   4. urine pH-altering medications.

6. Which are possible causes of AKI? Select all that apply.
   1. Decreased blood flow to the glomeruli
   2. A systolic BP of 70 mm Hg or greater
   3. Kidney infections
   4. Prostate cancer
   5. Nephrotoxic antibiotics
   6. Trauma
   7. Renal insufficiency

7. Which are symptoms of a patient with cystitis? Select all that apply.
   1. Hypertension
   2. Dark, tea-colored, or cloudy urine
   3. Frequency and urgency of urination
   4. Bladder spasms
   5. Low-grade fever

8. What are the signs of hypervolemia (increased blood volume)?
   1. Dementia
   2. Increased respiratory rate
   3. Increased urine volume
   4. Elevated blood pressure and edema

9. Which musculoskeletal changes are characteristic of chronic kidney disease? Select all that apply.
   1. Metastatic calcification
   2. Osteoarthritis
   3. Bone demineralization
   4. Fibromyalgia
   5. Osteitis fibrosa

10. Untreated or recurring UTIs can result in:
    1. enlarged prostate.
    2. seizures.
    3. renal scarring that may lead to renal failure.
    4. diabetes.

11. Patients in renal failure have a deficiency of erythropoietin, which causes them to have:
    1. pneumonia.
    2. anemia.
    3. seizures.
    4. hypertension.

12. Which are common risk factors for UTIs? Select all that apply.
    1. Renal calculi
    2. Incontinence
    3. Female gender
    4. Lack of testosterone
    5. Prolonged immobility
    6. Urinary diversion
    7. Indwelling urinary catheters

13. If crystals on the skin are observed during the examination of patients with urinary disorders, this is recorded as:
    1. ashen skin.
    2. edema.
    3. uremic frost.
    4. scaly skin.

14. Tissue turgor is evaluated in patients with urinary disorders to detect:
    1. uremic frost.
    2. Kussmaul respirations.
    3. infection.
    4. dehydration.

15. Patients with urinary disorders who have potassium imbalances may have:
    1. uremic frost.
    2. cardiac dysrhythmias.
    3. hypertension.
    4. rapid respirations.

16. The edema found in renal failure is described as:
    1. dependent.
    2. peripheral.
    3. pitting.
    4. generalized.

17. In patients with chronic kidney disease, the skin is likely to be described as:
    1. warm and moist.
    2. dry and yellow or pale gray.
    3. pink and intact.
    4. red and flushed.

18. Normally, urine is sterile and slightly:
    1. alkaline.
    2. acidic.
    3. pyuric.
    4. hematuric.

19. A diagnostic test for the identification of microorganisms present in urine is:
    1. BUN.
    2. urinalysis.
    3. urine culture.
    4. creatinine clearance.

20. The most common health care-associated infections are:
    1. skin infections.
    2. wound infections.
    3. UTIs.
    4. blood infections.

21. A patient has urethritis. Which are common symptoms the nurse would expect to find? Select all that apply.
    1. Dysuria
    2. Frequency
    3. Dull flank pain
    4. Hematuria
    5. Bladder spasms
    6. Urgency

22. The pain of urethritis may be reduced by:
    1. antiemetics.
    2. back massage.
    3. sitz baths.
    4. meditation.

23. The passage of renal calculi is facilitated by:
    1. bedrest.
    2. opiates.
    3. restricted fluids.
    4. ambulation.

24. Which is a common symptom of pyelonephritis?
    1. Polyuria
    2. Hypotension
    3. Bradycardia
    4. Flank pain

25. The most common type of glomerulonephritis follows a respiratory tract infection caused by:
    1. staphylococcus.
    2. a virus.
    3. a fungus.
    4. streptococcus.

26. A patient has acute glomerulonephritis. Which medications may be used in the treatment of this patient? Select all that apply.
    1. Diuretics
    2. Antihistamines
    3. Anticholinergics
    4. Antibiotics
    5. Antivirals

27. A patient is in the acute phase of glomerulonephritis. Bedrest is prescribed to prevent or treat heart failure and severe hypertension that result from:
    1. fluid volume deficit.
    2. fluid overload.
    3. potential for inadequate circulation.
    4. inadequate oxygenation.

28. In which group is the incidence of renal calculi high?
    1. Non-Hispanic whites
    2. Asian females
    3. African-American females
    4. Hispanic males

29. A major nursing concern for patients with renal calculi is:
    1. frequent ambulation.
    2. emotional support.
    3. range-of-motion exercises.
    4. pain relief.

30. The treatment of choice for renal cancer is:
    1. lithotripsy.
    2. radical nephrectomy.
    3. cystectomy.
    4. nephrostomy.

31. Which is the most common malignancy of the urinary tract?
    1. Cancer of the kidney
    2. Cervical cancer
    3. Bladder cancer
    4. Liver cancer

32. The most frequent symptom of bladder cancer is intermittent:
    1. glycosuria.
    2. proteinuria.
    3. pyuria.
    4. hematuria.

33. When the bladder is removed completely, urinary diversion is sometimes provided, which allows urine to be excreted through the:
    1. urethra.
    2. ileal conduit.
    3. ureter.
    4. cystoscopy.

34. Which is the most effective means of assessing changes in the fluid status of patients in acute renal failure?
    1. Monitoring edema
    2. Recording intake and output
    3. Weighing daily
    4. Taking vital signs

35. In chronic kidney disease, what percentage of nephrons can be lost before kidney function is impaired?
    1. 80%
    2. 90%–95%
    3. 10%
    4. 50%

36. The most life-threatening effect of renal failure is:
    1. hypernatremia.
    2. hyponatremia.
    3. hyperkalemia.
    4. hypokalemia.

37. Which medication is the transplant recipient given to control the body's response to foreign tissue?
    1. Analgesics
    2. Immunosuppressants
    3. Anticholinergics
    4. Antihistamines

38. Risk factors for bladder cancer include:
    1. obesity.
    2. cigarette smoking.
    3. a high-purine diet.
    4. a sedentary lifestyle.

39. After a nephrectomy, the position of the flank incision causes pain with expansion of which body part?
    1. Lungs
    2. Bladder
    3. Thorax
    4. Diaphragm

PART III: CHALLENGE YOURSELF!

G. Getting Ready for NCLEX

Choose the most appropriate answer or select all that apply.

1. A patient has a UTI. Which are the kinds of drugs that may be used to treat the UTI? Select all that apply.
   1. Antibiotics
   2. Urinary tract antiseptics
   3. Diuretics
   4. Analgesics
   5. Topical estrogen
   6. Antispasmodic agents

2. The eyes of a patient with a urinary disorder are examined and periorbital edema is present. What is the reason for periorbital edema in this patient?
   1. Dehydration
   2. Fluid retention
   3. Uremic frost
   4. Kussmaul respirations

3. A patient with a urinary disorder has dyspnea. The nurse recognizes that this may be a sign of:
   1. dehydration.
   2. uremic frost.
   3. potassium imbalance.
   4. fluid volume excess.

4. A patient is recovering from a streptococcal infection and experiencing decreased urine output that is tea-colored. What urinary condition commonly follows a streptococcal infection?
   1. Glomerulonephritis
   2. UTI
   3. Pyelonephritis
   4. Dyspnea

5. Management of renal disorders requires the nurse to pay attention to: (Select all that apply.)
   1. catheter maintenance.
   2. pain management.
   3. fluid balance.
   4. uremic frost.
   5. decreased activity.
   6. patient education.

6. Following urologic surgery, which output should be reported to the health care provider?
   1. Less than 30 mL/hour
   2. Less than 50 mL/hour
   3. Less than 70 mL/hour
   4. Less than 100 mL/hour

7. An older patient with pyelonephritis experiences a sudden increase in fluid volume. Which complication may develop for which the nurse must monitor?
   1. Hypotension
   2. Congestive heart failure
   3. Seizures
   4. Thrombophlebitis

8. When a patient with renal calculi is discharged, what will the nurse teach about prevention of renal calculi? Select all that apply.
   1. Continue appropriate fluid intake.
   2. Drink most of the fluids during the day to prevent nocturia.
   3. Advise the patient to drink two glasses of water before bed and two glasses when awakening at night.
   4. Watch for signs of heart failure.
   5. Follow a low-calcium diet.

9. A patient has had a nephrectomy and is protecting his chest by not breathing deeply. For which related complication must the nurse monitor?
   1. Hemorrhage
   2. Infection
   3. Pneumonia and atelectasis
   4. Shock

10. Urinary calculi form in the urinary tract and may move spontaneously through the tract by what method?
    1. Antibiotics
    2. Diuretics
    3. Flow of urine
    4. Lithotripsy

11. Which signs of dehydration would the nurse monitor in the patient who has had a renal transplant? Select all that apply.
    1. Thready pulse
    2. Bounding pulse
    3. Poor tissue turgor
    4. Hypertension
    5. Hypotension
    6. High fever

12. Which diet is recommended for patients with chronic kidney disease that will reduce the accumulation of urea? Select all that apply.
    1. High calcium
    2. High carbohydrates
    3. Low fat
    4. Low protein
    5. Low sodium

H. Nursing Care Plan

Refer to Nursing Care Plan, The Patient with Renal Calculi, in the textbook and answer questions 1-4.

A 43-year-old man was admitted to the hospital with excruciating abdominal pain radiating to the groin. He experienced nausea and vomiting with the pain. He has a history of hypertension controlled with captopril. He has had repeated urinary tract infections (UTIs), most recently 1 month ago. His symptoms subsided with antibiotic treatment.

A renal calculus was found in the right ureter. Extracorporeal shock wave lithotripsy (ESWL) was done to shatter the calculus. He returned to his hospital room 3 hours ago, complaining of soreness in his right lower abdomen.

Physical examination: BP 138/74 mm Hg; pulse 88 bpm; respiration 20 per minute; temperature 100° F. No bladder distention. He voided 350 mL of pink-tinged urine. IV fluids are infusing at 150 mL/ hour.

1. What are four abnormal findings on the physical examination for this patient?

2. How does this patient describe his pain after lithotripsy?

3. Which is a factor in this patient's history that fosters the development of calculi?

4. What are the nursing interventions to alleviate pain in this patient? Select all that apply.
    1. Administer analgesics as prescribed.
    2. Strain all urine to collect calculi fragments.
    3. Position changes to enhance analgesia.
    4. Administer antispasmodics as prescribed.
    5. Administer antiemetics as prescribed.
    6. Assess the abdomen and groin area for bruising.

I. Next-Generation NCLEX® Examination-Style Questions

A 30-year-old female client presents to the Emergency Department. The nurse reviews the past medical history physical assessment. The client presents with excruciating flank and abdominal pain that radiates to the groin. She complains of nausea, vomiting, and hematuria. Past medical history includes frequent urinary tract infections (UTIs). Radiologic studies showed a calculus lodged in the left ureter. Vital signs: blood pressure 130/70 mm Hg, pulse 90 beats/min, respiration 18 breaths/min, oral temperature 101°F. She is oriented to time, place, person, and situation. Her abdomen is soft; no bladder distention is noted. She has just voided 250 mL of pink-tinged urine, and reports soreness in her right lower abdomen at a level of "6" on a 1–10 pain scale.

Past Medical History:
The client has history of frequent urinary tract infections (UTIs). Radiologic studies showed a calculus lodged in the left ureter.

Physical Assessment:
The client presents with excruciating flank and abdominal pain that radiates to the groin. She complains of nausea, vomiting, and hematuria. Blood pressure 130/70 mm Hg, pulse 90 beats per minute, respiration 18 breaths per minute, oral temperature 101°F. She is oriented to time, place, person, and situation. Her abdomen is soft; no bladder distention is noted. She has just voided 250 mL of pink-tinged urine, and reports soreness in her right lower abdomen at a level of "6" on a 1–10 pain scale.

---

1. Highlight the assessment findings that indicate renal calculi.

A 63-year-old female client admitted to the surgical unit post L4-L5 spinal fusion is preparing for discharge. When receiving her discharge instructions, she tells the nurse that she has voided three times in the past hour. She states, "It hurts when I try to use the bathroom and it feels like I cannot empty my bladder completely." The discharge nurse reviews the nurse's notes and vital signs.

Nurse's Notes:
4/22/21 1600: The client is oriented to time, place, person, and situation. Preparing for discharge. Assisted to bathroom. Client voided 25 cc dark, tea-colored urine. *J. Hope, RN*

Vital Signs:

Blood Pressure	128/70 mm Hg
Pulse	88 beats/minute
Respirations	18 breaths/minute
Temperature	101°F oral

---

2. Based on the client information provided, which of the following patient teaching instructions does this client need? Select all that apply.
   1. Avoid coffee and tea.
   2. Maintain a high fluid intake.
   3. Empty the bladder twice per shift.
   4. Drink cranberry juice.
   5. Wipe from back to front after voiding.
   6. Stop the antimicrobial therapy once you begin to feel better.
   7. Wear satin undergarments because they keep the perineum drier than synthetic materials.
   8. Avoid tight-fitting clothing in the perineal area.
   9. Take vitamin B12 daily to prevent future infections.

Musculoskeletal System Introduction

Go to http://evolve.elsevier.com/Linton/medsurg/ for additional activities and exercises.

NCLEX CATEGORIES

Safe and Effective Care Environment:
Coordinated Care, Safety and Infection Control

Health Promotion and Maintenance

Psychosocial Integrity

Physiological Integrity: Pharmacological
Therapies

PART I: MASTERING THE BASICS

A. Key Terms

Match the definition in the numbered column with the most appropriate term in the lettered column. Some terms may be used more than once.

1. _____ Instrument used to measure joint range of motion
2. _____ Use when symptoms are not general
3. _____ Crackling sound
4. _____ Listen for when assessing joints
5. _____ Injection type that can be used when one or two joints are affected

A. Intraarticular
B. Crepitus
C. Goniometer

B. Diagnostic Tests

Match the purpose or description in the numbered column with the appropriate diagnostic test in the lettered column. Some tests may not be used.

1. _____ Determines presence of inflammation; increased with rheumatoid arthritis (RA) and decreased with osteoarthritis (OA)

2. _____ Detection of blood dyscrasias; decreased values in RA and systemic lupus erythematosus (SLE)
3. _____ Increased values with infection, tissue necrosis, and inflammation; sometimes decreased values in SLE
4. _____ Determines the presence of antibodies; present in patients with RA
5. _____ Assesses renal function; elevated values in SLE, scleroderma, and polyarteritis
6. _____ Detects active inflammation, as in RA and disseminated lupus erythematosus
7. _____ Measures presence of antibodies that are positive in SLE, RA, SSc, Raynaud phenomenon, and Sjögren syndrome

A. C-reactive protein
B. Rheumatoid factor (RF)
C. Erythrocyte sedimentation rate (ESR)
D. White blood cell count (WBC)
E. Antinuclear antibodies (ANA)
F. Red blood cell count (RBC)
G. Platelet count
H. Creatinine

C. Radiologic Tests

Match the purpose or description in the numbered column with the appropriate radiologic test in the lettered column. Some tests may not be used.

1. _____ Bone scan used to detect bone malignancies, osteoporosis, osteomyelitis, and some fractures
2. _____ Determines density, texture, and alignment of bones; assesses soft tissue involvement

3. _____ Detects tumors and some spinal fractures; instruct the patient that this may be a lengthy procedure

4. _____ Uses contrast medium to show soft-tissue joint structures; prepare the patient for some needle insertion discomfort and temporary swelling

5. _____ Contrast medium injected directly into vertebral disk being examined

6. _____ Sound waves used to determine the presence of pulses in the extremities

7. _____ Visualizes soft tissue; may detect avascular necrosis, disk disease, tumors, osteomyelitis, and torn ligaments

A. Doppler ultrasound
B. Magnetic resonance imaging (MRI)
C. Radiography
D. Discography
E. Nuclear scintigraphy (bone scan)
F. PET
G. Computed tomography (CT) scan
H. Arthrography

D. Drug Therapy

Match the description in the numbered column with the drug classification(s) in the lettered column. Some answers may have more than one drug classification. Some answers may be used more than once.

1. _____ Example is Indocin.

2. _____ Example is methotrexate (Folex).

3. _____ Examples are allopurinol and probenecid.

4. _____ Examples are etanercept (Enbrel) and infliximab (Remicade).

5. _____ Examples are Fosamax, calcitonin (Miacalcin), and raloxifene (Evista).

6. _____ Examples are hydrocortisone and prednisone.

7. _____ Example is celecoxib (Celebrex).

8. _____ Examples are aspirin, naproxen, and ibuprofen.

9. _____ Main side effect is GI bleeding.

10. _____ Indicated for treatment of RA and psoriatic arthritis.

11. _____ A monoclonal antibody that neutralizes activity of tumor necrosis factor, decreasing inflammation. Used to treat RA. Has serious side effects.

12. _____ Drugs that inhibit synthesis of uric acid or increase urinary excretion of uric acid.

13. _____ Antiinflammatory drugs that suppress normal immune response.

14. _____ Adverse effects may include increased risk of stroke and myocardial infarction (MI).

15. _____ Reduces joint destruction and slows disease progression.

A. First-generation nonsteroidal antiinflammatory drugs (NSAIDs)
B. Second-generation nonsteroidal antiinflammatory drugs: COX-2 inhibitors
C. Antigout agents
D. Glucocorticoids
E. Disease-modifying antirheumatic drugs (DMARDs); nonbiologic
F. Biologic response modifiers (BRMs), antiarthritic
G. Bone resorption inhibitors

PART II: PUTTING IT ALL TOGETHER

E. Multiple Choice/Multiple Response

Choose the most appropriate answer or select all that apply.

1. Important changes in the connective tissue of the body that occur with aging include loss of bone strength and bone:
   1. nutrients.
   2. mass.
   3. vitamins.
   4. minerals.

2. Age-related joint changes are related primarily to changes in:
   1. blood volume.
   2. bone strength.
   3. bone mass.
   4. cartilage.

3. When assessing patients for joint pain and range of motion, the nurse watches for signs of pain and listens for the crackling sound called:
   1. bursitis.
   2. grinding.
   3. crepitus.
   4. scraping.

4. Which blood test results would the nurse expect to see increase in patients with RA and decrease in patients with OA?
   1. C-reactive protein
   2. Creatinine
   3. WBC count
   4. ESR

5. Which categories of drugs are used in the treatment of arthritis? Select all that apply.
   1. NSAIDs
   2. Glucocorticoids
   3. DMARDs
   4. Diuretics
   5. Bisphosphonates

6. Often the pain in OA can be controlled with:
   1. beta blockers.
   2. salicylates.
   3. anticholinergics.
   4. opioids.

7. Which antiinflammatory drugs slow the progression of RA?
   1. COX-2 inhibitors
   2. DMARDs
   3. BRMs
   4. Glucocorticoids

8. What functions does the musculoskeletal system support? Select all that apply.
   1. Stores fat
   2. Supports lymphatic system
   3. Provides protection
   4. Prevents infectious disease

9. Match the purpose or description in the numbered column with the musculoskeletal system component in the lettered column.
   1. _____ Stores calcium and other ions
   2. _____ Also called *chondrocytes*
   3. _____ Yellow ones stretch, unlike white ones
   4. _____ Anchors muscle to bones
   5. _____ Classified as fixed, slightly movable, or freely movable

6. _____ Protects both skeletal structure and internal organs

   A. Ligaments
   B. Joints
   C. Bone
   D. Tendons
   E. Skeletal muscle
   F. Cartilage

PART III: CHALLENGE YOURSELF!

F. Getting Ready for NCLEX
Choose the most appropriate answer or select all that apply.

1. Why does the nurse assessing a patient with a musculoskeletal complaint ask the patient about previous sports injuries?
   1. To determine if the patient is or ever has been physically active
   2. To know what types of movement the patient is capable of making
   3. Previous sports injuries can result in OA
   4. Determine whether the musculoskeletal system is intact

2. What are some of the symptoms a patient might present with when seeking medical care related to the musculoskeletal system? Select all that apply.
   1. Febrile in evenings
   2. Stomach cramping when passing stool
   3. Skin rash
   4. Joint swelling
   5. General weakness
   6. Difficulty in performing activities of daily living

3. When examining a patient, what does the nurse look at to help identify insufficient blood supply to an area of concern? Select all that apply.
   1. Color of skin
   2. Temperature of skin
   3. Appetite
   4. Palpation of legs to detect circulatory differences
   5. Skin lesions and drainage
   6. Change in bowel habits, particularly change in color of stool

4. What types of questions would the nurse ask a patient with a musculoskeletal disorder to determine his or her functional status? Write at least three questions in the space below.

5. What is the reason a health care provider might be reluctant to prescribe the second-generation NSAID celecoxib to a patient with OA?
   1. Can increase risk of stomach ulcers
   2. Can impact blood sugar of patients with type II diabetes
   3. Can impair production of RBCs
   4. Can increase risk of myocardial infarction

Connective Tissue Disorders

Go to http://evolve.elsevier.com/Linton/medsurg/ for additional activities and exercises.

NCLEX CATEGORIES

Safe and Effective Care Environment:
Coordinated Care, Safety, and Infection Control

Health Promotion and Maintenance

Psychosocial Integrity

Physiological Integrity: Basic Care and Comfort, Pharmacological Therapies, Reduction of Risk Potential, Physiological Adaptation

PART I: MASTERING THE BASICS

A. Key Terms
Match the definition in the numbered column with the most appropriate term in the lettered column.

1. _____   Elevated level of uric acid in the blood
2. _____   Deposit of sodium urate crystals under the skin
3. _____   Firm, nontender masses that develop on the fingers, elbows, base of the spine, back of the head, sclera, and lungs
4. _____   Total joint replacement
5. _____   Inflammation of blood vessels
6. _____   Joint immobility

A. Hyperuricemia
B. Ankylosis
C. Tophi
D. Vasculitis
E. Rheumatoid nodule
F. Arthroplasty

B. Osteoarthritis and Rheumatoid Arthritis
Match the statement in the numbered column with the most appropriate term in the lettered column. Some terms may be used more than once, and some terms may not be used.

1. _____   The most common form of arthritis, which is also called *degenerative joint disease*
2. _____   The surgical treatment of choice for OA
3. _____   Disorder that breaks down joint cartilage; can be primary or secondary depending on the cause
4. _____   The primary indication for total joint replacement in patients with OA
5. _____   A condition that most frequently affects hands, hips, and knees

A. Total joint replacement
B. Physical therapy
C. Continuous passive motion machine (CPM)
D. Osteoarthritis (OA)
E. Ankylosing spondylitis
F. Intractable pain of joints

Match the statement in the numbered column with the most appropriate term in the lettered column. Some terms may be used more than once, and some terms may not be used.

6. _____   Disorder in which the synovium thickens and fluid accumulates in the joint spaces
7. _____   A loss of joint mobility occurring in rheumatoid arthritis (RA)

8. _____ Disorder in which morning stiffness lasting more than 1 hour is a common symptom

9. _____ Inflammation of blood vessels affected by RA

10. _____ Subcutaneous nodules over bony prominences, which are often present in RA

11. _____ Inflammation of sacs at joints treated by lidocaine injections for temporary relief

12. _____ Compression of the median nerve in the wrist, causing pain and tenderness

13. _____ A chronic, progressive inflammatory disease

A. RA
B. OA
C. Rheumatoid nodules
D. Bursitis
E. Vasculitis
F. Polymyositis
G. Ankylosis
H. Carpal tunnel syndrome

C. Connective Tissue Disorders
Complete the statements in the numbered column with the most appropriate term in the lettered column. Some terms may be used more than once, and some terms may not be used.

1. _____ A disease characterized by dry mouth, dry eyes, and dry vagina

2. _____ A condition in which there is loss of bone mass, making the patient susceptible to fractures

3. _____ A common site of fractures due to osteoporosis, in addition to the wrist and vertebrae

4. _____ A technique for measuring bone mass

5. _____ A systemic disease characterized by the deposition of urate crystals in the joints and other body tissues

6. _____ An excessive rate of uric acid production or decreased uric acid excretion by the kidneys

7. _____ The joint commonly affected by gout

8. _____ Substance not recommended in the diet for patients with gout

A. Absorptiometry
B. Hyperuricemia
C. Purine
D. Hip
E. Systemic lupus erythematosus
F. Sjögren syndrome
G. Osteoporosis
H. Gout
I. Big toe

Complete the statement or match the numbered column with the most appropriate term in the lettered column. Some terms may be used more than once.

9. _____ Decreased elasticity, stenosis, and occlusion of vessels

10. _____ An inflammatory disease that primarily affects the vertebral column, causing spinal deformities

11. _____ The management of the Raynaud phenomenon is aimed at elimination of anything that causes _____

12. _____ Disorder that may be brought into remission with high doses of immunosuppressants or steroids

13. _____ A condition characterized by inflammation and damage to blood vessels caused by rheumatoid arthritis

14. _____ A condition characterized by degeneration of articular cartilage

15. _____ Symptom of polymyositis

16. _____ A chronic multisystem disease that is named for the characteristic hardening of the skin

A. Muscle weakness
B. OA
C. Vasculitis
D. Scleroderma
E. Progressive systemic sclerosis (scleroderma)
F. Ankylosing spondylitis
G. Vasospasm
H. Dermatomyositis
I. Polymyositis

PART II: PUTTING IT ALL TOGETHER

D. Multiple Choice/Multiple Response
Choose the most appropriate answer or select all that apply.

1. When a patient complains of oral and genital ulcers and large-joint arthritis, which disease may be suspected as the cause?
   1. Sjögren syndrome
   2. Gout
   3. Behçet syndrome
   4. Periarteritis nodosa

2. Which types of drugs are usually given to a patient diagnosed with polymyalgia rheumatica?
   1. Corticosteroids
   2. NSAIDs
   3. DMARDs
   4. Lidocaine injections

3. A patient who has recently been treated for *Chlamydia trachomatis* currently has arthritis, urethritis, and conjunctivitis. What connective tissue disease is suspected?
   1. Sjögren syndrome
   2. Reiter syndrome
   3. Behçet syndrome
   4. Periarteritis nodosa

4. What response should a nurse give to a patient asking whether there is a cure for her rheumatoid arthritis?
   1. The nurse should not respond to questions regarding potential cures as every case is different.
   2. The nurse should assure the patient that her health care provider is doing everything possible to cure the disease.
   3. The nurse should indicate that it is up to the patient to lose enough weight to change her outcome.
   4. The nurse should inform the patient that RA is a chronic disease, but with medicine and therapy it can be kept under control.

5. Which is a patient problem that patients with OA often may have related to pain and limited range of motion?
   1. Inadequate coping
   2. Impaired self-concept
   3. Inadequate circulation
   4. Mobility

6. A patient has had knee replacement surgery. Which are interventions that reduce the risk of deep vein thrombosis? Select all that apply.
   1. Antiembolic stockings
   2. Pneumatic compression devices
   3. Anticoagulants
   4. Placement of pillows under legs
   5. Exercises to flex and extend the toes, feet, and ankles hourly

7. A patient who has had hip surgery is showing signs of cerebral blood vessel occlusion, headache, confusion, and loss of consciousness. The nurse will monitor this patient for:
   1. deep vein thrombosis.
   2. hemorrhage.
   3. fat embolus.
   4. neuropathy.

8. How should the nurse document the manifestation of pressure caused by edema or constrictive dressings following joint replacement surgery that is causing nerve damage?
   1. Paresthesia
   2. Infection
   3. Positive Homan sign
   4. Hemorrhage

9. Which drugs are administered to patients with joint replacements who are at risk for infection?
   1. Antihistamines
   2. Antimicrobials
   3. Antiemetics
   4. Anticoagulants

10. Which factor promotes bone formation and improves strength, balance, and reaction time (reducing the risk of falls and fractures)?
    1. Vitamin D
    2. Increased fluid intake
    3. Regular exercise
    4. Protein

11. Patients with gout may have altered urinary elimination related to:
    1. dehydration.
    2. restricted fluid intake.
    3. kidney stones.
    4. edema.

12. To prevent the complication of kidney stones in patients with gout, patients are advised to:
    1. protect affected joints from trauma.
    2. keep walking pathways lighted and free from obstacles.
    3. obtain assistance with activities of daily living.
    4. drink at least eight glasses of fluid daily.

13. When a patient is taking NSAIDs for RA, the nurse monitors the patient for:
    1. fatigue.
    2. edema.
    3. bruising.
    4. infection.

14. Which are symptoms of RA? Select all that apply.
    1. Fatigue
    2. Morning stiffness lasting more than 1 hour
    3. Muscle aches
    4. Increased temperature
    5. Hypotension
    6. Tingling in extremities

PART III: CHALLENGE YOURSELF!

E. Getting Ready for NCLEX

Choose the most appropriate answer or select all that apply.

1. When mobility is severely impaired following hip replacement surgery, which are complications for which the patient is at risk? Select all that apply.
   1. Contractures
   2. Pulmonary and circulatory complications
   3. Urinary retention
   4. Constipation
   5. Hemorrhage
   6. Skin breakdown

2. Which patient problems are common in patients with gout? Select all that apply.
   1. Pain related to joint inflammation
   2. Pain related to swelling and tenderness
   3. Potential for trauma related to loss of bone strength
   4. Potential injury related to improper alignment
   5. Pain with motion related to loss of smooth joint surfaces
   6. Impaired fluid balance related to urate kidney stones

3. The nurse is taking care of an 80-year-old patient with RA. This patient is exhibiting symptoms of salicylate toxicity. A symptom for which the nurse is monitoring in this patient is:
   1. drowsiness.
   2. confusion.
   3. malaise.
   4. hypotension.

4. The nurse is taking care of a 75-year-old female patient with poor hip mobility. The nurse plans to promote independence and safety for this patient when she goes home. What should the nurse include in discharge teaching? Select all that apply.
   1. Bathroom grab bars
   2. Seat in the shower
   3. Antiembolic stockings
   4. Raised toilet seat
   5. Use of sterile technique

5. A patient has had a total joint replacement. Which patient problem is related to improper alignment, dislocated prosthesis, and weakness?
   1. Inadequate circulation
   2. Potential injury
   3. Potential infection
   4. Inadequate self-care

6. A patient with uncontrolled pain is reluctant to participate in rehabilitation measures following total joint replacement surgery. Which intervention may improve patient participation?
   1. Assess nerve and circulatory status before exercises.
   2. Check vital signs at least every 4 hours.
   3. Assist the patient in and out of bed.
   4. Administer analgesics 30 minutes to 1 hour before exercises.

7. Prosthetic joints can become dislocated if they are not maintained in proper alignment. After hip replacement surgery, the affected leg must be kept in a position of:
   1. abduction.
   2. adduction.
   3. slight elevation.
   4. supination.

8. A patient has had a knee replacement. Body areas distal to the operative joint are monitored for circulatory adequacy by assessing warmth, color, and:
    1. peripheral pulses.
    2. ulceration.
    3. skin necrosis.
    4. wound drainage.

9. The nurse is assisting with teaching a class about rehabilitation for patients with joint replacements. The nurse emphasizes in the class that pillows and pads should not be placed under the legs of patients with joint replacements to reduce the risk of:
    1. ulceration.
    2. gangrene.
    3. deep vein thrombosis.
    4. infection.

10. After joint replacement, the patient often has inadequate circulation and is at risk for:
    1. headache.
    2. hemorrhage.
    3. seizure.
    4. pneumonia.

11. If the nurse suspects that a dressing is too tight and is causing nerve damage, the nurse monitors sensations:
    1. at the wound site.
    2. proximal to the joint.
    3. distal to the joint.
    4. within the joint.

12. A nursing intervention related to the patient's potential for infection is that the nurse will:
    1. place the call light in easy reach.
    2. instruct patient to keep legs slightly abducted.
    3. use strict sterile technique for dressing changes.
    4. assess nerve and circulatory status.

13. In a community health clinic, the nurse is teaching a class for patients with RA. The nurse explains that a measure to control morning pain and stiffness in patients with RA is to:
    1. take a warm shower.
    2. increase intake of fluids.
    3. eat foods low in purines.
    4. apply ice.

14. The nurse is taking care of a patient with gout who has come to the community health clinic. The nurse recognizes that an important teaching point for patients taking antigout medications is to:
    1. increase potassium intake.
    2. avoid foods high in vitamin K.
    3. rise slowly from a sitting position.
    4. increase fluids.

15. A patient with gout asks the nurse whether there are any food restrictions. Which food should be avoided in patients with acute gout?
    1. Sardines
    2. Aged cheese
    3. Bananas
    4. Orange juice

F. Nursing Care Plan

Refer to Nursing Care Plan, The Patient with a Total Hip Replacement, in the book and answer questions 1–4.

A 74-year-old homemaker has had OA for 10 years, with progressive loss of function in both legs. She had a total hip replacement 2 days ago.

1. What are the four priority problems for which this patient is at risk?

    1. _____

    2. _____

    3. _____

    4. _____

2. What are this patient's risk factors related to OA that resulted in the need for total hip replacement surgery?

    1. _____

    2. _____

3. What are three interventions related to prevention of injury concerning dislocation for this patient?

    1. _____

    2. _____

    3. _____

4. What tasks for this patient could be assigned to unlicensed assistive personnel?

   1. _____

   2. _____

   3. _____

   4. _____

   5. _____

G. Next-Generation NCLEX® Examination-Style Questions

A 54-year-old male client is admitted to the surgical unit post right total knee arthroplasty related to osteoarthritis. The nurse reviews the client's past medical history and physical assessment.

Past Medical History:
Osteoarthritis of both knees
Rheumatoid arthritis
Plantar fasciitis

Physical Assessment:
The client has an ace bandage covering the right knee incision. The dressing is clean, dry, and intact. The client rates his right knee pain 6/10 on a numeric pain scale. The client has firm, nontender masses on his fingers and bilateral elbows. He rates the pain in his fingers and elbows 5/10 on a numeric scale with movement. In the mornings he complains of morning stiffness that lasts approximately 2 hours and swelling of the joints in the upper and lower extremities.

1. Click to specify which assessment finding is most likely associated with each of the listed client's health problems. Some findings may be consistent with more than one condition.

Assessment Finding	Osteoarthritis (OA)	Rheumatoid Arthritis (RA)
Acute Pain		
Swelling of joints		
Firm, nontender nodules		
Morning stiffness lasting approximately 2 hours		

A 64-year-old female is admitted to the surgical unit post left total hip arthroplasty. The nurse reviews the physical assessment and vital signs.

Physical Assessment:
The client rates her left hip pain 8/10 on a numeric pain scale. Her surgical dressing has a dime-sized amount of serosanguineous drainage. The physician has instructed the nursing staff to continue to monitor the site. The client states, "I just want to lay in bed. I need to rest." The client denies numbness or tingling to bilateral lower extremities. She has antiembolic stockings to her bilateral lower extremities.

Vital Signs:

Blood Pressure	172/84 mm Hg
Pulse	90 beats/minute
Respirations	22 breaths/minute
Temperature	99°F

2. The assessment finding that requires immediate follow-up is _____.

   Assessment Findings:
   Blood pressure 172/84 mm Hg
   Respirations 22 breaths/minute
   Pulse 90 beats/minute
   Temperature 99°F
   Dime-sized amount of serosanguineous drainage
   Left hip pain rated 8/10

Fractures

Go to http://evolve.elsevier.com/Linton/medsurg/ for additional activities and exercises.

NCLEX CATEGORIES

Safe and Effective Care Environment:
Coordinated Care, Safety, and Infection Control

Health Promotion and Maintenance

Psychosocial Integrity

Physiological Integrity: Basic Care and Comfort, Pharmacological Therapies, Reduction of Risk Potential, Physiological Adaptation

PART I: MASTERING THE BASICS

A. Key Terms
Match the definition in the numbered column with the most appropriate term in the lettered column.

1. _____ Fracture in which the fragments of the broken bone break through the skin

2. _____ Fracture in which the break extends across the entire bone, dividing it into two separate pieces

3. _____ Fracture in which the bone breaks only partially across, leaving some portion of the bone intact

4. _____ Fracture caused by either sudden force or prolonged stress

5. _____ Break or disruption in the continuity of a bone

6. _____ Fracture in which the bone is broken or crushed into small pieces

7. _____ Fracture in which the bone is broken on one side but only bent on the other; most common in children

A. Incomplete fracture
B. Fracture

C. Complete fracture
D. Stress fracture
E. Open or compound fracture
F. Comminuted fracture
G. Greenstick fracture

B. Complications and Medical Treatment
Match the definition in the numbered column with the most appropriate term in the lettered column.

1. _____ Condition in which fat globules are released from the marrow of the broken bone into the bloodstream, migrate to the lungs, and cause pulmonary edema

2. _____ Serious complication of a fracture caused by internal or external pressure on the affected area, resulting in decreased blood flow, pain, and tissue damage

3. _____ Failure of a fracture to heal

4. _____ Procedure done during the open reduction surgical procedure to attach the fragments of the broken bone together when reduction alone is not feasible

5. _____ Process of bringing the ends of the broken bone into proper alignment

6. _____ Nonsurgical realignment of the bones to their previous anatomic position; may be done before using traction, angulation, rotation, or a combination of these

7. _____ Surgical procedure in which an incision is made at the fracture site, usually on patients with open (compound) or comminuted fractures, to clean the area of fragments and debris

8. _____   Process in which immature bone cells are gradually replaced by mature bone cells

9. _____   Healing of fracture does not occur in the normally expected time

10. _____   Unsatisfactory alignment of bone; results in external deformity and dysfunction

A. Compartment syndrome
B. Open reduction
C. Fixation
D. Delayed union
E. Nonunion
F. Bone remodeling
G. Closed reduction or manipulation
H. Fat embolism
I. Reduction
J. Malunion

C. Casts

Refer to Table 45.1 in your book. Complete the statements in the numbered column with the most appropriate term in the lettered column. Some terms may be used more than once.

1. _____   A cast used for breaks in the forearm, elbow, or humerus

2. _____   A cast used for fracture of the distal femur, knee, or lower leg

3. _____   A cast that encircles the trunk; used for stable spine injuries of the thoracic or lumbar spine

4. _____   A cast that encases the trunk plus two extremities; used for fractures of the femur, acetabulum, or pelvis

5. _____   Used for fractures of the foot, ankle, or distal tibia or fibula

6. _____   Used for injury to the knee or knee dislocation

7. _____   Used for fracture of the hand or wrist

A. Body jacket cast
B. Short arm cast
C. Short leg cast
D. Bilateral long leg hip spica cast
E. Long leg cast
F. Long arm cast

D. Traction

In Figure 45.8 from the book, label each type of traction (A–E) using the following list.

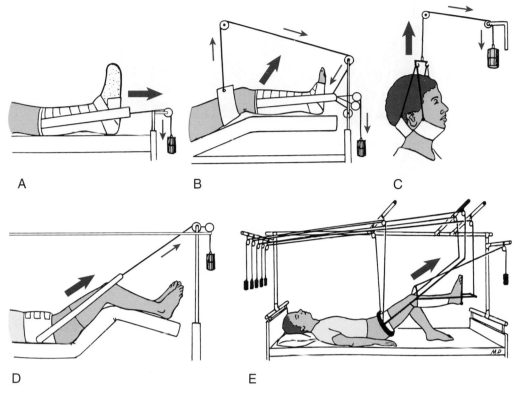

A   B   C

D   E

1. _____ Head halter traction
2. _____ Pelvic traction
3. _____ Russell traction

4. _____ Buck traction
5. _____ Balanced suspension traction

Match the statements in the numbered column with the most appropriate term in the lettered column. Some terms may be used more than once.

6. _____ A pulling force on a fractured extremity to provide alignment of the broken bone fragments
7. _____ Traction applied directly to a bone
8. _____ Traction applied directly to the skin
9. _____ A type of skeletal traction used for immobilization of fractures of the cervical vertebrae
10. _____ A type of skin traction used for hip and knee contractures, muscle spasms, and alignment of hip fractures
11. _____ A type of skeletal traction in which tongs are inserted into either side of the skull

A. Skin traction
B. Buck traction
C. Crutchfield traction
D. Skeletal traction
E. Traction

12. What are the purposes of traction? Select all that apply.
    1. Prevent or correct deformity
    2. Decrease muscle spasm
    3. Promote rest
    4. Clean the area of fragments and debris
    5. Use of rods, pins, and metal plates to align bone fragments and keep them in place for healing
    6. Maintain the position of the diseased or injured part

E. Fracture Healing

Place the stages of fracture healing in the correct order. Refer to Figure 45.3 in the book.

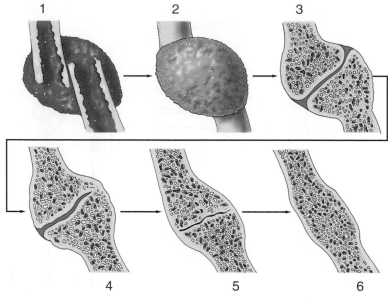

A. _____   Granulation tissue

B. _____   Consolidation and bone remodeling

C. _____   Callus formation

D. _____   Osteoblastic proliferation; ossification

E. _____   Hematoma formation

F. _____   Bone healing completed

F. Signs and Symptoms of Fracture

Match the cause of the signs and symptoms of fracture in the numbered column with the most appropriate sign or symptom in the lettered column.

1. _____   Strong muscle pull may cause bone fragments to override

2. _____   Edema may appear rapidly from localization of serous fluid at the fracture site and extravasation of blood into adjacent tissues

3. _____   Caused by subcutaneous bleeding

4. _____   Involuntary muscle contraction near the fracture

5. _____   Occurs over fracture site due to underlying injuries

6. _____   Severe at the time of injury; following injury, this symptom may result from muscle spasm or damage to adjacent structures

7. _____   Results from nerve damage

8. _____   Grating sensations or sounds felt or heard if the injured part is moved; results from broken bone ends rubbing together

9. _____   Results from blood loss or other injuries

A. Muscle spasm
B. Crepitus
C. Pain
D. Hypovolemic shock
E. Swelling
F. Impaired sensation (numbness)
G. Bruising (ecchymosis)
H. Deformity
I. Tenderness

G. Types of Fractures

1. *In Figure 45.2 from the book, label each type of fracture (A–L) with numbers from the following list.*

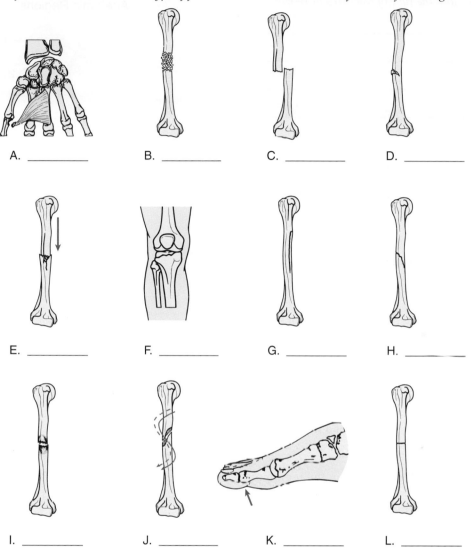

A. _____ B. _____ C. _____ D. _____

E. _____ F. _____ G. _____ H. _____

I. _____ J. _____ K. _____ L. _____

1. Greenstick	7. Comminuted (fragmented)
2. Oblique	8. Interarticular
3. Transverse	9. Spiral
4. Displaced	10. Avulsion
5. Longitudinal	11. Impacted
6. Stress	12. Pathologic

2. Which type of fracture is caused by a tumor in the bone?

3. Which type of fracture occurs most frequently in children?

4. Which type of fracture is often related to a sports injury, such as track?

H. Hip Fractures

Using Figure 45.1 on this page, label the anatomic regions in A, 1–2 and the type of fractures in B–E.

A. 1. _____

    2. _____

B. _____

C. _____

D. _____

E. _____

1. Where do most hip fractures occur? Select all that apply.
   1. Femoral head
   2. Femoral neck
   3. Intertrochanteric region
   4. Subtrochanteric region
   5. Intracapsular region

2. What percentage of women by the age of 90 have sustained a hip fracture?
   1. 10%
   2. 20%
   3. 30%
   4. 40%

3. What are signs and symptoms of a hip fracture? Select all that apply.
   1. History of a fall
   2. Severe pain and tenderness in the region of the fracture site
   3. Bleeding at the fracture site
   4. Internal rotation of the hip on the affected side
   5. Compartment syndrome

4. What is the standard treatment for hip fractures? Select all that apply.
   1. Traction
   2. External fixation
   3. Femoral head replacement
   4. Total hip replacement
   5. Increased calcium intake

Anatomic Regions

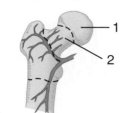

A

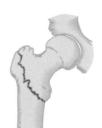

B

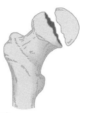

C

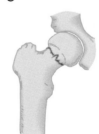

D

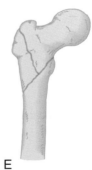

E

PART II: PUTTING IT ALL TOGETHER

I. Multiple Choice/Multiple Response
Choose the most appropriate answer or select all that apply.

1. In adults, the bones most commonly fractured are:
    1. femurs.
    2. ribs.
    3. pelvic bones.
    4. wrists.

2. In young and middle-aged adults, the most common fractures are those of the:
    1. femur.
    2. rib.
    3. wrist.
    4. pelvis.

3. The most common fractures in older adults are fractures of the wrist and:
    1. femur.
    2. rib.
    3. hip.
    4. shoulder.

4. Which is a characteristic of fat embolism following a fracture?
    1. Bradycardia
    2. Decreased respirations
    3. Oliguria
    4. Petechiae

5. The most common diagnostic test used to reveal bone disruption, deformity, or malignancy following a fracture is:
    1. myelography.
    2. standard radiography.
    3. ultrasonography.
    4. bone scan.

6. The use of rods, pins, nails, screws, or metal plates to align bone fragments is called:
    1. external fixation.
    2. closed reduction.
    3. internal fixation.
    4. mechanical reduction.

7. Which are used for external fixation of extensive fractures and fractures of the extremities?
    1. External frames
    2. Rods
    3. Pins
    4. External metal plates

8. What is a condition caused by compression of a portion of the duodenum between the superior mesenteric artery and the aorta and vertebral column?
    1. Compartment syndrome
    2. Cardiac shock
    3. Cast syndrome
    4. Fat embolus

9. Following total hip replacement, which patient teaching is contraindicated?
    1. Do not extend the affected hip more than 90°.
    2. Use an elevated toilet seat.
    3. Sit in supportive chairs.
    4. Avoid crossing the legs.

10. Crutch use may not be appropriate for older or frail patients because it requires good:
    1. lower extremity function.
    2. cardiac function.
    3. lung expansion.
    4. upper body strength.

11. When walking with crutches, patients should put their weight on the:
    1. top of the crutches.
    2. hand grips.
    3. lower extremities.
    4. shoulders.

12. The type of gait pattern used with bilateral lower extremity prostheses is called:
    1. four-point.
    2. swing-to.
    3. swing-through.
    4. two-point.

13. When a patient is climbing stairs using crutches, which body part goes up the step first while the body is supported by the crutches?
    1. Unaffected leg
    2. Affected leg
    3. Upper extremities
    4. Spine

14. Which gait is used with a walker?
    1. Two-point
    2. Four-point
    3. Modified swing-to
    4. Modified swing-through

15. Canes should be held close to the body on the:
    1. left side.
    2. right side.
    3. affected side.
    4. unaffected side.

16. When the nurse is assessing the patient with a fracture, the affected extremity is compared with the:
    1. proximal body parts.
    2. distal body parts.
    3. unaffected extremity.
    4. normal skeleton.

17. To assess circulation and sensation in the affected and unaffected extremity, the nurse should perform neurovascular checks in the areas:
    1. distal to the wound.
    2. proximal to the wound.
    3. surrounding the wound.
    4. inside the wound.

18. A good indication of circulation to the extremity in patients with a fracture is:
    1. size of the wound.
    2. edema.
    3. skin color.
    4. infection.

19. If pallor is observed in the extremity of patients with fractures, this may be an indication of:
    1. infection.
    2. poor circulation.
    3. hemorrhage.
    4. skin breakdown.

20. The primary method of pain relief for patients with fractures is:
    1. application of cold to the affected part.
    2. application of heat to the affected part.
    3. wrapping the affected part with a blanket.
    4. immobilization of the affected part.

21. An appropriate intervention for patients with fractures who have impaired mobility is:
    1. strict aseptic technique.
    2. monitor for fever.
    3. isolation precautions.
    4. gait training.

22. Patients with fractures have a potential for skin breakdown; treatment measures such as casts or traction to immobilize parts may result in:
    1. pressure sores.
    2. petechiae.
    3. palmar erythema.
    4. paralysis.

23. For older patients with hip fractures, the treatment of choice is:
    1. immobilization.
    2. antibiotic therapy.
    3. surgical repair.
    4. traction.

24. Colles fracture is a break in the distal:
    1. humerus.
    2. tibia.
    3. radius.
    4. fibula.

25. Colles fractures frequently occur in older adults when they use their hands to:
    1. sew or knit.
    2. break a fall.
    3. write letters.
    4. reach for objects above their heads.

26. Interventions for Colles fractures are aimed at relieving pain and preventing edema; for the first few days, the extremity should be:
    1. below the heart.
    2. exercised.
    3. elevated.
    4. flat.

27. Patients with Colles fractures are encouraged to move their fingers and thumb to promote circulation and reduce:
    1. temperature.
    2. swelling.
    3. infection.
    4. dyspnea.

28. Patients with Colles fractures are encouraged to move their shoulders to prevent:
    1. infection.
    2. circulation.
    3. cyanosis.
    4. stiffness.

29. The most common cause of pelvic fractures in young adults is:
    1. head injury.
    2. motor vehicle accidents.
    3. falls.
    4. myocardial infarction.

30. The main cause of pelvic fractures in older adults is:
    1. motor vehicle accidents.
    2. head injury.
    3. falls.
    4. heart attacks.

31. The nurse needs to observe the patient with a pelvic fracture closely for signs of:
    1. internal trauma.
    2. bone infection.
    3. kidney failure.
    4. dyspnea.

32. What is the primary reason for taking extreme care when handling patients with a pelvic facture?
    1. Prevent increased pain
    2. Prevent additional breaks
    3. Prevent nausea
    4. Prevent displacement of fracture fragments

33. Which are short-term complications of a fracture that the nurse should monitor during the first 3 days postsurgery? Select all that apply.
    1. Deep vein thrombosis
    2. Fat embolism
    3. Delayed union
    4. Joint stiffness and contractures
    5. Compartment syndrome
    6. Shock

34. Which are common causes of osteomyelitis associated with fractures? Select all that apply.
    1. Indwelling hardware used to repair the bone
    2. Wound contamination
    3. Fat embolism
    4. Compartment syndrome
    5. Joint contractures

PART III: CHALLENGE YOURSELF!

J. Getting Ready for NCLEX

Choose the most appropriate answer.

1. The nurse is taking care of a patient with a lumbar spine fracture. Which is the proper positioning for this patient?
   1. Before medical treatment, keep patient supine and immobilize patient's neck; after treatment, turn with head well-supported.
   2. Avoid high sitting positions; log-roll.
   3. When fracture is stable or after fixation, turn to side opposite fracture.
   4. Elevate head of bed to comfort; turn to side opposite fracture.

2. An appropriate intervention for patients with fractures who have inadequate circulation is:
   1. strict aseptic technique.
   2. gait training.
   3. elevation of the affected part above the heart.
   4. rest periods to preserve strength.

3. The nurse is taking care of a patient with a fracture of the femur. The nurse observes that the patient has a low-grade fever and is beginning to be short of breath. The nurse recognizes that this patient has which complication?
   1. Fat embolism
   2. Compartment syndrome
   3. Pneumonia
   4. Osteomyelitis

4. If the nurse suspects that the patient with a hip fracture is developing a fat embolism, what is the priority nursing action?
   1. Turn the patient on the right side.
   2. Raise the head of the bed 45°.
   3. Take the vital signs.
   4. Contact the health care provider immediately.

5. The nurse is presenting an in-service program about the care of older patients with hip fractures. Which problem is particular to older patients?
   1. Skin breakdown
   2. Pain
   3. Delirium
   4. Impaired circulation

K. Nursing Care Plan

Refer to Nursing Care Plan, The Patient with a Fracture, in the book and answer questions 1–3.

An 80-year-old woman was admitted to the hospital for a Colles fracture in the left wrist 2 days ago. She lived alone, cared for herself, and was active, alert, and independent. Since the fracture repair, she has reported some pain over the area of the break, with no signs of infection. She is ready to be discharged to her home.

Physical examination: BP 165/95 mm Hg; pulse 98 bpm; respiration 20 per minute; temperature 97.4°F. Needs assistance with activities of daily living (ADLs), especially bathing, dressing, and toileting. Cast on left arm from above her elbow to her fingers.

1. What is the priority patient problem for this patient?

2. What are risk factors for this patient to have a fracture?

3. What tasks can be assigned to unlicensed assistive personnel?

L. Next-Generation NCLEX® Examination-Style Questions

A 25-year-old male client admitted with a left radius fracture has a short arm cast in place. The nurse reviews the physical assessment.

During the nurse's initial nursing assessment, the client is tearful and states, "The cast is too tight. It hurts so bad." He rates the pain to his left arm a 10/10 on a numeric scale. Upon further assessment, the nurse notes edema, pallor, and weakness to the left arm. The client complains of numbness and tingling.

> Physical Assessment:
> The client is tearful and states, "The cast is too tight. It hurts so bad." He rates the pain to his left arm a 10/10 on a numeric scale. Observed edema, pallor, and weakness to the left arm. The client complains of numbness and tingling.

1. Complete the diagram by dragging from the choices below to specify one potential condition the client is most likely experiencing, two actions the nurse would take to address that condition, and two parameters the nurse would monitor to assess the client's progress.

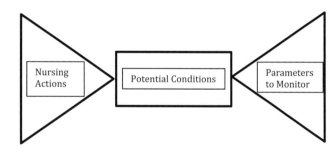

Actions to Take	Potential Conditions	Parameters to Monitor
Obtain an x-ray	Infection	Oxygen saturation
Notify the physician	Compartment syndrome	Point of care glucose level
Obtain supplies for cast removal	Fat embolism	Pain level
Administer oxygen 2 L/min NC	Shock	Neurological status
Insert a peripheral IV	Contracture	Bowel patterns

A 26-year-old female client presents to the Emergency Department with swelling, bruising, and pain to the right wrist. The nurse reviews the physician's progress notes and vital signs.

Physician's Progress Notes:
A 26-year-old female client presents with swelling, bruising, and pain to the right wrist. She states that she fell during her morning workout and heard a "crackling" sound, followed by pain when she landed on her wrist. She rates the pain to her wrist an 8/10 on a numeric pain scale. X-ray reveals fracture of the right wrist. Recommend application of a short arm plaster cast.

Vital Signs:

Blood Pressure	160/76 mm Hg
Pulse	92 beats/minute
Respirations	22 breaths/minute
Temperature	98.7°F

2. Which of the following patient teaching instructions will this client need related to cast care? Select all that apply.
   1. You may wash the cast daily to remove debris
   2. Do not remove any padding
   3. Do not insert any foreign object inside the cast.
   4. Do not cover the cast with plastic for prolonged periods
   5. If swelling and discoloration of fingers occurs, apply ice to the site
   6. Report burning or tingling under the cast
   7. You may remove the cast with blunt scissors when the pain has subsided

Amputations

Go to http://evolve.elsevier.com/Linton/medsurg/ for additional activities and exercises.

NCLEX CATEGORIES

Safe and Effective Care Environment:
Coordinated Care, Safety, and Infection Control

Health Promotion and Maintenance

Psychosocial Integrity

Physiological Integrity: Basic Care and Comfort, Pharmacological Therapies, Reduction of Risk Potential, Physiological Adaptation

PART I: MASTERING THE BASICS

A. Key Terms

Match the definition in the numbered column with the most appropriate term in the lettered column. Some terms may be used more than once.

1. _____ Type of amputation in which a limb or portion of a limb is severed from the body and the wound is left open; a type of open amputation

2. _____ Amputation in which the severed bone is uncovered by skin flap until the infection is resolved

3. _____ Performed to create a weight-bearing residual limb or stump

4. _____ Individual who has undergone an amputation

5. _____ Death of tissue due to inadequate blood supply and bacterial destruction

6. _____ Deformity or absence of a limb or limbs occurring during fetal development in the uterus

7. _____ The sensation that a limb still exists following amputation of the limb

8. _____ Amputation in which the wound is left open; usually done in cases of gangrene or trauma

9. _____ Partial limb remaining after amputation

10. _____ Another term for residual limb

11. _____ Removal of a limb, part of a limb, or an organ; may be done by surgical means or may be the result of an accident

12. _____ Surgical reattachment of a limb to its original site

A. Phantom limb
B. Amputee
C. Guillotine amputation
D. Staged amputation
E. Gangrene
F. Open amputation
G. Replantation
H. Closed amputation
I. Congenital amputation
J. Amputation
K. Residual limb
L. Stump

B. Indications for Amputation

1. Which are diseases leading to impaired circulation that may result in the need for an amputation? Select all that apply.
   1. Osteoporosis
   2. Peripheral vascular disease
   3. Diabetes mellitus
   4. Arteriosclerosis
   5. Osteoarthritis

C. Types of Amputations

Match or complete the statement in the numbered column with the most appropriate term in the lettered column.

1. _____ The removal of the lower leg at the middle of the shin

2. _____ Removal of part or all of a limb during a serious accident

3. _____ In addition to trauma and disease, a condition that leads to the need for an amputation

4. _____ An amputation through the joint

A. Tumors
B. Traumatic amputation
C. Disarticulation
D. Below-knee amputation

D. Complications

Match the description in the numbered column with the most appropriate term in the lettered column.

1. _____ Swelling due to discomfort or positioning

2. _____ Invasion of tissue by pathogens at the residual limb site

3. _____ Caused by inadequate blood supply and bacterial destruction

4. _____ Bleeding into tissue in and around the residual limb due to inadequate hemostasis

5. _____ Flexion of joints with loss of range of motion

6. _____ Opening of suture line because of early removal of sutures or trauma

7. _____ Tissue destruction and death because of ongoing disease

8. _____ Caused by scar formation on nerve fibers

A. Hematoma and hemorrhage
B. Necrosis
C. Wound dehiscence
D. Gangrene
E. Edema
F. Contracture
G. Pain
H. Infection

PART II: PUTTING IT ALL TOGETHER

E. Multiple Choice/Multiple Response

Choose the most appropriate answer or select all that apply.

1. Replantation surgery is most likely to be performed on the:
   1. shoulder.
   2. hand.
   3. forearm.
   4. upper arm.

2. The purpose of giving heparin to a postoperative replantation patient is to reduce the risk of:
   1. thrombosis.
   2. edema.
   3. infection.
   4. hypersensitivity.

3. A complication of amputation due to inadequate hemostasis is:
   1. necrosis.
   2. hemorrhage.
   3. gangrene.
   4. contracture.

4. A complication of amputation manifested by redness, warmth, swelling, and exudate formation at the residual limb site due to invasion of tissues by pathogens is called:
   1. contracture.
   2. infection.
   3. edema.
   4. necrosis.

5. Which may be prevented by frequent position changes and range-of-motion exercises?
   1. Infection
   2. Hemorrhage
   3. Necrosis
   4. Contractures

6. Which is an opening of the suture line (caused by early removal of sutures or falling) that requires reclosure?
   1. Gangrene
   2. Necrosis
   3. Wound dehiscence
   4. Contracture

7. Which person is most likely to request that an amputated body part be present for burial?
   1. Roman Catholic
   2. Mormon
   3. Orthodox Jew
   4. Muslim

8. Which patient problem is a priority in the postoperative period for a patient after surgical amputation?
   1. Altered body image
   2. Loss of protective barrier: skin
   3. Pain
   4. Potential infection

9. Which treatment for venous congestion of a replanted limb utilizes the saliva of parasites to extract excess blood?
   1. Anticoagulants
   2. Vasodilators
   3. Leeches
   4. Local anesthetics

10. What complication can occur if pillows are placed continuously under a below-knee amputation?
    1. Infection
    2. Necrosis
    3. Phantom limb sensation
    4. Hip contractures

11. Which complications are associated with amputations? Select all that apply.
    1. Urinary retention
    2. Hemorrhage and hematoma
    3. Wound dehiscence
    4. Gangrene
    5. Hyperglycemia
    6. Contracture
    7. Infection
    8. Constipation
    9. Pulmonary complications
    10. Necrosis
    11. Phantom limb sensation
    12. Phantom limb pain

12. What are signs that indicate the medical emergency of inadequate arterial circulation following replantation? Select all that apply.
    1. No peripheral pulse
    2. Warm skin
    3. Pallor
    4. Slow capillary refill
    5. Excessive swelling

13. Which medications may be helpful for phantom limb pain? Select all that apply.
    1. Beta blockers
    2. Anticonvulsants
    3. Antidepressants
    4. Benzodiazepines
    5. Opioids
    6. NSAIDs

14. Which are reasons for doing an open amputation instead of a closed amputation? Select all that apply.
    1. To create a weight-bearing residual limb
    2. When an actual or potential infection exists
    3. Done in the case of gangrene or trauma
    4. For nonweight-bearing residual limb amputations
    5. For surgical reattachment of parts

15. Which are complementary therapies that are used with analgesics to control pain in patients after surgical amputation? Select all that apply.
    1. Imagery
    2. Relaxation
    3. Aerobic exercises
    4. Meditation
    5. Acupuncture

16. A patient has an amputation with no complications. How soon after surgery can this patient bear full weight on a permanent prosthesis?
    1. 1 month
    2. 3 months
    3. 6 months
    4. 1 year

17. What accounts for the majority of lower extremity amputations?
    1. Vascular diseases
    2. Trauma
    3. Tumors
    4. Bone diseases

PART III: CHALLENGE YOURSELF!

F. Getting Ready for NCLEX

Choose the most appropriate answer or select all that apply.

1. A patient had a lower extremity amputation in the hospital. The nurse is providing instruction for residual limb and prosthesis care when the patient is getting ready to be discharged. Which statements are true regarding patient instruction for residual limb and prosthesis care? Select all that apply.
   1. Wash the residual limb with soap and water every night. Rinse and dry the skin thoroughly.
   2. Do not expose the residual limb to air.
   3. Keep the prosthetic socket and residual limb sock clean. Use a clean sock every day.
   4. Lotions, ointments, and powders may be applied once a day.
   5. If redness or irritation develops on the residual limb, discontinue use of prosthesis and have area checked.
   6. The residual limb may shrink in size for up to 2 years after surgery. Annual visits to the prosthetist are recommended.

2. The nurse is taking care of a postoperative patient who has an amputation. What is the indication that this patient would experience desire for enhanced self-care?
   1. Surgical incision, scar formation on a severed nerve
   2. Surgical disruption of skin integrity
   3. Expressed need to function independently after loss of limb
   4. Perceived threat of disability

3. A patient had an above-knee amputation 1 week ago. Which nursing interventions related to impaired mobility are indicated for this patient to prevent contractures? Select all that apply.
   1. Active and passive range-of-motion exercises
   2. Check temperature; watch for foul or unpleasant odor from stump
   3. Use of overbed trapeze
   4. Whirlpool, massage, or transcutaneous electrical nerve stimulation (TENS) if prescribed
   5. Wrap bandage smoothly; elevate residual limb
   6. Avoid prolonged flexion of the hip

4. The nurse is taking care of a postoperative patient following amputation. Which are appropriate outcome criteria for this patient? Select all that apply.
   1. Patient accepts limb loss; demonstrates proper care of residual limb.
   2. Bright-red bleeding is expected at first in Hemovac, followed by reddish-brown drainage.
   3. Patient carries out daily activities without excessive fatigue.
   4. Treatment for phantom limb pain includes diversional activities and TENS.
   5. Reinforce dressing, apply pressure, and elevate residual limb.

5. A 75-year-old man with diabetes has had an amputation. Which are nursing interventions that are appropriate for this patient? Select all that apply.
   1. Emphasize a high-calorie and high-protein diet.
   2. Skip unnecessary details when teaching.
   3. Provide a prosthesis with extra padding and support to patients with diabetes.
   4. Recognize that poor vision and decreased sensation may keep older people from recognizing complications.
   5. Explain that phantom pain is a serious complication that should be reported to the health care provider.

6. The nurse is taking care of a patient with a replanted limb. Which are nursing measures that promote circulation to the replanted limb? Select all that apply.
   1. Elevate limb above the level of the heart.
   2. Avoid caffeine for 7–10 days postoperatively.
   3. Enforce no smoking.
   4. Maintain room temperature at 80°F to prevent vasoconstriction.
   5. Wear loose clothing.

G. Nursing Care Plan

Refer to Nursing Care Plan, The Patient with an Upper Extremity Amputation, in the book, and answer questions 1–4.

A 32-year-old man sustained an injury in an industrial accident that required amputation of his right forearm just below the elbow. The patient's right hand was his dominant hand. He has had no other serious physical injuries or illnesses. He is a machinist who is a senior employee in his department. He is married and is the father of three children. His wife is a homemaker who has never worked outside the home. Physical examination: BP 126/68, pulse 80, respiration 16 breaths/min, oral temperature 98.2°F. Alert. A bulky dressing is in place on the residual limb of the right arm; dressing is dry and intact. A Jackson-Pratt drain is in place and the receptacle contains about 30 mL of sanguineous fluid. The client has IV fluids infusing into a 20 gauge peripheral IV located in his left arm. Up in a chair for breakfast. Uses left arm for self-feeding. Expresses intent to remain independent.

1. What is the priority problem for this patient?

2. What were risk factors that led to this patient's need for an upper extremity amputation?

3. What is the most common reason for upper extremity amputations?
   1. Congenital defects
   2. Tumors
   3. Disease
   4. Trauma

4. Name three tasks that can be assigned to unlicensed assistive personnel.

H. Next-Generation NCLEX® Examination-Style Questions

A 65-year-old male client is admitted to the surgical unit post right below-the-knee amputation. The nurse reviews the health history, physical assessment, and vital signs.

Health History:
Diabetes
Hypertension

Physical Assessment:
There is blood draining around the right lower extremitiy surgical dressing and under the patient. Foul odor observed. The client states, "Is it supposed to smell like that?" The client rates the pain to the right lower extremity 8/10 on a numeric pain scale.

Vital Signs:

Blood Pressure	186/88 mm Hg
Pulse	88 beats/minute
Respirations	20 breaths/minute
Temperature	102°F

1. Highlight the assessment findings that require immediate follow-up by the nurse.

A 55-year-old female client with a history of diabetes mellitus type 1 presents to the Emergency Department with complaints of loss of sensation to her right foot. The nurse reviews the physician's progress notes.

Physician's Progress Notes:
A 55-year-old female client with a history of diabetes mellitus type 1 presents with complaints of loss of sensation to her right foot. She states, "It started as severe pain that came on suddenly, followed by a feeling of numbness." Blisters on the sole of the client's right foot with a foul-smelling discharge observed. The client's skin appears pale and feels cool to the touch. Recommend right lower extremity amputation. The client appears tearful and anxious, stating "My life will never be the same!"

2. **Complete the following sentence by choosing from the lists of options.**

   Based on the client's response, the priority

   patient problems include _____ and

   _____.

Patient Problems:
Activity intolerance
Anxiety
Acute pain
Anticipatory grief
Impaired physical mobility

Endocrine System Introduction

Go to http://evolve.elsevier.com/Linton/medsurg/ for additional activities and exercises.

NCLEX CATEGORIES

Safe and Effective Care Environment:
Coordinated Care, Safety and Infection Control

Health Promotion and Maintenance

Psychosocial Integrity

Physiological Integrity: Basic Care and Comfort, Pharmacological Therapies, Reduction of Risk Potential, Physiological Adaptation

PART I: MASTERING THE BASICS

A. Key Terms
Match the definition in the numbered column with the most appropriate term in the lettered column.

1. _____ Part of the system that creates, stores, and secretes hormones that are delivered to tissues through the bloodstream

2. _____ Type of hormone secreted by the adrenal cortex and involved in the regulation of fluid and electrolyte levels in the body

3. _____ Class of hormones produced by the zona reticularis and zona fasciculata; the most abundant and potent is cortisol

4. _____ Chemical (dopamine, epinephrine, norepinephrine) released at sympathetic nerve endings in response to stress

5. _____ Hormones produced by the ovaries and adrenal glands in females that are responsible for the development and maturation of females

6. _____ Hormones produced by the adrenal cortex and testes that stimulate the development of male characteristics

7. _____ Also known as epinephrine; produced by the medulla and along with norepinephrine helps maintain homeostasis

8. _____ When the face is tapped over the facial nerve, the facial muscle spasms

9. _____ Bulging of the eyes

10. _____ Carpopedal spasm occurring when BP cuff is inflated above the patient's BP and left in place for several minutes

A. Adrenaline
B. Androgens
C. Catecholamines
D. Chvostek sign
E. Endocrine gland
F. Estrogens
G. Exophthalmos
H. Glucocorticoids
I. Mineralocorticoids
J. Trousseau sign

B. Pituitary and Adrenal Hormones

Match the definition or description in the numbered column with the most appropriate term in the lettered column. Some terms may be used more than once, and some may not be used.

1. _____ Stimulates the growth and development of bone, muscles, or organs

2. _____ Controls ovulation or egg release in the female and testosterone production in the male

3. _____ Controls the release of glucocorticoids and adrenal androgens

4. _____ Stimulates the development of eggs in the ovary of the female and the production of sperm in the testes of the male

5. _____ Another name for the somatotropic hormone

6. _____ Stimulates breast milk production in the female

7. _____ Promotes pigmentation

8. _____ Another name for the lactogenic hormone

9. _____ Causes the reabsorption of water from the renal tubules of the kidney

10. _____ Causes contractions of the uterus in labor and the release of breast milk

11. _____ Another name for vasopressin

12. _____ Controls the secretory activities of the thyroid gland

A. Luteinizing hormone
B. Thyroid-stimulating hormone
C. Oxytocin
D. Melanocyte-stimulating hormone
E. Growth hormone
F. Antidiuretic hormone
G. Adrenocorticotropic hormone (ACTH)
H. Prolactin
I. Follicle-stimulating hormone

C. Diagnostic Tests

Match the description in the numbered column with the name of the procedure in the lettered column. Some terms may be used more than once.

1. _____ Used to detect diabetes mellitus.

2. _____ Material from thyroid nodules is aspirated, guided by ultrasonography.

3. _____ Provides high-quality images of thyroid and any nodules.

4. _____ Used to diagnose adrenal hyperfunction and its cause.

5. _____ An elevated T_3 serum level indicates Graves' disease.

6. _____ Assesses response of the pituitary to thyroid-releasing hormone (TRH); differentiates types of hypothyroidism.

7. _____ Uses radiographs to create images of internal structures and detect tumors.

8. _____ After radioactive iodine is given and the amount of iodine taken up is measured, a high uptake indicates hyperthyroidism.

9. _____ After iodine isotope is given, a scanner detects the pattern of uptake by the thyroid gland.

10. _____ Elevated T_4 serum levels indicate hyperthyroidism.

A. Cerebral computed tomography scan
B. Glucose tolerance test
C. Dexamethasone suppression tests
D. Radioactive iodine uptake test
E. Thyroid scan
F. Thyroid ultrasonography
G. Serum T_3 and T_4 measurements
H. Fine needle aspiration biopsy
I. TRH stimulation test

D. Endocrine System

Using Figure 47.1 from the book, label the organs of the endocrine system (A–G).

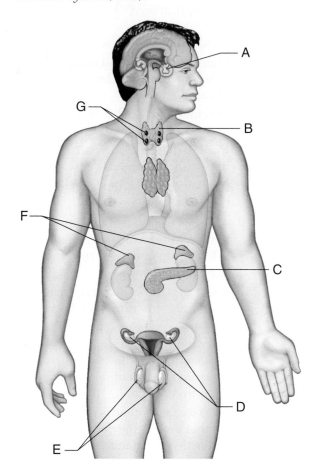

A. _____

B. _____

C. _____

D. _____

E. _____

F. _____

G. _____

PART II: PUTTING IT ALL TOGETHER

E. Multiple Choice/Multiple Response

Choose the most appropriate answer or select all that apply.

1. One drug commonly prescribed for patients with acromegaly is:
   1. octreotide (Sandostatin).
   2. furosemide (Lasix).
   3. levothyroxine (Synthroid).
   4. digoxin.

2. If there is a lack of melanocyte-stimulating hormone, the skin exhibits decreased:
   1. sensory perception.
   2. immunity.
   3. pigmentation.
   4. thermoregulation.

3. In postmenopausal women, the primary source of endogenous estrogen is the:
   1. hypothalamus.
   2. thyroid gland.
   3. adrenal cortex.
   4. ovarian follicle.

4. Which of the following describes the function of the adrenal glands in older persons?
   1. Increased response to ADH
   2. Function remains adequate
   3. At risk for fluid volume excess
   4. Decreased aldosterone levels

5. Which of the following is secreted when serum calcium levels are high to limit the shift of calcium from the bones into the blood?
   1. Calcitonin
   2. Thyroxine
   3. Thymine
   4. Phosphorus

6. Results of two tests that are indicative of hypocalcemia are:
   1. positive Chvostek and Trousseau signs.
   2. increased blood urea nitrogen and potassium levels.
   3. increased WBC and decreased RBC levels.
   4. increased phosphorus and decreased iodine levels.

7. Which drug stains the teeth and should be sipped through a straw?
   1. Calcium salts
   2. Saturated solution of potassium iodide (SSKI)
   3. Levothyroxine (Synthroid)
   4. Propylthiouracil

8. Thyroxine (T_4), triiodothyronine (T_3), and calcitonin are hormones produced by the:
   1. adrenal gland.
   2. thymus gland.
   3. thyroid gland.
   4. parathyroid gland.

9. Which drug is used to treat hypothyroidism?
   1. SSKI
   2. Synthroid
   3. Methimazole (Tapazole)
   4. Lugol's solution

F. Matching
Match the description in the numbered column with the drug classification in the lettered column. Answers may be used more than once.

1. _____ Used to treat hyperthyroidism by interfering with synthesis of thyroid hormones

2. _____ Concentrates in thyroid tissue for diagnostic scans

3. _____ Treat hypothyroidism and thyroiditis (increases the metabolic rate)

4. _____ Reduces the size and vascularity of thyroid gland in hyperthyroidism

5. _____ Prevents vitamin D deficiency

6. _____ Used with vitamin D to treat hypoparathyroidism

7. _____ Increases the metabolic rate

A. Thyroid hormone replacement drugs
B. Antithyroid drugs
C. Iodides
D. Radioactive iodine
E. Calcium salts
F. Vitamin D

Match the descriptions of drugs used for adrenal disorders in the numbered column with the drug classification in the lettered column. Answers may be used more than once.

8. _____ Used to suppress adrenocortical function

9. _____ Stimulate reabsorption of sodium and excretion of potassium and hydrogen ions

10. _____ Stimulate the formation of glucose and promote the storage of glucose as glycogen

11. _____ Used to treat adrenal insufficiency

12. _____ Example of this category is Florinef

13. _____ Example of this category is dexamethasone (e.g., Decadron)

A. Glucocorticoids
B. Mineralocorticoids
C. Adrenocortical cytotoxic agents

PART III: CHALLENGE YOURSELF!

G. Getting Ready for NCLEX
Choose the most appropriate answer or select all that apply.

1. Which functions are related to hormones? Select all that apply.
   1. Reproduction
   2. Fluid and electrolyte balance
   3. Regulate blood pressure
   4. Response to CNS activity
   5. Energy metabolism

2. What is the most abundant and potent hormone of the glucocorticoids?
   1. Epinephrine
   2. Aldosterone
   3. Cortisol
   4. Catecholamine

3. Which of the following applies to the thyroid gland? Select all that apply.
    1. Increases protein catabolism
    2. Regulates growth and development
    3. Maintains intravascular volume in shock states
    4. Stimulated by TSH
    5. Increases body's metabolic rate
    6. Regulates serum calcium level

4. What changes may occur in older adults when homeostasis is impacted by illness? Select all that apply.
    1. Diminished response to ADH
    2. Increased protein synthesis
    3. Decreased cortisol metabolism
    4. Hypothyroidism risk is diminished
    5. Reduced immune function

5. What is a simple test used to elicit Chvostek sign?
    1. Palpate skin texture and turgor
    2. Test reflexes for slowness
    3. Inflate over a patient's systolic BP and leave in place for 2–3 minutes
    4. Tapping over the facial nerve

6. What is the general purpose of endocrine drug therapy? Select all that apply.
    1. Manage hormone deficiency
    2. Manage hormone secretion
    3. Control mood disorders due to hormone deficiency
    4. Manage symptoms of endocrine disorders

7. What should the nurse know when monitoring a patient taking thyroid hormone replacement drugs? Select all that apply.
    1. Older patients can be more susceptible to toxic effects of the drug.
    2. Monitor pulse and BP of older patients.
    3. Thyroid hormone replacement drugs are only given temporarily.
    4. Warn the patient to consult health care provider before receiving vaccinations.
    5. Metabolism of other drugs may be affected.
    6. Advise patient to avoid pregnancy or breastfeeding.

8. What is the primary purpose of oral hypoglycemic agents?
    1. Treatment of hypoparathyroidism
    2. Stimulates pancreatic secretion of insulin in patients with diabetes mellitus
    3. Reduces size and vascularity of the thyroid gland
    4. Treats hyperthyroidism by interfering with the synthesis of thyroid hormones

Pituitary and Adrenal Disorders

Go to http://evolve.elsevier.com/Linton/medsurg/ for additional activities and exercises.

NCLEX CATEGORIES

Safe and Effective Care Environment:
Coordinated Care, Safety, and Infection Control

Health Promotion and Maintenance

Psychosocial Integrity

Physiological Integrity: Basic Care and Comfort, Pharmacological Therapies, Reduction of Risk Potential, Physiological Adaptation

PART I: MASTERING THE BASICS

A. Key Terms
Match the definition in the numbered column with the most appropriate term in the lettered column.

1. _____ Disease resulting from a deficiency of adrenocorticotropic hormone (ACTH) caused by destruction or dysfunction of the adrenal glands; characterized by increased pigmentation of the skin and mucous membranes, weakness, fatigue, hypotension, nausea, weight loss, and hypoglycemia

2. _____ Disease caused by inadequate secretion of antidiuretic hormone (ADH) by the posterior pituitary gland; symptoms include excessive urination, thirst, and dehydration

3. _____ Disease of middle-aged adults resulting from overproduction of growth hormone (GH) by the anterior pituitary gland; characterized by enlargement of the facial bones, nose, lips, and jaw; also associated with decreased libido, moodiness,

fatigue, muscle pains, sweating, and headache

4. _____ Disorder resulting from excessive glucocorticoids in the body as a result of a tumor or hypersecretion of the pituitary; may also be caused by the prolonged administration of large doses of exogenous steroids; symptoms include fat deposits in the neck and abdomen, fatigue, weakness, edema, excess hair growth, glucose intolerance, skin discoloration, and mood swings

5. _____ One of several drugs that can be used to treat hypercalcemia by inhibiting the release of calcium from bones

6. _____ Disease caused by excessive growth hormone in children and young adolescents, resulting in excessive proportional growth

7. _____ Disease caused by the hypersecretion of glucocorticoids as a result of the excessive release of adrenocorticotropic hormone by the pituitary gland

8. _____ Syndrome related to an inadequate secretion of GH occurring during preadolescence

A. Acromegaly
B. Addison disease
C. Cushing disease
D. Cushing syndrome
E. Diabetes insipidus (DI)
F. Estrogen
G. Gigantism

B. Pituitary Gland Disorders

Match or complete the statements in the numbered column with the most appropriate term in the lettered column.

1. _____   Often the first symptom of a problem in hyperpituitarism

2. _____   Radiographic films of the skull of people with hyperpituitarism may show a large sella turcica and increased _____

3. _____   The treatment of choice for patients with a diagnosis of pituitary tumor

4. _____   A disease that occurs in early childhood or puberty in which the diaphyses of the long bones grow to great lengths stimulated by excess GH

5. _____   A disease that appears when adults are in their 30s and 40s in which bones increase in thickness and width after epiphyseal closure

A. Gigantism
B. Hypophysectomy
C. Bone density
D. Acromegaly
E. Visual deficit

C. SIADH

Complete or match the statements in the numbered column with the most appropriate term in the lettered column. Some terms may be used more than once.

1. _____   A syndrome characterized by a water imbalance related to an increase in ADH secretion

2. _____   Kidneys retain fluid due to the elevation of _____

3. _____   Plasma volume expands when ADH is elevated in SIADH, causing an increased _____

4. _____   Dilution of the body's sodium

5. _____   Condition in which weight gain without edema occurs as one of the main symptoms

6. _____   The treatment of SIADH promotes the elimination of _____

7. _____   In patients with SIADH, fluids are restricted and patients are given _____

8. _____   Patients with SIADH have fluid volume excess related to excess secretion of _____

A. Blood pressure
B. Excess water
C. SIADH
D. Hyponatremia
E. ADH
F. Sodium chloride

D. Addison Disease

Complete or match the statements in the numbered column with the most appropriate term in the lettered column. Some terms may be used more than once.

1. _____   Addison disease results in the loss of aldosterone and _____

2. _____   A test that is necessary for a definitive diagnosis of hypoadrenalism, such as Addison disease

3. _____   The mainstay of the treatment of patients with Addison disease is replacement therapy with mineralocorticoids and _____

4. _____   A condition that results when potassium excretion is decreased when cortisol is not secreted

5. _____   Secondary adrenal insufficiency is a result of dysfunction of the hypothalamus or the _____

6. _____   Decreased levels of aldosterone alter the clearance of potassium, water, and _____

7. _____   When sodium and water excretion rates accelerate, the resulting problems are hyponatremia and _____

8. _____   Another name for acute adrenal crisis

9. _____   Impaired secretion of cortisol results in decreased liver and muscle glycogen and decreased _____

10. _____   Secondary adrenal insufficiency leads to the decreased production of cortisol and _____

11. _____   Another name for primary adrenal insufficiency

12. _____   Decreased supply of available glucose that occurs as a result of the impaired secretion of cortisol

13. _____ Patients with either primary or secondary adrenal insufficiency are at risk for episodes of _____

14. _____ A condition that occurs because hyperkalemia promotes hydrogen ion retention

A. Hypovolemia
B. Pituitary gland
C. Addison disease
D. Gluconeogenesis
E. Glucocorticoids
F. ACTH stimulation test
G. Hypoglycemia
H. Hyperkalemia
I. Metabolic acidosis
J. Sodium
K. Androgen
L. Cortisol
M. Addisonian crisis

E. Diabetes Insipidus
Complete or match the statements in the numbered column with the most appropriate term in the lettered column.

1. _____ Increased plasma osmolarity stimulates the osmoreceptors, which in turn relay information to the cerebral cortex, causing the person to experience _____

2. _____ Type of severe imbalance that results from massive dehydration

3. _____ With ADH deficiency, massive dehydration occurs, which leads to decreased intravascular volume, circulatory collapse, and _____

4. _____ Electrolyte imbalances contribute to circulatory collapse by causing arrhythmias and impaired contractility of the _____

5. _____ Massive diuresis results in increased plasma _____

A. Thirst
B. Hypotension
C. Heart
D. Electrolyte
E. Osmolarity

PART II: PUTTING IT ALL TOGETHER

F. Multiple Choice/Multiple Response
Choose the most appropriate answer or select all that apply.

1. An increased secretion of ADH may lead to:
   1. fluid imbalance.
   2. dyspnea.
   3. hypertension.
   4. hypopituitarism.

2. The production of excess GH may lead to the development of:
   1. atherosclerosis and hyperglycemia.
   2. edema and congestive heart failure.
   3. dyspnea and pneumonia.
   4. oliguria and kidney failure.

3. GH antagonizes insulin and interferes with its effects, thus leading to:
   1. hyperkalemia.
   2. hypokalemia.
   3. hyperglycemia.
   4. hypoglycemia.

4. Because growth hormone mobilizes stored fat for energy, levels of free fatty acids are elevated in the bloodstream, leading to the development of:
   1. pneumonia.
   2. kidney failure.
   3. hypotension.
   4. atherosclerosis.

5. Visual problems occur in hyperpituitarism due to pressure on the:
   1. occipital lobe.
   2. optic nerves.
   3. frontal lobe.
   4. oculomotor nerves.

6. Patients with gigantism and acromegaly initially present with increased strength, progressing rapidly to complaints of:
   1. hypotension and syncope.
   2. weakness and fatigue.
   3. edema and dry skin.
   4. dehydration and bradycardia.

7. A common problem for patients with hyperpituitarism is:
   1. inadequate circulation.
   2. loss of protective barrier: skin.
   3. potential infection.
   4. altered body image.

8. Strict documentation of intake and output and measurement of specific gravity are important because postoperative hypophysectomy patients are at risk for:
   1. congestive heart failure.
   2. kidney failure.
   3. pneumonia.
   4. Diabetes insipidus (DI).

9. A lab test can be done to detect whether drainage in a postoperative hypophysectomy patient is cerebrospinal fluid (CSF) because CSF has a high concentration of:
   1. glucose.
   2. protein.
   3. white blood cells.
   4. red blood cells.

10. Decreased pigmentation of the skin results in:
    1. edema.
    2. pallor.
    3. pruritus.
    4. erythema.

11. The patient who has a total hypophysectomy requires hormone replacement:
    1. preoperatively.
    2. during the postoperative recovery period.
    3. for 6 months to 1 year.
    4. for a lifetime.

12. In patients with hypopituitarism, insufficient thyroid hormone is available for normal metabolism and:
    1. visual acuity.
    2. muscle tone.
    3. heat production.
    4. bone growth.

13. To produce or maintain libido, secondary sexual characteristics, and well-being, males with hypopituitarism should receive:
    1. testosterone.
    2. estrogen.
    3. levothyroxine (Synthroid).
    4. bromocriptine (Parlodel).

14. Which drug may be a cause of diabetes insipidus (DI)?
    1. Bromocriptine (Parlodel)
    2. Lithium carbonate (Eskalith)
    3. Levothyroxine (Synthroid)
    4. Digitalis

15. A 24-hour urine output of greater than 4 liters of fluid suggests a diagnosis of:
    1. hypertension.
    2. kidney infection.
    3. congestive heart failure.
    4. Diabetes insipidus (DI).

16. To maintain adequate blood pressure in patients with diabetes insipidus (DI), two measures that are required include intravenous fluid volume replacement and:
    1. diuretics.
    2. vasopressors.
    3. anticholinergics.
    4. antihistamines.

17. The level of consciousness deteriorates and the patient may have seizures or lapse into a coma when water intoxication affects the:
    1. respiratory system.
    2. urinary system.
    3. cardiovascular system.
    4. central nervous system.

18. What is a common sign of diabetes insipidus (DI)?
    1. Massive diuresis
    2. Edema
    3. Hyperglycemia
    4. Oliguria

19. Which is the most common exogenous cause of the Cushing syndrome?
    1. Prolonged administration of high doses of corticosteroids
    2. Corticotropin-secreting pituitary tumor
    3. Truncal obesity
    4. Protein wasting

20. In the immediate postoperative period after adrenalectomy, which medication is needed to maintain blood pressure?
    1. Glucocorticoids
    2. Vasopressors
    3. Beta blockers
    4. Oxytocin

21. Indicate whether the following laboratory study results would be expected to (A) increase or (B) decrease in patients with Addison disease.
    1. _____ Serum cortisol level
    2. _____ Fasting glucose
    3. _____ Sodium
    4. _____ Potassium
    5. _____ Blood urea nitrogen

22. Which are problems for patients with the Cushing syndrome? Select all that apply.
    1. Potential for injury (fracture)
    2. Potential for disrupted skin integrity
    3. Altered body image
    4. Risk for fluid volume deficit
    5. Altered thought processes
    6. Potential for infection

23. The nurse is caring for a patient postoperatively who is recovering from pheochromocytoma removal. Which are potential risks that the nurse should monitor postoperatively?
    1. Water retention
    2. Hyperglycemia
    3. Fluctuations in blood pressure
    4. Hypoglycemia

24. The nurse is monitoring the postoperative hypophysectomy patient for signs and symptoms of infection. Which are signs and symptoms that may be indications of meningitis? Select all that apply.
    1. Decreased white blood cell (WBC) count
    2. Sudden rise in temperature
    3. Headache
    4. Neck rigidity
    5. Slow pupil response

25. Which medications are given as hormone replacement therapy following a complete hypophysectomy? Select all that apply.
    1. Pituitary hormone suppressants
    2. Dopamine receptor antagonists
    3. Glucocorticoids
    4. Thyroid medications
    5. Beta blockers

26. The postoperative hypophysectomy patient is instructed to avoid any activities that can cause the Valsalva maneuver. Which activities may create enough intracranial pressure to disrupt the surgical site and cause CSF leakage? Select all that apply.
    1. Passive range-of-motion exercises
    2. Coughing
    3. Straining
    4. Vomiting
    5. Eating

27. Which are the manifestations of acute adrenal crisis (addisonian crisis)? Select all that apply.
    1. Bradycardia
    2. Dehydration
    3. Confusion
    4. Hyponatremia
    5. Hypoglycemia
    6. Hypertension

28. Which types of stressors can initiate an addisonian crisis? Select all that apply.
    1. Infection
    2. Illness
    3. Steroid therapy use
    4. Trauma
    5. Fatigue

29. Which are diagnostic test results used to determine the presence of Addison disease? Select all that apply.
    1. Decreased fasting glucose
    2. Decreased BUN
    3. Hyponatremia
    4. Hyperkalemia
    5. Decreased eosinophil count after ACTH administration

G. Matching

Match the problems for patients with the Cushing syndrome in the numbered column with the most appropriate "related to" statements in the lettered column.

1. _____ Potential for infection
2. _____ Ineffective management of condition
3. _____ Potential for disrupted skin integrity
4. _____ Potential for injury (fracture)
5. _____ Altered body image

A. Changes in skin and connective tissue and edema
B. Changes in physical appearance and function
C. Lack of understanding of disease, drug therapy, diet, and self-care
D. Osteoporosis
E. High serum cortisol levels

PART III: CHALLENGE YOURSELF!

H. Getting Ready for NCLEX

Choose the most appropriate answer or select all that apply.

1. A patient has been admitted to the hospital with Addison disease. Which problem would the nurse expect to see in this patient?
   1. Fluid volume excess related to excess ADH secretion
   2. Potential for infection related to high serum cortisol levels
   3. Ineffective peripheral circulation related to electrolyte imbalances
   4. Fluid volume deficit related to excessive urine output

2. A patient has had a hypophysectomy. Changes in assessment findings following hypophysectomy that may reflect edema due to the manipulation of tissues or bleeding intracranially include:
   1. unequal pupil size.
   2. decreasing alertness.
   3. decreasing blood pressure.
   4. rising body temperature.

3. Following hypophysectomy, the nurse asks the patient to place the chin to the chest to assess for nuchal rigidity. This is associated with:
   1. bone density.
   2. meningeal irritation.
   3. cerebral edema.
   4. impaired circulation.

4. The nurse is taking care of a postoperative hypophysectomy patient. Because CSF leaks sometimes occur in postoperative hypophysectomy patients, the nurse should check:
   1. intake and output.
   2. pupil reactivity.
   3. nasal packing.
   4. vital signs.

5. A postoperative hypophysectomy patient has a deficiency of thyroid-stimulating hormones. This necessitates thyroid replacement with a drug such as:
   1. octreotide acetate (Sandostatin).
   2. bromocriptine (Parlodel).
   3. levothyroxine (Synthroid).
   4. vasopressin (Pitressin Synthetic).

6. The nurse is taking care of a patient with SIADH. A problem for this patient is potential for injury related to confusion. This problem is associated with:
   1. acute adrenal insufficiency.
   2. impaired physiologic response to stress.
   3. water intoxication.
   4. decreased ADH secretion.

7. The nurse is taking care of a patient with SIADH. To prevent progressive cerebral edema in this patient, what is the appropriate position for this patient in bed?
   1. 30–45°
   2. Flat
   3. 90°
   4. Side-lying

8. The nurse is taking care of a patient with Addison disease. Signs and symptoms of hyperkalemia that should be reported to the health care provider by patients with Addison disease include:
   1. dyspnea and coughing.
   2. oliguria and flank pain.
   3. constipation and fatty stools.
   4. weakness and paresthesia.

9. A patient with Addison disease is getting ready to go home from the hospital. Which substance may be used freely in the diet of patients with Addison disease?
   1. Carbohydrates
   2. Salt
   3. Saturated fats
   4. Caffeine

10. A patient has had an adrenalectomy. What is a priority problem specific to the patient?
    1. Ineffective peripheral circulation related to fluid volume deficit
    2. Potential for injury related to acute adrenal insufficiency
    3. Fatigue related to fluid and electrolyte imbalance
    4. Potential for infection related to corticosteroid use

11. The nurse is taking care of a patient with the Cushing syndrome. Which are appropriate nursing interventions for this patient? Select all that apply.
    1. Avoid exposure to infections.
    2. Report minor signs such as low-grade fever, sore throat, or aches, to the provider.
    3. Seek a psychiatric referral if mood swings continue to be a problem.
    4. Avoid eating green, leafy vegetables.
    5. Protect patient from falls or trauma.
    6. Discuss bruises, abnormal fat distribution, and hirsutism with the patient if they cause embarrassment.

I. Nursing Care Plan
Refer to Nursing Care Plan, The Patient with Addison Disease, in the book.

A 52-year-old Caucasian man is admitted with Addison disease. He considers himself healthy but has had some joint pain in his knees. He had an appendectomy 20 years ago. The patient complains of weight loss, anorexia, weakness, and darkening of the skin on his face and arms. His usual weight is 170 lb. He has had bouts of nausea, vomiting, and diarrhea accompanied by vague abdominal pain. He is a salesman and reports that his symptoms are making it difficult for him to keep up with his work. He is embarrassed about the change in his skin color. Physical examination: BP 110/80 mm Hg (sitting), and 88/42 mm Hg (standing). Pulse 102, respiration 20 breaths/min, oral temperature 98°F. Oriented, but somewhat lethargic. Skin on face, arms, and abdominal scar are darkly pigmented. His body hair is sparse. Oral mucous membranes are slightly dry.

1. What is the priority problem for this patient?

2. What is the most common cause of primary Addison disease?

3. What are the manifestations of adrenal insufficiency exhibited by this patient? Select all that apply.
   1. Hypoglycemia
   2. Nausea, vomiting, and diarrhea
   3. Weight loss
   4. Weakness
   5. Darkening of the skin on his face and arms
   6. Irritability
   7. Dehydration
   8. Hypokalemia
   9. Hypotension

4. What type of diet should this patient follow?

5. Name four tasks that can be assigned to unlicensed assistive personnel for this patient.

J. Next-Generation NCLEX® Examination-Style Questions

A 45-year-old female is admitted with Cushing syndrome. The nurse reviews the physician's progress notes and physical assessment.

> Physician's Progress Notes:
> A 45-year-old female admitted with Cushing syndrome presents with truncal obesity, slender extremities, moon face, and excess facial hair. Her husband states that the client has had insomnia, irritability, and anxiety the past month. The client states that her symptoms are making it difficult for her to keep up with her work. She is embarrassed about the change in her appearance.
>
> Physical Assessment:
> Blood pressure 108/62 mm Hg, pulse 90, respiration 20 breaths/minute, oral temperature 98.3° F. Oriented to person, place, time, and situation. Skin on left lower extremity is red and inflamed, with purulent drainage to site. The client states she injured her leg at work 2 weeks ago.

1. **Complete the following sentence by choosing from the lists of options.**

   The assessment finding that requires

   immediate follow-up includes

   _____ 1 (Select).

> **Assessment Findings:**
> insomnia
> irritability
> anxiety
> truncal obesity
> moon face
> excess facial hair
> purulent drainage to left lower extremity

A 35-year-old male client presents to the Emergency Department with complaints of a severe, pounding headache, and profuse sweating. The client states that the symptoms began after completing his morning workout. The nurse reviews the physical assessment and vital signs.

> Physical Assessment:
> The client alert and oriented times 4. The client reports severe, pounding headache rated 8/10 on a numeric scale. Profuse sweating, pallor and dilated pupils observed. The client complains of blurred vision.
>
> Vital Signs:
>
> | Blood Pressure | 200/115 mm Hg |
> |---|---|
> | Pulse | 108 beats/minute |
> | Respirations | 22 breaths/minute |
> | Temperature | 98.9°F |
>
> Physician's Progress Notes:
> Symptoms indicate pheochromocytoma.
>   *K. Sahn, MD*

2. Based on the client information provided, what would be the nurse's first action?
   1. Administer Tylenol for headache.
   2. Administer phenoxybenzamine.
   3. Obtain an ophthalmologist consult.
   4. Check the patient's blood glucose levels.
   5. Encourage the client to turn, cough, deep breathe.
   6. Obtain surgical consent.

Thyroid and Parathyroid Disorders

Go to http://evolve.elsevier.com/Linton/medsurg/ for additional activities and exercises.

NCLEX CATEGORIES

Safe and Effective Care Environment:
Coordinated Care, Safety, and Infection Control

Health Promotion and Maintenance

Psychosocial Integrity

Physiological Integrity: Basic Care and Comfort, Pharmacological Therapies, Reduction of Risk Potential, Physiological Adaptation

PART I: MASTERING THE BASICS

A. Key Terms
Match the definition in the numbered column with the most appropriate term in the lettered column.

1. _____   Facial edema that develops with severe, long-term hypothyroidism; sometimes used as a synonym for hypothyroidism

2. _____   Enlargement of the thyroid gland, causing the neck to appear swollen

3. _____   Steady muscle contraction caused by hypocalcemia

4. _____   Small mass that may be malignant or benign

5. _____   Paralysis of vocal cords may cause spasms that close the airway

6. _____   Permanent mental and physical retardation caused by congenital deficiency of thyroid hormones

7. _____   Excessive metabolic stimulation caused by elevated thyroid hormone level

8. _____   Inflammation of the parotid (salivary) gland

9. _____   Inflammation of the thyroid gland

10. _____   Substance that suppresses thyroid hormone production

11. _____   Protrusion of the eyeballs associated with Graves disease

A. Goiter
B. Goitrogen
C. Exophthalmos
D. Myxedema
E. Nodule
F. Cretinism
G. Parotiditis
H. Tetany
I. Laryngospasm
J. Thyroiditis
K. Thyrotoxicosis

B. Hyperthyroidism/Hypothyroidism
For each of the following signs or symptoms, indicate whether it is characteristic of (A) hyperthyroidism or (B) hypothyroidism.

1. _____   Heat intolerance

2. _____   Apathy

3. _____   Increased appetite

4. _____   Tachycardia

5. _____   Cold intolerance

6. _____   Weight loss

7. _____   Anorexia

8. _____   Bradycardia

9. _____   Nervousness and restlessness

10. _____   Weight gain

11. _____   Coarse, dry skin and hair

12. _____   Systolic hypertension

C. Thyroid and Parathyroid Hormones

Complete the statements below with either (A) increases or (B) decreases.

1. _____ The effect on the pulse rate when thyroid hormones are elevated

2. _____ The effect on the body's metabolic rate when there is excess thyroid hormones such as thyroxine

3. _____ The effect on the retention of calcium caused by high levels of parathyroid hormone (parathormone, PTH)

4. _____ The effect on blood pressure when thyroid hormones are elevated

5. _____ The effect on the loss of phosphates by the kidneys when there are high levels of PTH

PART II: PUTTING IT ALL TOGETHER

D. Multiple Choice/Multiple Response

Choose the most appropriate answer or select all that apply.

1. Hyperthyroid patients often experience sleep disturbances and:
   1. sedation.
   2. bradycardia.
   3. restlessness.
   4. hypotension.

2. Poor tolerance of heat and excessive perspiration are symptoms of:
   1. hyperparathyroidism.
   2. hypoparathyroidism.
   3. hyperthyroidism.
   4. hypothyroidism.

3. If untreated, hyperthyroidism may lead to:
   1. thyrotoxic crisis (thyroid storm).
   2. hypotension.
   3. bradycardia.
   4. decreased metabolism.

4. Signs of iodine toxicity include:
   1. bradycardia and hypotension.
   2. urinary retention and oliguria.
   3. esophageal ulcers and pyloric sphincter spasms.
   4. swelling and irritation of mucous membranes and increased salivation.

5. Elevated thyroid hormones result in:
   1. decreased pulse and blood pressure.
   2. increased pulse and blood pressure.
   3. decreased temperature and susceptibility to infection.
   4. increased temperature and susceptibility to infection.

6. A problem for the patient with exophthalmos is:
   1. potential for infection.
   2. inadequate knowledge (of disease process).
   3. impaired tissue perfusion.
   4. altered body image.

7. A complication of thyroidectomies includes injury to the parathyroid glands, which results in:
   1. bradycardia.
   2. cyanosis.
   3. tetany.
   4. headache.

8. An early symptom of tetany is:
   1. flank pain with hematuria.
   2. difficulty breathing.
   3. a tingling sensation around the mouth, fingers, and toes.
   4. muscle cramps in leg and arm muscles.

9. Graves disease (toxic diffuse goiter) is characterized by:
   1. increased secretion of thyroid hormones.
   2. a decreased metabolic rate.
   3. intolerance to cold.
   4. constipation.

10. In patients with toxic diffuse goiter, there is a potential for injury related to:
    1. increased metabolic energy production.
    2. exophthalmos.
    3. increased thyroid hormone stimulation.
    4. intolerance to heat.

11. Lack of iodine is associated with:
    1. goiter.
    2. hypoparathyroidism.
    3. tetany.
    4. thyrotoxicosis.

12. If thyroid enlargement is mild and thyroid hormone production is normal, what treatment is required?
    1. No treatment
    2. Radioactive iodine
    3. Antithyroid medication
    4. Thyroid replacement therapy

13. Which statements are true about hyperparathyroidism? Select all that apply.
    1. PTH plays a critical role in regulating sodium.
    2. The most notable effect of hyperparathyroidism is hypercalcemia.
    3. People who undergo kidney transplantation after being on dialysis for a long time may experience hyperparathyroidism.
    4. A spasm of the facial muscle when the face is tapped over the facial nerve is called Chvostek sign.
    5. Supporting a diagnosis of hyperparathyroidism are Chvostek sign and Trousseau sign.
    6. Potassium is an element that is an important component of strong bones and plays a vital role in the functions of nerve and tissue cells.

14. Which are manifestations of hyperparathyroidism? Select all that apply.
    1. Cramps
    2. Poor muscle tone
    3. Bone pain
    4. Demineralization
    5. Weakness
    6. Fractures

15. Which are signs and symptoms of poor oxygenation due to airway obstruction that may occur after thyroidectomy? Select all that apply.
    1. Restlessness
    2. Increased pulse
    3. Increased temperature
    4. Petechiae
    5. Dyspnea
    6. Cold intolerance

16. Which are signs of laryngeal nerve damage that may occur after thyroidectomy? Select all that apply.
    1. Tachycardia
    2. Exophthalmos
    3. Inability to speak
    4. Hoarseness
    5. Hypertension

17. Which are signs of thyroid crisis (thyroid storm) that may occur approximately 12 hours after thyroidectomy? Select all that apply.
    1. Tetany
    2. Fever
    3. Confusion
    4. Tachycardia
    5. Hypercalcemia

18. Which are true statements about complications following thyroidectomy? Select all that apply.
    1. A complication involving injury to parathyroid glands results in tetany.
    2. Symptoms of infection that should be reported after thyroidectomy include fever, wound swelling, and foul discharge.
    3. The most serious side effect of hypocalcemia is dyspnea.
    4. Laryngospasm can be prevented by preoperative treatment with parathyroid drugs.

PART III: CHALLENGE YOURSELF!

E. Getting Ready for NCLEX
Choose the most appropriate answer or select all that apply.

1. The nurse is taking care of a patient who is having a thyroidectomy. Which should be placed at the bedside before this patient returns from surgery?
    1. Thromboembolic stockings
    2. Incentive spirometer
    3. Emergency tracheotomy tray
    4. Continuous passive motion (CPM) machine

2. The nurse is taking care of a patient who has had a thyroidectomy, and is monitoring the respirations carefully. Which are reasons that respiratory distress can result following thyroidectomy? Select all that apply.
   1. Compression of the trachea
   2. Aspiration leading to atelectasis
   3. Spasms of the larynx due to nerve damage or hypocalcemia
   4. Bronchospasm
   5. Dyspnea

3. Following thyroidectomy surgery, where should the nurse check the patient for bleeding? Select all that apply.
   1. Inspect the dressing on the front of the neck.
   2. Check behind the neck.
   3. Check the upper back.
   4. Observe the oral cavity.
   5. Check the pharynx.

4. The nurse is assisting with teaching a class about thyroid disorders. Which statements are true about hyperthyroidism? Select all that apply.
   1. Symptoms of thyrotoxicosis include tachycardia, heart failure, and hyperthermia.
   2. The two classes of drugs commonly used as antithyroid drugs are iodides and thyroid hormones.
   3. When a patient is taking drugs that interfere with thyroxine (T_4) secretion, the nurse should monitor for edema, weight gain, and cold intolerance.
   4. Examples of antithyroid thioamides are methimazole (Tapazole) and propylthiouracil (PTU).
   5. One main disadvantage of the thioamides is that they can cause agranulocytosis.

5. A patient comes to the community health clinic with hyperthyroidism. The nurse expects to see which problems this patient may have? Select all that apply.
   1. Heat intolerance related to increased metabolic energy production
   2. Inadequate oxygenation related to laryngeal spasm
   3. Potential skin breakdown related to dryness and edema
   4. Potential for injury related to hypocalcemia
   5. Potential for injury related to exophthalmos
   6. Decreased cardiac output related to excessive thyroid hormone stimulation

6. The nurse is taking care of a patient who has had a thyroidectomy. Which problems is the nurse likely to observe in this patient? Select all that apply.
   1. Cold intolerance related to slow metabolism
   2. Urinary incontinence related to urinary calculi
   3. Decreased cardiac output related to dysrhythmias and heart failure secondary to hypocalcemia
   4. Decreased cardiac output related to blood loss
   5. Potential for airway obstruction related to laryngeal spasm

F. Nursing Care Plan
Refer to Nursing Care Plan, The Patient with Hypothyroidism, in the book, and answer questions 1–5.

A 53-year-old woman comes to the health care provider's office complaining of fatigue and irritability. The review of symptoms reveals frequent headaches, anorexia, constipation, menstrual irregularity, numbness and tingling in her legs, and intolerance to cold. Her BP is 90/60 mm Hg and her pulse is 74 bpm. She has noticed a 10-pound weight gain over the past 6 months. She is oriented but lethargic. Her medical diagnosis is hypothyroidism. The provider is planning to start her on Synthroid.

1. What is the priority problem for this patient?

2. What data collected for this patient indicate the presence of hypothyroidism?

3. When the patient starts taking Synthroid, for what should she be monitored, related to the problem of decreased cardiac output?

4. The patient returns home and calls the nurse at the provider's office to report that she is having palpitations. What is the appropriate nursing intervention?

5. What tasks for this patient can be assigned to unlicensed assistive personnel?

Patient Problem	Client Assessment Finding
Inadequate nutrition	Decreased peristalsis
Pain	Slow metabolic rate
Infection	Tissue trauma
Cold Intolerance	Increased metabolic requirements
Constipation	Decreased metabolic requirements

A 50-year-old male client presents to his primary care provider with complaints of forgetfulness and frequent headaches. The nurse reviews the past medical history and physical assessment.

Past Medical History:
History of Hyperthyroidism. The client has been treated with propylthiouracil (PTU) for the past 3 years.

Physical Assessment:
Client states, "I do not know what is going. I keep forgetting things and I'm always cold these days". Examination reveals dry, thick skin; bruising to all four extremities; and thin, coarse hair. Laboratory testing reveals low Free T4 levels.

2. Based on the client information provided, highlight the probable cause of the hypothyroidism.

G. Next-Generation NCLEX® Examination-Style Questions

A 44-year-old woman comes to the health care provider's office complaining of restlessness, irritable behavior, and sleep disturbances. The nurse reviews the physician's progress notes.

Physician's Progress Notes:
A 44-year-old woman presents with reports of restlessness, irritable behavior, and sleep disturbances. She states that she has lost 8 lbs in one month, despite no changes to her diet. The review of symptoms reveals warm, moist, velvety skin and fine tremors of the hands. Her blood pressure is 180/80 mm Hg and her pulse is 115 beats/minute. Laboratory findings reveal decreased TSH and elevated serum T4 levels. Findings indicate Graves disease. *L. Lawson, MD*

1. Drag one patient problem and one client assessment finding to fill in each blank in the following sentence.

The client is at risk for _____, due to _____.

Diabetes and Hypoglycemia

chapter

50

Go to http://evolve.elsevier.com/Linton/medsurg/ for additional activities and exercises.

NCLEX CATEGORIES

Safe and Effective Care Environment:
Coordinated Care, Safety, and Infection Control

Health Promotion and Maintenance

Psychosocial Integrity

Physiological Integrity: Basic Care and Comfort, Pharmacological Therapies, Reduction of Risk Potential, Physiological Adaptation

PART I: MASTERING THE BASICS

A. Key Terms

Match or complete the statement in the numbered column with the most appropriate term in the lettered column. Some terms may not be used.

1. _____ Condition that occurs when insulin is absent, and the blood becomes thick with glucose

2. _____ Lumps that should be avoided as injection sites

3. _____ Microvascular complications of the eyes

4. _____ Insulin produced within one's body

5. _____ Hollowing or pitting of the subcutaneous tissue

6. _____ Abnormally increased urine volume caused by osmotic force

7. _____ Causes ketoacidosis in individuals with type 1 diabetes mellitus (DM)

8. _____ Insulin comes from an external source

9. _____ Complications that are accelerated atherosclerotic changes associated with DM

10. _____ Feeling of excessive hunger

11. _____ High concentrations along with hypertension gradually destroy the capillaries

12. _____ Deficiency of insulin and elevated hormones that constitute a life-threatening emergency

13. _____ Poor glucose control resulting in pathologic changes in nerve tissue

14. _____ Elevated blood glucose that occurs in patients who have DM

15. _____ Complications occurring in both types of DM resulting from changes in small blood vessels

16. _____ Abnormally low level of glucose in the blood

17. _____ Microvascular complications to the kidneys

A. Endogenous
B. Exogenous
C. Glycosuria
D. Hyperglycemia
E. Hypoglycemia
F. Ketoacidosis
G. Ketone bodies
H. Lipoatrophy
I. Lipohypertrophy
J. Macrovascular
K. Microvascular
L. Nephropathy
M. Neuropathy
N. Polydipsia
O. Polyphagia
P. Polyuria
Q. Retinopathy

B. Complications of Diabetes

Match the description in the numbered column with the complication in the lettered column. Answers may be used more than once.

1. _____ Nerve tissue involvement that affects the sympathetic and parasympathetic nervous systems

2. _____ Complication in which signs and symptoms are classified as adrenergic and neuroglycopenic

3. _____ Complication caused by rough shoe linings, burns, or chemical irritation

4. _____ Symptoms range from tingling, numbness, and burning to complete loss of sensation caused by sensory and autonomic nerve impairment

5. _____ Glycosuria, along with hypertension, gradually destroy the capillaries that supply the renal glomeruli

6. _____ Characterized by macular edema

7. _____ Dangerous drop in blood glucose caused by taking too much insulin, not eating enough food, or not eating at the right time

8. _____ Results from inadequate blood supply and is experienced as sharp, stabbing pain in muscles

9. _____ Patient goes into a coma from extremely high glucose levels with no evidence of elevated ketones

A. Retinopathy
B. Nephropathy
C. Neuropathy
D. Polyneuropathy
E. Autonomic neuropathy
F. Neuropathic foot ulcers
G. Acute hypoglycemia
H. Hyperglycemic hyperosmolar nonketotic syndrome (HHNS)

Complete the statement in the numbered column with the most appropriate term in the lettered column.

10. _____ DM is the leading cause of _____.

11. _____ With diabetic retinopathy, the vitreous humor becomes cloudy and vision is lost as a result of _____.

12. _____ A symptom of eye problems for patients with DM is the presence of spots, which are called _____.

13. _____ People with DM account for a large percentage of patients with renal disease, which is called _____.

14. _____ Elevated insulin levels circulating in the blood of patients with DM contribute to the premature development of _____.

A. Floaters
B. Hemorrhage
C. Atherosclerosis
D. Nephropathy
E. End-stage renal disease (ESRD)

A patient with DM has signs of foot complications. Indicate which changes occur (A) when the nerve function is impaired and (B) when the blood supply is impaired.

15. _____ The foot is warm and pink.

16. _____ There are no pedal pulses.

17. _____ Sensation is impaired.

18. _____ The foot is cold; foot is pale when raised and red when lowered.

19. _____ The pedal pulses are good and can be felt.

20. _____ The sensation is normal.

C. Ketoacidosis

Complete the statement in the numbered column with the most appropriate term in the lettered column.

1. _____ Treatment of ketoacidosis is aimed at correction of three main problems, which are acidosis, dehydration, and _____.

2. _____ The patient with ketoacidosis may have lost a large volume of fluid as the result of vomiting, hyperventilation, and _____.

3. _____ Replacement of potassium is vital in patients with ketoacidosis because hypokalemia can lead to severe _____.

4. _____ A life-threatening emergency caused by lack of insulin or inadequate amounts of insulin is called diabetic _____.

5. _____ Air hunger, seen in patients with ketoacidosis, is observed as _____.

6. _____ The movement of potassium from the extracellular compartment into the cells is enhanced by _____.

7. _____ Ketoacidosis results in disorders in the metabolism of carbohydrates, fats, and _____.

8. _____ The electrolyte of primary concern in ketoacidosis is _____.

A. Ketoacidosis
B. Insulin
C. Electrolyte imbalance
D. Potassium
E. Cardiac dysrhythmias
F. Kussmaul respirations
G. Protein
H. Polyuria

D. Hypoglycemia

1. Which are initial signs and symptoms of hypoglycemia? Select all that apply.
    1. Blurred vision
    2. Slurred speech
    3. Shakiness
    4. Nervousness
    5. Bradycardia
    6. Anxiety
    7. Lightheadedness
    8. Hunger
    9. Drowsiness
    10. Tingling or numbness of the lips or tongue
    11. Diaphoresis
    12. Disorientation

E. Insulin

Indicate whether insulin (A) increases or (B) decreases each of the following actions or conditions.

1. _____ Rate of metabolism of carbohydrates
2. _____ Conversion of glucose to glycogen
3. _____ Conversion of glycogen to glucose
4. _____ Fatty acid synthesis and conversion of fatty acids into fat

5. _____ Breakdown of adipose tissue
6. _____ Rate of glucose utilization
7. _____ Mobilization of fat
8. _____ Conversion of fats to glucose
9. _____ Protein synthesis in tissue
10. _____ Conversion of protein into glucose

Match the description in the numbered column with the drug in the lettered column. Answers may be used more than once. Refer to Drug Therapy Table 50.1 in the textbook.

11. _____ Category that includes NPH and lente insulin
12. _____ Category that includes ultralente and insulin glargine (Lantus)
13. _____ Category that includes Humalog and NovoLog
14. _____ Category that includes regular insulin
15. _____ Onset occurs in 10–30 minutes
16. _____ The peak occurs in 4–12 hours
17. _____ Duration is up to 24 hours
18. _____ The onset is 30 minutes to 1 hour

A. Rapid-acting
B. Short-acting
C. Intermediate-acting
D. Long-acting

F. . Diagnostic Tests

Match the description in the numbered column with the diagnostic test in the lettered column.

1. _____ A reading greater than 200 mg/dL indicates a diagnosis of DM.
2. _____ Reflects glucose levels over the past few months.
3. _____ A diagnosis of DM is indicated if the 2 hours postprandial glucose level is greater than or equal to 200.

A. Serum glucose levels
B. Oral glucose tolerance test (OGTT)
C. Glycosylated hemoglobin (HgbA$_{1C}$) levels

PART II: PUTTING IT ALL TOGETHER

G. Multiple Choice/Multiple Response
Choose the most appropriate answer or select all that apply.

1. Which inhibits the conversion of glycogen to glucose?
   1. Fatty acids
   2. Insulin
   3. Triglycerides
   4. Ketones

2. Which herbal supplement may lower blood glucose?
   1. Ginseng
   2. Ginkgo
   3. Kava kava
   4. Ephedra

3. The diagnosis of diabetes is based on:
   1. amylase levels.
   2. red blood cell count.
   3. hemoglobin.
   4. serum glucose levels.

4. Which represents normal fasting serum glucose level?
   1. 30–50 mg/dL
   2. 70–100 mg/dL
   3. 150–200 mg/dL
   4. 205–300 mg/dL

5. The American Diabetes Association recommends that the intake of which nutrient should not be less than 130 g/day?
   1. Protein
   2. Saturated fats
   3. Carbohydrates
   4. Polyunsaturated fats

6. The most commonly used insulin concentration is:
   1. U-40.
   2. U-80.
   3. U-100.
   4. U-500.

7. Regular insulin should be given:
   1. at bedtime.
   2. before meals.
   3. during meals.
   4. after meals.

8. Which injection site has the fastest rate of absorption for insulin?
   1. Upper arm
   2. Upper buttocks
   3. Abdomen
   4. Thighs

9. The two oral sulfonylurea hypoglycemic agents that are recommended for older patients are glipizide (Glucotrol) and:
   1. chlorpropamide (Diabinese).
   2. glyburide (Diabeta, Micronase).
   3. tolbutamide (Orinase).
   4. acetohexamide (Dymelor).

10. When mixing short- and long-acting insulins, which should be drawn into the syringe first?
    1. Short-acting insulin
    2. Protamine zinc insulin
    3. Ultralente U insulin
    4. Lente L insulin

11. What is the most frequent cause of hypoglycemia?
    1. Liver deficiency
    2. Alcohol
    3. Oral hypoglycemic agents
    4. Insulin

12. Which is a side effect of sulfonylureas used in the treatment of DM?
    1. Hyperglycemia
    2. Hypoglycemia
    3. Hyperkalemia
    4. Hypokalemia

13. Patients who require insulin injections need to self-monitor levels of:
    1. serum cholesterol.
    2. red blood cells.
    3. amylase.
    4. blood glucose.

14. Late signs of hypoglycemia include:
    1. palpitations and dyspnea.
    2. oliguria and hypotension.
    3. peripheral edema and tachypnea.
    4. disorientation and unconsciousness.

15. To detect possible changes in the eyes associated with DM, the nurse inquires whether the patient has had floaters, blurred vision, or:
    1. hemorrhage.
    2. infection.
    3. diplopia.
    4. conjunctivitis.

16. Weakness in diabetic patients, including dehydration and lethargy with stomach pain, may be due to:
    1. neuropathy.
    2. nephropathy.
    3. ketoacidosis.
    4. hyperglycemia.

17. *Hypoglycemia* is defined as a syndrome that develops when the blood glucose level falls to less than:
    1. 15 mg/dL.
    2. 70 mg/dL.
    3. 120 mg/dL.
    4. 300 mg/dL.

18. When blood glucose levels fall rapidly, the four substances that are secreted by the body in an attempt to increase glucose levels are cortisol, glucagon, growth hormone, and:
    1. antidiuretic hormone.
    2. epinephrine.
    3. aldosterone.
    4. thyroxine.

19. Early signs of hypoglycemia include:
    1. bradycardia and edema.
    2. oliguria and constipation.
    3. infection and red skin.
    4. weakness and hunger.

20. Which group of oral antidiabetic agents does not cause hypoglycemia as a side effect when used alone?
    1. Biguanide (Metformin)
    2. Alpha-glucosidase inhibitors (Precose)
    3. Sulfonylureas
    4. Thiazolidinediones (Avandia)

21. Patients with hypoglycemia have potential for injury related to:
    1. oliguria and nephropathy.
    2. polydipsia and polyphagia.
    3. dizziness and weakness.
    4. retinopathy and hypotension.

22. Hyperosmolar nonketotic coma is loss of consciousness caused by extremely high serum:
    1. ketones.
    2. glucose.
    3. calcium.
    4. potassium.

23. When a patient's serum glucose is elevated and ketosis is present, the patient should:
    1. administer glucagon.
    2. drink 8 ounces of skim milk.
    3. drink 4 ounces of concentrated orange juice.
    4. avoid exercise.

24. To treat hypoglycemia, follow the 15/15 rule, which involves 15 g of quick-acting carbohydrate. Which are examples of 15 g of carbohydrates? Select all that apply.
    1. 8 oz of skim milk
    2. 4–5 Life savers or other hard candies
    3. 2 oz of chicken or beef
    4. 1 cup of leafy green vegetables

25. The goal of the diabetic diet is to:
    1. limit carbohydrate intake.
    2. increase protein intake.
    3. limit total calorie intake.
    4. normalize plasma glucose levels.

26. What are areas of injection sites for insulin? Select all that apply.
    1. Buttocks
    2. Upper arm
    3. Abdomen
    4. Thighs
    5. Shoulder

27. Which statement is true regarding the administration of insulin?
    1. It is best to rotate sites from one area of the body to another.
    2. The site with the fastest absorption rate is the abdomen.
    3. Exercise decreases the absorption rate of insulin.
    4. Heat and massage do not affect the absorption rate of insulin.

28. Which insulin is cloudy in appearance?
    1. Rapid-acting (Humalog)
    2. Short-acting (Regular)
    3. Intermediate-acting (NPH)
    4. Long-acting (Lantus)

29. Which are exogenous causes of hypoglycemia? Select all that apply.
    1. Tumors
    2. Insulin
    3. Alcohol
    4. Exercise
    5. Severe liver deficiency

30. Which organs of the body do not depend on insulin for the transport of glucose into them? Select all that apply.
    1. Kidneys
    2. Brain and nerve cells
    3. Lens of the eye
    4. Lungs
    5. Heart
    6. Exercising muscles

31. Indicate whether (A) too much or (B) not enough of the following factors causes serum glucose levels to drop.
    1. _____ Insulin
    2. _____ Food
    3. _____ Exercise

PART III: CHALLENGE YOURSELF!

H. Getting Ready for NCLEX

Choose the most appropriate answer or select all that apply.

1. The nurse is presenting an educational program on risk factors for type 2 DM. Which will the nurse include as risk factors for type 2 DM? Select all that apply.
   1. Obesity
   2. Family history of diabetes
   3. People younger than age 40
   4. Hispanic/Latino ethnicity
   5. Asian ethnicity
   6. Presence of acanthosis nigricans or insulin resistance condition

2. The nurse is taking care of a patient with DM at the community health clinic. Which are causes of foot problems in the person with DM? Select all that apply.
   1. Impaired hormone supply
   2. Impaired blood supply
   3. Impaired nerve supply
   4. Decreased weight
   5. Decreased glucose

3. A patient with DM asks the nurse: "How could it be that I have a large ulcer on my foot and yet I didn't even know it was there? I don't feel anything, and my foot looks normal." The nurse's most appropriate response would be:
   1. "It is common for people with diabetes to have ulcers on their feet. Just elevate your feet at the end of the day."
   2. "When the nerve supply to the foot is impaired, the foot remains warm and pink, but the sensation is impaired."
   3. "This is an emergency situation. I will contact your health care provider."
   4. "The ulcer will heal within a week. It is important to keep it clean."

4. The nurse is explaining to the patient with DM the risk factors for ketoacidosis. Which situations put the patient with DM at risk for ketoacidosis? Select all that apply.
   1. The patient eats too much food and does not take enough insulin.
   2. The patient does not get enough exercise.
   3. The patient experiences stress such as infection or surgery.
   4. The patient has DM that has not been diagnosed.
   5. The patient is obese.

5. Which statements explain why patients receiving total parenteral nutrition or dialysis have increased risk for hyperosmolar nonketotic coma? Select all that apply.
   1. IV solutions containing large amounts of glucose are administered to the patient.
   2. The digestive system is bypassed.
   3. There is no stimulus to trigger the pancreas to release insulin.
   4. Patients can go into a coma from extremely low glucose levels.
   5. Wound healing is decreased.

6. The nurse reads a provider's written prescription for a patient with DM that states: "Give regular insulin, 20 units, PO, bid." What is the nurse's most appropriate response?
   1. Explain to the patient that insulin cannot be given PO and that she will call the provider to get a prescription to give it IM.
   2. Give the insulin PO as prescribed, making sure that it's given before meals.
   3. Call the provider to clarify the prescription, since the nurse knows that regular insulin is made ineffective in the gastrointestinal tract and cannot be given PO.
   4. Explain to the patient that the peak effect of regular insulin will be in 2–3 hours.

7. A reason for avoiding long-acting oral sulfonylurea hypoglycemic agents in older patients is that decreased renal function makes them more prone to:
   1. hyponatremia.
   2. hypernatremia.
   3. hypoglycemia.
   4. hyperglycemia.

8. The nurse is taking care of a patient who has just been diagnosed with type 1 DM. As the nurse collects data about this patient, he inspects the feet carefully for lesions, discoloration, and:
   1. edema.
   2. ability to dorsiflex.
   3. ability to evert.
   4. dehydration.

9. The nurse is taking care of a patient with DM who has come to the clinic complaining of chronic pain. The nurse recognizes that chronic pain in this patient is related to:
   1. abnormal blood glucose levels.
   2. adverse effects of drugs.
   3. neuropathy.
   4. alterations in urine output.

10. The nurse is assisting with a staff development program in the hospital on patients with DM who have disrupted skin integrity. The nurse explains that disrupted skin integrity in patients with DM is related to:
    1. dietary restrictions.
    2. anxiety and fear.
    3. imbalance between food intake and activity expenditure.
    4. neurologic and circulatory changes.

11. The nurse is assisting with developing a teaching plan for a patient with DM who is being discharged from the hospital to home. A safety precaution that the nurse explains to the patient is that alterations in tactile sensations in diabetic patients may result in:
    1. burns or frostbite.
    2. floaters or diplopia.
    3. altered urine output or oliguria.
    4. abnormal blood glucose levels.

I. Nursing Care Plan
Refer to Nursing Care Plan, The Patient with Type 1 Diabetes Mellitus, in the book, and answer questions 1–5.

A 17-year-old girl who has recently been diagnosed with type 1 DM is hospitalized to begin her insulin therapy and stabilize her blood glucose. She sought medical attention because of persistent thirst and increased urination. She has no other health problems. The review of symptoms reveals periodic blurred vision, itching, increased appetite, weight loss of 7 lb in 3 months, and fatigue.

1. What is the priority problem for this patient?

2. What data collected in the health history and physical examination indicate the presence of type 1 DM?

3. Which statements are correct and should be included in this patient's teaching plan about reduced activity tolerance and exercise? Select all that apply.
   1. It is important to avoid trauma.
   2. Inspect your feet daily.
   3. Exercise must be done as part of a regular routine.
   4. Avoid injecting insulin into a body area that will be affected by exercise soon after the injection.
   5. Do not exercise during peak insulin activity.
   6. Eat a snack before or during exercise if the blood glucose is less than 100 mg/dL.

4. This patient is experiencing fluid volume deficit related to altered urine output. Which is the appropriate nursing intervention for this problem?
   1. Teach the patient and family members to recognize and respond to hypoglycemia.
   2. Instruct the patient to take concentrated sugar if hypoglycemia occurs.
   3. Point out that excessive urine output may indicate hypoglycemia.
   4. Stress the importance of drinking at least eight glasses of water daily.

Refer to Nursing Care Plan, The Patient with Type 2 Diabetes Mellitus, in the book, and answer questions 6–9.

An 80-year-old Hispanic woman was seen in her provider's office and diagnosed with type 2 DM. A referral has been made to a home health agency. Her provider prescribed glyburide (Micronase), 2.5 mg daily before breakfast. She has a history of hypertension and venous insufficiency. Her toenails are unevenly cut. A reddened area is seen on one heel, but she says it is not painful.

5. What is the priority problem for this patient?

6. What data collected in the health history and physical examination are related to the presence of type 2 DM?

7. This patient is experiencing reduced activity tolerance. Which are factors that contribute to reduced activity tolerance for this patient? Select all that apply.
   1. Inadequate coping
   2. Fatigue
   3. Venous insufficiency
   4. Circulatory impairment
   5. Increased susceptibility to infection

8. Which nursing intervention is a safety priority for this patient related to her potential for injury?
   1. Emphasize the importance of protecting the feet from injury by wearing tight-fitting shoes and trimming her own nails correctly.
   2. Avoid heating pads and test bath water with a thermometer.
   3. Monitor weight carefully.
   4. Assess her energy level and discuss ways to conserve energy.

J. Next-Generation NCLEX® Examination-Style Questions

A 50-year-old female client presents to her primary care provider (PCP) with complaints of pink-tinged urine. The nurse reviews the past medical history, physical assessment, vital signs, and lab results.

Past Medical History:
Diabetes Mellitus Type I
Hypertension
Obesity

Physical Assessment:
The client is alert and oriented ×4. She states that she voids frequently during the day. Assessment reveals a reddened, non-blanchable area to her right foot with diminished pedal pulses. Skin in bilateral upper extremities is warm to touch. The client states, "I did not know that was there. I have not been having any pain to the area." The client states that she recently ran out her insulin prescription and has not been able to afford her medications.

Vital Signs:

Blood Pressure	130/82 mm Hg
Pulse	100 beats/minute
Respirations	20 breaths/minute
Temperature	99.7°F

Lab Results:

Blood Glucose	220 mg/dL
HbA1C	10
Urine	Positive hematuria

1. For each body system, select the client findings below that are of immediate concern to the nurse.

Body System	Assessment Findings
Renal _____ 1 (Select) _____	Options for 1: Voids frequently pink-tinged urine
Integumentary _____ 2 (Select) _____	Options for 2: Reddened, non-blanchable area to her right foot Skin in bilateral upper extremities warm to touch
Neurological _____ 3 (Select) _____	Options for 3: Alert and oriented × 4 Diminished pedal pulses

2. Which physician orders would the nurse anticipate being prescribed? Select all that apply.
   1. Soft diet
   2. Complete bedrest
   3. Abdominal CT scan
   4. IV infusion 1000 mL NS bolus
   5. Continuous insulin IV drip
   6. Kayexalate oral suspension TID
   7. 50% Dextrose IV bolus
   8. 15 g glucose tab STAT

A 40-year-old male client presents to the Emergency Department with reports of nausea, headache, and loss of appetite. The nurse reviews the physical assessment and lab results.

Physical Assessment:
The client reports nausea, headache, and loss of appetite. The client states that he has been voiding frequently and feels very thirsty. Assessment reveals fruity breath, blood pressure 100/54 mm Hg, pulse 122 beats/minute, temperature 98.7°F, respirations 26 breaths/minute.

Lab Results:

Blood Glucose	310 mg/dL
pH	7.10
Bicarbonate	12 mEq/L
Potassium	3.9 mEq/L
Urinalysis	3+ ketones

Female Reproductive System Introduction

Go to http://evolve.elsevier.com/Linton/medsurg/ for additional activities and exercises.

NCLEX CATEGORIES

Health Promotion and Maintenance

Physiological Integrity: Pharmacological Therapies, Reduction of Risk Potential

PART I: MASTERING THE BASICS

A. Key Terms
Match the definition in the numbered column with the most appropriate term in the lettered column.

1. _____ Surgical removal of the uterus
2. _____ Cessation of menstruation
3. _____ Age at which the first menstrual period occurs

A. Hysterectomy
B. Menarche
C. Menopause

B. Diagnostic Procedures
Match the definition or description in the numbered column with the most appropriate term in the lettered column. Some terms may be used more than once, and some terms may not be used.

1. _____ A type of invasive surgical procedure in which a large amount of cervical tissue is removed to treat cancer
2. _____ An invasive surgical procedure that provides direct visualization of the female pelvic cavity
3. _____ A test for which specimens are collected routinely to detect cervical cancer and dysplasia

4. _____ Procedure in which the cervix is dilated and the uterine lining scraped to diagnose uterine cancer and causes of abnormal uterine bleeding
5. _____ A type of biopsy done in a provider's office or an outpatient clinic in which several specimens of cervical tissue are obtained to rule out cervical cancer
6. _____ Specimens collected to identify infections
7. _____ The procedure that is done to identify ectopic pregnancy, causes of irregular uterine bleeding, and pelvic masses
8. _____ A test performed to study fertility or to detect cancer
9. _____ A procedure in which an instrument is used to inspect the cervix under magnification and to identify abnormal and potentially cancerous tissue; usually done before cervical biopsy
10. _____ Deliberate tissue destruction by means of heat, electricity, or chemicals during pelvic examination
11. _____ Visualization of abdominal organs to perform minor surgery such as tubal ligation

A. Multiple punch biopsy
B. Papanicolaou (Pap) test
C. Dilation and curettage
D. Culture tests
E. Cone biopsy or conization
F. Aspiration biopsy
G. Endometrial biopsy
H. Culdoscopy
I. Breast biopsy
J. Colposcopy
K. Laparoscopy
L. Cauterization

C. Drug Therapy

1. Which descriptions of drug actions and uses described below are related to ovulatory stimulants? Select all that apply.
   1. Treat uterine bleeding and endometriosis
   2. Promote secretory function in endometrium
   3. Initially increase and then decrease testosterone levels
   4. Stimulate ovarian follicular growth
   5. Used as fertility drugs
   6. Clomid and repronex are examples

2. Which descriptions of drug actions and uses below are related to selective estrogen receptor modulators (SERMs)? Select all that apply.
   1. Used to replace natural hormones after menopause and to treat advanced breast cancer
   2. Influence contractile activity of the uterus
   3. Inhibit production of pituitary gonadotropins
   4. Initially increase and then decrease testosterone levels; used to treat endometriosis
   5. Used to treat breast cancer
   6. Tamoxifen and raloxifene (Evista) are examples

D. Female Genitalia

Using Figure 51.1 from the book, label the external female genitalia (A–L) from the terms (1–12) below.

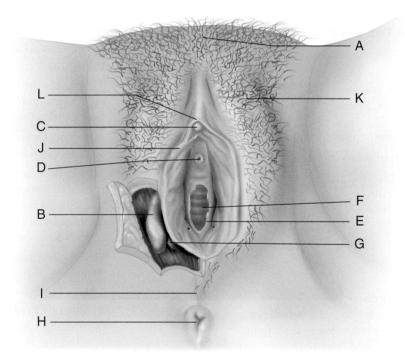

1. _____	Labium minus	7. _____	Vaginal orifice (introitus)
2. _____	Hymen	8. _____	External urinary meatus
3. _____	Labium majus	9. _____	Perineum
4. _____	Vestibular (clitoral) bulb	10. _____	Prepuce
5. _____	Clitoris glans	11. _____	Anus
6. _____	Mons pubis	12. _____	Greater vestibular (Bartholin) gland

PART II: PUTTING IT ALL TOGETHER

E. Multiple Choice/Multiple Response

Choose the most appropriate answer or select all that apply.

1. Which is a main hormone produced by the ovaries?
   1. Estrogen
   2. Prolactin
   3. Oxytocin
   4. Follicle-stimulating hormone

2. In which position is the patient placed for a pelvic exam?
   1. Lithotomy
   2. Right side-lying
   3. Knee-chest
   4. Supine

3. Advise the patient that air entering the pelvic cavity during the culdoscopy procedure may cause pain in the:
   1. abdomen.
   2. heart.
   3. thigh.
   4. shoulder.

4. A method of deliberate tissue destruction through use of heat, electricity, or chemicals is called:
   1. culdoscopy.
   2. colposcopy.
   3. cauterization.
   4. dilation and curettage.

5. Which is a particularly helpful type of heat application for small areas such as the vulva or perineum?
   1. Sitz baths
   2. An electric heating pad
   3. Aquathermia (K-pad)
   4. Hot compresses

6. For which signs of complications must the nurse observe in patients taking sitz baths? Select all that apply.
   1. Dyspnea
   2. Faintness
   3. Dermatitis
   4. Headache
   5. Severe pain
   6. Shock

7. Dilation of large pelvic vessels during sitz baths may cause:
   1. hypertension.
   2. hypotension.
   3. pneumonia.
   4. seizures.

8. Following the administration of vaginal suppositories, the patient is asked to remain in which position for at least 15 minutes to allow the medication to be absorbed?
   1. Prone
   2. Supine
   3. Sitting
   4. Right side-lying

9. Which are common side effects of danazol, which may be given to patients with endometriosis? Select all that apply.
   1. Irregular bleeding
   2. Fever and chills
   3. Voice deepening
   4. Hirsutism
   5. Decreased breast size
   6. Acne

10. Which type of drug is given to patients with endometriosis because it inhibits endometrial proliferation?
    1. Oral contraceptive
    2. Ovulatory stimulant
    3. Androgen
    4. SERM

PART III: CHALLENGE YOURSELF!

F. Getting Ready for NCLEX

Choose the most appropriate answer or select all that apply.

1. What is an appropriate opening question for an obstetric history?
   1. "How many times have you been pregnant?"
   2. "What is the number of term and preterm births?"
   3. "What is the number of living children you have?"
   4. "How many abortions have you had?"

2. What are subjects that a gynecologic history would address? Select all that apply.
   1. Infections and sexually transmitted infections (STIs)
   2. Cancer
   3. Cysts and tumors
   4. Diabetes mellitus
   5. Structural and functional abnormalities
   6. Birth control
   7. Infertility
   8. Sexual trauma and rape
   9. Stress incontinence
   10. Psychiatric disorders

3. Why should a douche only be used for therapeutic treatment and not for regular hygiene?
   1. Douching washes away tissue and microorganisms from entering the uterus.
   2. Douching prevents contraception.
   3. Douching can wash away the normal acidic pH of the vagina.
   4. Douching can interfere with radiation therapy.

4. Which professional would be responsible for cauterization of small growths and polyps during a pelvic examination?
   1. Nurse
   2. LPN/LVN
   3. Pathologist
   4. Physician or nurse practitioner

5. A 28-year-old patient is concerned that her menstrual cycle lasts an average of 34–40 days. She knows a normal cycle is usually 28–30 days. What could the nurse suggest as a possible cause for this discrepancy?
   1. A Papanicolaou (Pap) test can delay your cycle.
   2. Stress, illness, or physical activity can affect your menstrual cycle.
   3. Low-dose hormone therapy would be needed to regulate the menstrual cycle.
   4. Hot compresses and sitz baths often affect your menstrual cycle.

6. Short-term, low-dose hormonal therapy is appropriate for managing menopausal symptoms. What is the only acceptable indication for long-term therapy according to Lehne (2016)?
   1. Postmenopausal osteoporosis
   2. Advanced breast cancer
   3. Menopause resulting from surgery, chemotherapy, or radiation treatments
   4. Postmenopausal spotting or bleeding

7. A pregnant patient asks what the age of viability is for her fetus. What should be the nurse's response to that question?
   1. 3 months
   2. 9 weeks
   3. 7 months
   4. 20 weeks

8. The nurse is taking care of a patient who will be receiving estrogen replacement therapy. The nurse recognizes which contraindications for estrogen replacement therapy? Select all that apply.
   1. Certain types of cancer (such as estrogen receptor breast cancer)
   2. Hot flashes
   3. Undiagnosed uterine bleeding
   4. Thromboembolism
   5. Uterine prolapse

9. When a patient comes to a clinic with a female reproductive system problem, the opening question the nurse should ask is:
   1. "What is wrong with you today?"
   2. "What is the problem that made you come in?"
   3. "Why did you come to the clinic today?"
   4. "What is the reason for your visit today?"

Female Reproductive Disorders

Go to http://evolve.elsevier.com/Linton/medsurg/ for additional activities and exercises.

NCLEX CATEGORIES

Health Promotion and Maintenance

Physiological Integrity: Pharmacological Therapies, Reduction of Risk Potential, Physiological Adaptation

PART I: MASTERING THE BASICS

A. Key Terms

Match the definition in the numbered column with the most appropriate term in the lettered column.

1. _____ Surgical excision of a fallopian tube and ovary

2. _____ Difficult or painful sexual intercourse in women

3. _____ A condition in which endometrial tissue is abnormally located outside the uterus

4. _____ Inflammation of breast tissue

5. _____ Menstrual periods characterized by profuse or prolonged bleeding

6. _____ Herniation of the urinary bladder into the vagina

7. _____ Bleeding or spotting between menstrual periods

8. _____ Surgical removal of the uterus

9. _____ Changes in cells

10. _____ A backward tilt of the uterus with the cervix pointed downward toward the anterior vaginal wall

11. _____ Herniation of part of the rectum into the vagina

12. _____ Painful menstruation

A. Cystocele
B. Dysmenorrhea
C. Dyspareunia
D. Dysplasia
E. Endometriosis
F. Hysterectomy
G. Mastitis
H. Menorrhagia
I. Metrorrhagia
J. Rectocele
K. Retroversion
L. Salpingo-oophorectomy

B. Uterine Displacement

Match the definition or description in the numbered column with the most appropriate term in the lettered column.

1. _____ The body of the uterus bends posteriorly

2. _____ A forward tilt (anteriorly) of the uterus

3. _____ The uterus bends anteriorly

4. _____ A backward tilt (posteriorly) of the uterus

A. Anteflexion
B. Retroversion
C. Retroflexion
D. Anteversion

C. Menstruation

Match the term in the numbered column with the most appropriate numerical range in the lettered column. (These terms refer to the variations within normal menstrual periods.) Some ranges may be used more than once, and some may not be used.

1. _____   Length of cycle (days)
2. _____   Duration of menstruation (days)
3. _____   Amount of blood loss (mL)

A. 2–8
B. 10–14
C. 21–40
D. 40–100
E. 150–200

D. Female Reproductive System Disorders

1. Which two groups of women are especially prone to developing pelvic inflammatory disease not associated with sexually transmitted infections? Select two that apply.
    1. Women in low socioeconomic groups
    2. Women who are poorly nourished
    3. Women with compromised resistance to infection

E. Menopause

1. How do these structures change after menopause without estrogen present? Select all that apply.
    1. The uterus becomes enlarged.
    2. The vagina shortens.
    3. Vaginal tissues become drier.
    4. Pubic and axillary hair become sparse.
    5. Bone mass increases and becomes less flexible.
    6. Osteoporosis risk increases.

F. Mastectomy

Complete the statement in the numbered column with the most appropriate term in the lettered column.

1. _____   Mastectomy patients have potential for injury related to _____.
2. _____   The removal of the tumor with a margin of surrounding healthy tissue but preserving most of the breast is called _____.
3. _____   A low-incidence cancer of the nipple and areola is _____.
4. _____   The implantation of a tissue expander injected with saline is a type of _____.
5. _____   The removal of all breast tissue, overlying skin, axillary lymph nodes, and underlying pectoral muscles is called _____.
6. _____   If breast cancer cells removed during surgery need estrogen for cell replication, they are said to be _____.
7. _____   Removal of the entire breast is called _____.

A. Paget's disease
B. Radical mastectomy
C. Simple mastectomy
D. ER-positive
E. Breast reconstruction
F. Lumpectomy
G. Lymphedema

G. Endometriosis

Using Figure 52.1, label the sites of endometriosis (A–I) from the terms provided (1–9) below.

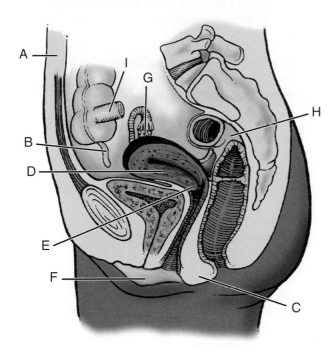

1. _____ Ileum
2. _____ Perineum
3. _____ Cervix
4. _____ Vulva
5. _____ Umbilicus
6. _____ Ovary
7. _____ Appendix
8. _____ Pelvic colon
9. _____ Uterine wall

PART II: PUTTING IT ALL TOGETHER

H. Multiple Choice/Multiple Response

Choose the most appropriate answer or select all that apply.

1. Deviations from normal menstrual cycles are viewed as:
    1. uterine bleeding disorders.
    2. vaginal hemorrhage problems.
    3. endometrial cancers.
    4. pelvic inflammatory diseases.

2. Which are signs and symptoms of vaginitis? Select all that apply.
    1. Local swelling
    2. Itching
    3. Redness
    4. Hemorrhage
    5. Ulcers
    6. Significant discharge

3. A potential complication of vaginitis is:
    1. hypotension.
    2. ascending infection.
    3. seizures.
    4. thrombophlebitis.

4. When Bartholin glands are infected, the resultant edema and pus formation occlude the duct and form:
    1. tumors.
    2. cysts.
    3. warts.
    4. abscesses.

5. The most noticeable symptom of bartholinitis that causes patients to seek medical attention is:
    1. edema.
    2. pain.
    3. discharge.
    4. itching.

6. The portal of entry for organisms that cause mastitis is the:
    1. areola.
    2. mammary gland.
    3. nipple.
    4. lactating duct.

7. The most serious complication of pelvic inflammatory disease is:
    1. peritonitis.
    2. pneumonia.
    3. hemorrhage.
    4. hypertension.

8. Which are methods of treatment for pelvic inflammatory disease? Select all that apply.
    1. Application of heat
    2. Antibiotics
    3. Diuretics
    4. Antispasmodics
    5. Rest

9. Which are major symptoms of endometriosis? Select all that apply.
   1. Pain
   2. Sudden weakness
   3. Difficulty breathing
   4. Pelvic heaviness
   5. Dysmenorrhea

10. Women who are given androgenic steroids for treatment of endometriosis often experience the common side effect of:
    1. masculinizing characteristics.
    2. palpitations.
    3. insomnia.
    4. diuresis.

11. Severe and sudden abdominal pain may occur as a complication of follicular ovarian cysts due to:
    1. infection.
    2. rupture.
    3. muscle spasms.
    4. vaginitis.

12. A serious complication of a very large fibroid tumor is that it may compress the urethra, obstructing urine flow and causing secondary:
    1. vaginitis.
    2. pelvic inflammatory disease.
    3. hydronephrosis.
    4. diuresis.

13. For women with fibroid tumors who desire to become pregnant, a procedure that can be done by laser surgery to remove only the tumor is:
    1. hysterectomy.
    2. myomectomy.
    3. dilation and curettage.
    4. culdoscopy.

14. Women at risk for developing rectoceles and cystoceles are those who have experienced a weakened pubococcygeal muscle due to:
    1. extended antibiotic treatment.
    2. repeated pregnancies.
    3. effects of herpes infection.
    4. poor nutrition.

15. A treatment of small cystoceles that is aimed at improving the tone of the pubococcygeal muscle is:
    1. pelvic floor (Kegel) exercises.
    2. surgical intervention (A & P repair).
    3. vaginal hysterectomy.
    4. increased fluid intake.

16. Which is an established risk factor for breast cancer?
    1. Age of first baby 24 years or older
    2. Age 12 years or older at menarche
    3. Radiation exposure
    4. Age over 50

17. The American Cancer Society (ACS, 2013) recommends that mammograms be done every year beginning at age:
    1. 35.
    2. 40.
    3. 50.
    4. 65.

18. A common problem for mastectomy patients is:
    1. sleep disturbance.
    2. inadequate circulation.
    3. urinary incontinence.
    4. body image disturbance.

19. An important aspect of postoperative care after mastectomy is directed toward the prevention and minimization of:
    1. lymphedema.
    2. hemorrhage.
    3. hypertension.
    4. nausea.

20. The high mortality from ovarian cancer is due to the fact that:
    1. symptoms are multiple and serious.
    2. it is asymptomatic in early stages.
    3. abnormal cell growth occurs in one ovary.
    4. it is diagnosed around the time of menopause concurrent with ascites.

21. Diminished ovarian function associated with aging causes cessation of ovulation as well as decreased production of:
    1. thyroxine.
    2. estrogen.
    3. epinephrine.
    4. prolactin.

22. A woman is said to be menopausal when she has not had a menstrual period for:
    1. 3 months.
    2. 1 year.
    3. 2 years.
    4. 5 years.

23. Some women experience surgical menopause, which occurs as a result of surgical removal of the:
    1. ovaries.
    2. uterus.
    3. vagina.
    4. cervix.

24. The type of drug therapy prescribed promptly for surgical menopause to decrease menopausal symptoms is:
    1. diuretics.
    2. steroids.
    3. estrogen.
    4. analgesics.

25. The symptom of hot flashes that may accompany menopause is due to:
    1. increased menstrual bleeding.
    2. vasodilation.
    3. abdominal cramps.
    4. increased body temperature.

26. The treatment of choice for large and symptomatic cystoceles and rectoceles is:
    1. hysterectomy.
    2. myomectomy.
    3. Kegel exercises.
    4. A & P repair.

27. The incidence of fibroid tumors is increased among women who are:
    1. African American.
    2. Caucasian.
    3. Asian.
    4. Hispanic.

28. Recent findings from the Women's Health Initiative indicate that combination estrogen–progestin therapy increases the risk of breast cancer and:
    1. osteoporosis.
    2. endometriosis.
    3. coronary heart disease.
    4. amenorrhea.

29. Mastectomy patients have potential for injury related to:
    1. infectious drainage.
    2. tissue trauma.
    3. possible abscess formation.
    4. lymphedema.

30. Which are the signs and symptoms of menopause? Select all that apply.
    1. Vaginal dryness
    2. Drowsiness
    3. Headache
    4. Hot flashes
    5. Depression

31. Which are signs and symptoms of pelvic inflammatory disease? Select all that apply.
    1. Nausea and vomiting
    2. Abdominal pain
    3. Fever and chills
    4. Hypotension
    5. Dysuria
    6. Irregular bleeding
    7. Foul-smelling vaginal discharge
    8. Dyspareunia

32. In addition to lower back and pelvic discomfort and recurrent bladder infections, what are symptoms that women with cystoceles are likely to experience? Select all that apply.
    1. Dyspareunia
    2. Stress incontinence
    3. Irregular bleeding
    4. Incomplete bladder emptying
    5. Fever and chills

33. What are ways ovarian cancer metastasizes? Select all that apply.
    1. Direct invasion
    2. Pleural fluid
    3. Lymphatic and venous systems
    4. Peritoneal fluid
    5. Vaginal secretions

PART III: CHALLENGE YOURSELF!

I. Getting Ready for NCLEX
Choose the most appropriate answer or select all that apply.

1. The nurse is assisting with a staff development program about patients with cystocele and rectocele diagnoses. The nurse asks the participants to complete the following matching exercise. Match the problem for patients with cystocele and rectocele in the numbered column with the appropriate nursing intervention in the lettered column. Some interventions may be used more than once for one problem statement.

   1. _____ Urinary incontinence
   2. _____ Constipation
   3. _____ Potential for infection
   4. _____ Pain

   A. Initial application of cold to reduce pain and swelling
   B. Teaching the patient Kegel exercises
   C. Emphasizing the need for a high-fiber diet
   D. Sitz baths and heat lamps
   E. Instructing the patient to report signs of urinary frequency, burning, or foul odor

2. The nurse is conducting a community health program at the clinic on risk factors of breast cancer. Which influence a person's chance for getting breast cancer? Select all that apply.
   1. Female
   2. Increased chance if mother or aunt has had breast cancer
   3. Increases markedly from the age of 35 on
   4. Early menarche
   5. Late menopause
   6. Mutation of the BRCA genes

3. What are ways the nurse can intervene to prevent or minimize lymphedema in the patient with a mastectomy? Select all that apply.
   1. Keep the affected arm below the heart level.
   2. Take blood pressure on the unaffected arm.
   3. No venipuncture or IV fluid administration should be done in the affected arm.
   4. Deodorant may be applied in small amounts 3 days after surgery.
   5. Exercise arm on the affected side frequently.

4. The nurse is assisting with an educational program for women and their families at a community health clinic. The topic is cancer of the female reproductive system. Which are problems related to patients with cancer of the cervix, ovaries, vulva, or vagina? Select all that apply.
   1. Altered sexual function related to physical and emotional effects of cancer of the reproductive system
   2. Potential for injury related to trauma of the exposed uterus
   3. Pain related to inflammation
   4. Potential for injury (to patient and others) related to effects of radiotherapy and chemotherapy
   5. Incontinence related to pelvic muscle weakness

5. The nurse is taking care of a patient who has had a total abdominal hysterectomy. Which are common problems to anticipate for this patient? Select all that apply.
   1. Lack of knowledge related to the effect of hormone replacement therapy (HRT)
   2. Potential for fluid volume deficit related to postoperative bleeding
   3. Urinary retention related to surgical manipulation, local tissue edema, temporary sensory, or motor impairment
   4. Potential for injury related to trauma of the exposed uterus
   5. Constipation related to weakening of abdominal musculature, abdominal pain, decreased physical activity, dietary changes, environmental changes

J. Next-Generation NCLEX® Examination-Style Questions

A 48-year-old female client presents to her primary care provider (PCP) reporting periods of incontinence when going for her daily morning run. The nurse reviews the medical history, physical assessment, and vital signs.

Medical History:
A 48-year-old female client reports periods of incontinence when going for her daily morning run. She states that she has been wearing incontinence briefs since the symptoms began. The client also states that she has also had vaginal dryness and difficulty sleeping at night. Her last menstrual cycle was 13 months ago.

Physical Assessment:
Active bowel sounds in all four quadrants, clear lung sounds bilaterally, firm breast tissue, sparse axillary hair, and capillary refill less than 3 seconds.

Vital Signs:

Blood Pressure	108/68 mmHg.
Pulse	80 beats/minute
Respirations	16 breaths/minute
Temperature	98.8°F (37.1°C)

---

1. Highlight the assessment findings that indicate that the client may be experiencing menopause.

A 29-year-old female client presents to urgent care with complaints of abdominal pain. The nurse reviews the physician's progress notes and vital signs.

Physician's Progress Notes:
The client reports dull, steady, low abdominal pain rated a 7/10 on a numeric pain scale. She states, "It hurts when I urinate or try to have sexual intercourse and I have noticed a foul-smelling vaginal discharge." Symptoms indicate pelvic inflammatory disease (PID).
H. Hemming, MD

Vital Signs:

Blood Pressure	130/78 mmHg
Pulse	90 beats/minute
Respirations	20 breaths/minute
Temperature	100.8°F

---

2. Which physician orders would the nurse anticipate being prescribed? Select all that apply.
   1. Rest
   2. Application of heal via warm compress
   3. Soft diet
   4. Complete bedrest
   5. Stool specimen
   6. Analgesics
   7. Broad-spectrum antibiotics

Male Reproductive System Introduction

Go to http://evolve.elsevier.com/Linton/medsurg/ for additional activities and exercises.

NCLEX CATEGORIES

Health Promotion and Maintenance

Physiological Integrity: Pharmacological Therapies, Reduction of Risk Potential, Physiological Adaptation

PART I: MASTERING THE BASICS

A. Key Terms

Match the description or definition in the numbered column with the most appropriate term in the lettered column.

1. _____ A mass filled with serous fluid
2. _____ Failure of the testicles to descend from the abdomen into the cooler scrotum
3. _____ Tumor
4. _____ The result of sympathetic stimulation leaving the spinal cord at L1 and L2
5. _____ Expulsion of semen

A. Cryptorchidism
B. Ejaculation
C. Emission
D. Hematocele
E. Hydrocele

B. Anatomy and Physiology

Match the description or definition in the numbered column with the most appropriate term in the lettered column. Some terms may be used more than once.

1. _____ Male reproductive organs
2. _____ Extends from the bladder to the urinary meatus at the end of the penis
3. _____ The production of sperm
4. _____ Produces alkaline liquid that enhances motility and fertility of sperm
5. _____ A hormone necessary for the development of male reproductive organs, descent of the testicles, and production of sperm
6. _____ Provides outflow for semen during ejaculation

A. Testosterone
B. Urethra
C. Prostate
D. Spermatogenesis
E. Testes

C. Male Reproductive System

Refer to Figure 53.1 in your book. Label the parts of the male reproductive system (A–M) from the terms (1–13) below.

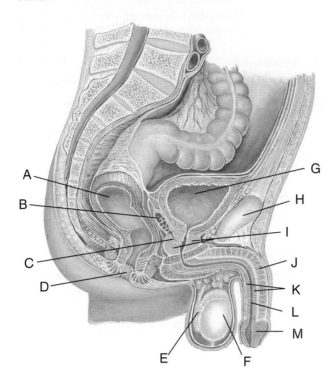

1. _____ Corpus cavernosum
2. _____ Ejaculatory duct
3. _____ Seminal vesicle
4. _____ Urethra
5. _____ Glans
6. _____ Urinary bladder
7. _____ Anus
8. _____ Rectum
9. _____ Symphysis pubis
10. _____ Testis
11. _____ Prostate gland
12. _____ Epididymis
13. _____ Corpus spongiosum

PART II: PUTTING IT ALL TOGETHER

D. Multiple Choice/Multiple Response

Choose the most appropriate answer or select all that apply.

1. Three normal changes that may occur in the male reproductive system due to aging are decreased testosterone, a longer refractory period between erections, and:
   1. penile discharge.
   2. pain with urination.
   3. slower arousal.
   4. descent of testicles.

2. Which factors may make assessment of the male reproductive system difficult for some patients? Select all that apply.
   1. Chronic disease
   2. Advanced age
   3. Defensiveness about sexual behavior
   4. Lack of sexual experience
   5. Health beliefs
   6. Need for privacy

3. Which test is done to document sterilization after a vasectomy?
   1. Ultrasonography
   2. Radiography
   3. Analysis of semen
   4. CBC

4. Medical history helps link the current male reproductive problem of a patient with previous problems and should include information about injuries, diseases, surgeries, allergies, medications, and:
   1. marital status.
   2. treatments.
   3. age and health of siblings.
   4. age and health of parents.

5. The health history should include information about medications the patient is taking because they may:
   1. impair his cognitive abilities.
   2. make him too tired to participate in the assessment.
   3. impair sexual function.
   4. impair gastrointestinal function.

6. Physical examination of the male reproductive system can be accomplished by inspection and:
   1. palpation.
   2. auscultation.
   3. percussion.
   4. radiography.

7. Which drug may cause cardiovascular collapse in patients who are taking organic nitrate therapy?
   1. Alprostadil
   2. Sildenafil
   3. Papaverine
   4. Testosterone

8. Which drug actions are related to tamsulosin (Flomax) and doxazosin (Cardura; an alpha-adrenergic blocking agent)?
   1. Relax smooth muscle in the bladder neck and prostate
   2. Decrease testosterone levels
   3. Suppress prostatic tissue growth
   4. Reduce obstruction to urinary flow
   5. Increase resistance to urinary flow

9. Which drug actions are related to sildenafil (Viagra), vardenafil (Levitra), tadalafil (Cialis), and avanafil (Stendra)? **Select all that apply.**
   1. Relax smooth muscle in the corpus cavernosum.
   2. Decrease testosterone levels.
   3. Suppress prostatic tissue growth.
   4. Increase blood flow with subsequent erection.
   5. Increase resistance to urinary flow.

E. Matching

Match characteristics of drugs used to treat disorders of the male reproductive system in the numbered column with the drugs in the lettered column. Some terms may be used more than once.

1. _____ Increases arterial blood flow to penis and decreases venous outflow

2. _____ Replacement for low hormone levels in men

3. _____ Palliative treatment of advanced prostate cancer

4. _____ Examples are sildenafil (Viagra), vardenafil (Levitra), and tadalafil (Cialis)

5. _____ Relaxes smooth muscle in corpus cavernosum, increasing blood flow

6. _____ Used with luteinizing-hormone-releasing hormone (LHRH) to treat prostate cancer, decreasing testosterone level

A. Testosterone
B. Agents used to treat erectile dysfunction
C. Estramustine (Emcyt)
D. Testosterone inhibitors

PART III: CHALLENGE YOURSELF!

F. Getting Ready for NCLEX

Choose the most appropriate answer or select all that apply.

1. A healthy, 76-year-old male patient is concerned about his sexual function as he ages. What is the appropriate teaching the nurse should give?
   1. Erectile dysfunction is common in males over 70 years old.
   2. Despite normal age-related changes in the reproductive systems, in a healthy male spermatogenesis and the ability to have erections last a lifetime.
   3. Testosterone therapy is recommended after age 50 to maintain sexual function.
   4. Males do experience symptoms similar to menopause.

2. A semen analysis is required for a 30-year-old male who has been trying with his wife to start a family for the last 12 months and wants to assess his fertility. What should the nurse instruct him to do before giving the specimen?
   1. Refrigerate the specimen, if obtained at home, for up to 24 hours before bringing it to the laboratory.
   2. Use a rubber condom to collect the sample
   3. Abstain from sexual activity and alcohol for 2–3 days then collect specimen in a clean container.
   4. Eat a high-protein diet for 2–3 days before collecting a specimen.

3. The prostate-specific antigen (PSA) of a 46-year-old man is elevated. He is anxious that this means he has prostate cancer. What is the appropriate teaching the nurse can give this patient?
   1. The patient should contact an oncologist.
   2. Three positive PSA results should be done before any action is taken.
   3. The PSA can be elevated by many factors other than prostate cancer.
   4. Drugs given for BPH can increase the PSA, which must be considered when interpreting PSA results.

4. What should a nurse assess for after a urethral smear or stain is performed before letting the patient rise?
   1. Bleeding
   2. Postprocedural incontinence
   3. Inability to void
   4. Hypotension, bradycardia, and pallor

5. What is the post procedure nursing care for a cystoscopy? Select all that apply.
   1. Measure the patient's urine output for 24 hours.
   2. Urine will be pink-tinged.
   3. Report excessive bleeding.
   4. Limit fluids for 24 hours.
   5. Report inability to void.
   6. Advise patient that burning and hesitancy are common.

6. What should a nurse assess for after a patient is administered testosterone?
   1. Hypotension and fainting
   2. Hypertension and edema
   3. Blood pressure
   4. Liver function

7. What is a nursing intervention for immunotherapy?
   1. Macrophages collected from venous blood before each dose
   2. Advise patient he must not have immunotherapy if he is taking nitroglycerin
   3. Advise patient to seek medical attention for priapism
   4. Monitor for heart failure, dyspnea, edema, and fatigue

Male Reproductive Disorders

Go to http://evolve.elsevier.com/Linton/medsurg/ for additional activities and exercises.

NCLEX CATEGORIES

Health Promotion and Maintenance

Physiological Integrity: Pharmacological Therapies, Reduction of Risk Potential, Physiological Adaptation

PART I: MASTERING THE BASICS

A. Key Terms
Match the definition or description in the numbered column with the appropriate term in the lettered column.

1. _____ The foreskin is retracted and cannot be moved over the glans

2. _____ Infertile

3. _____ A term used to describe couples who have had unprotected intercourse over a 12-month period and have been unable to become pregnant

4. _____ As a result of poor hygiene, the foreskin may become inflamed and swollen, preventing retraction

5. _____ Inflammation of the epididymis

6. _____ Surgical removal of all or part of the prostate

7. _____ The inability to produce and maintain an erection for sexual intercourse; impotence

8. _____ Inflammation of the prostate gland

A. Epididymitis
B. Erectile dysfunction
C. Infertility
D. Paraphimosis
E. Phimosis
F. Prostatectomy
G. Prostatitis
H. Sterile

B. Erectile Dysfunction
Complete the statement in the numbered column with the most appropriate term in the lettered column. Some terms may be used more than once, and some may not be used.

1. _____ In erectile dysfunction, atherosclerosis compromises the ability to fill with blood because of _____.

2. _____ Two conditions in patients with diabetes mellitus that may contribute to erectile dysfunction are autonomic neuropathy and _____.

3. _____ The type of erectile dysfunction likely to be caused by high blood pressure and its treatment is _____.

4. _____ Two treatments that may be recommended for treating erectile dysfunction in the diabetic patient are papaverine self-injection and _____.

5. _____ Spinal cord injuries that are more likely to cause erectile dysfunction are those that are located _____.

6. _____ The most likely drugs to cause erectile dysfunction are _____.

A. Failure to store
B. Low
C. Antihypertensives
D. Failure to initiate
E. Atherosclerosis
F. Penile implant
G. Vascular surgery

H. High
I. Failure to fill
J. Antihistamines
K. Reduced blood flow
L. Neurologic disorders

PART II: PUTTING IT ALL TOGETHER

C. Multiple Choice/Multiple Response
Choose the most appropriate answer or select all that apply.

1. What are the three most common parts of the male reproductive system that may be affected by cancer? Select all that apply.
   1. Epididymis
   2. Penis
   3. Testicles
   4. Scrotum
   5. Prostate gland

2. Erectile dysfunction related to diabetes mellitus may be caused by:
   1. spinal cord injury.
   2. atherosclerosis.
   3. low hormone levels.
   4. medication side effects.

3. Autonomic neuropathy inhibits muscle relaxation of lacunar spaces of the erectile chambers, which may make:
   1. the patient anxious about performance.
   2. adequate filling of the penis with blood for an erection impossible.
   3. testosterone levels abnormally low.
   4. the patient sterile.

4. Transurethral prostatectomy (TURP) is the most common surgical procedure for benign prostatic hyperplasia (BPH). In this procedure:
   1. the prostate is approached through the bladder by way of a low abdominal incision.
   2. portions of the prostate are cut away through a resectoscope inserted into the urethra.
   3. access to the prostate is gained through an incision between the scrotum and the anus.
   4. the surgeon reaches the prostate through a low abdominal incision and opens the front of the prostate.

5. Which is the most common patient problem for the patient with BPH?
   1. Potential infection
   2. Impaired sexual function
   3. Pain
   4. Urinary obstruction

6. A common obstructive symptom of BPH is:
   1. urine retention.
   2. nocturia.
   3. frequency.
   4. hematuria.

7. The reason for bladder irrigation following a TURP procedure is to:
   1. decrease postoperative infection.
   2. prevent constriction of the urethra.
   3. prevent clot formation and obstruction.
   4. decrease urinary retention.

8. If postvoid dribbling occurs in a postoperative TURP patient after removal of the catheter, the nurse should:
   1. suggest perineal exercises.
   2. recommend biofeedback.
   3. use isotonic fluid for irrigation.
   4. monitor for signs of infection.

9. Drugs most likely to interfere with erection are:
   1. antihistamines.
   2. decongestants.
   3. analgesics.
   4. antihypertensives.

10. Which herb is thought by some to increase penile blood flow, although research has shown that this may not be valid?
    1. Ginkgo biloba
    2. Kava kava
    3. Garlic
    4. Oil of jasmine

11. Which is an established risk factor for testicular cancer?
    1. Multiple sex partners
    2. African American
    3. Caucasian
    4. High-fat diet

12. A cancer that occurs much more frequently among African-American men than Caucasians is:
    1. prostatic cancer.
    2. testicular cancer.
    3. penile cancer.
    4. bladder cancer.

13. Which intervention is appropriate for a patient with BPH?
    1. Place a rolled towel across the patient's thighs to elevate the scrotum and reduce pain.
    2. Provide bedrest, scrotal support, and local heat to the scrotum.
    3. Drink at least eight glasses of fluids throughout the day.
    4. Eat a high-protein diet.

14. Which is an irritative symptom of BPH?
    1. Nocturia
    2. Urine retention
    3. Postvoid dribbling
    4. Decreased force of the urinary stream

15. Which drugs may cause urinary retention in patients with BPH?
    1. Smooth muscle relaxants
    2. Cold remedies
    3. Analgesics
    4. Antacids

16. Which drug is given to a postprostatectomy patient to relieve bladder spasms?
    1. Propantheline bromide (Pro-Banthine)
    2. Tamsulosin (Flomax)
    3. Phenoxybenzamine HCl (Dibenzyline)
    4. Finasteride (Proscar)

17. Which herb is believed (but not proven) to relieve urinary symptoms associated with benign prostatic hyperplasia?
    1. Garlic
    2. Ginkgo biloba
    3. Siberian ginseng
    4. Saw palmetto

18. Which are treatment methods for a patient with epididymitis? Select all that apply.
    1. Bedrest
    2. Local heat
    3. Ice packs
    4. Sitz baths
    5. Analgesics
    6. Scrotal support

19. Which are factors that may trigger urinary retention in a patient with BPH? Select all that apply.
    1. Infections
    2. Delayed voiding
    3. Bedrest
    4. Antiinflammatory agents
    5. Antihistamines
    6. Chilling

PART III: CHALLENGE YOURSELF!

D. Getting Ready for NCLEX
Choose the most appropriate answer or select all that apply.

1. The nurse is taking care of a patient with testicular cancer. The nurse recognizes which problems are anticipated for this patient? Select all that apply.
    1. Anxiety
    2. Pain
    3. Urinary obstruction
    4. Potential injury
    5. Potential for fluid volume deficit
    6. Impaired self-concept

2. Which are nursing interventions for a patient with a prostatectomy who is experiencing pain related to urinary obstruction and bladder spasms? Select all that apply.
    1. Reposition tubing if urine is not draining.
    2. Inspect urine, dressing, and wound drainage for excess bleeding.
    3. Watch for water intoxication.
    4. Monitor for signs of infection [temperature above 101°F (38.3°C)].
    5. Give antispasmodics and analgesics as prescribed.

3. Which are nursing interventions for a patient with a prostatectomy who is experiencing potential infection related to invasive procedures of the urinary tract or catheterization? Select all that apply.
    1. Maintain urine flow.
    2. Use strict aseptic technique.
    3. Keep closed urinary drainage systems intact.
    4. Monitor for signs of infection [temperature above 101°F (38.3°C); purulent wound drainage, and confusion].
    5. Monitor output.

4. A patient with BPH has been instructed by the nurse to void promptly when the urge is felt and to space fluid intake throughout the day. Two hours after being admitted to the hospital, the patient states he is unable to void and his bladder is distended. What is the appropriate nursing intervention?
   1. Restrict fluids.
   2. Notify the health care provider.
   3. Record a complete description of urinary symptoms.
   4. Observe the patient's urine for hematuria.

5. A patient with BPH is admitted to the hospital for a TURP procedure. The nurse notes that the catheter output is less than the irrigating fluid delivered. Which is the priority problem for this patient?
   1. Potential fluid volume deficit related to hemorrhage
   2. Potential infection related to invasive procedures of the urinary tract and surgical incision
   3. Pain related to tissue trauma and bladder spasms
   4. Urinary obstruction related to enlarged prostate

E. Nursing Care Plan

Refer to Nursing Care Plan, The Patient with a Prostatectomy, in the book, and answer questions 1–3.

A 77-year-old retired radio announcer underwent a TURP this morning. He returned to the nursing unit 3 hours ago. He complains of genital pain and states that he feels like he needs to empty his bladder. Intravenous fluids are infusing at 100 mL/h to a right forearm peripheral IV. A three-way Foley is in place, taped to his inner thigh, and draining freely into a collection bag. Irrigation fluid is set at the prescribed flow rate. Urine is pink, not viscous. Several clots observed in bag. Vital signs are within normal limits.

1. What is the priority problem for this patient?
   1. Potential fluid volume deficit
   2. Pain
   3. Potential infection
   4. Potential injury

2. The nurse is observing the patient for early signs of fluid volume deficit. Which is an early sign of fluid volume deficit?
   1. Blood in urine
   2. Drowsiness
   3. Increasing heart rate
   4. Confusion

3. The nurse notices that the urine is no longer draining freely. What is the action the nurse should take first?
   1. Notify the health care provider.
   2. Irrigate according to agency policy.
   3. Monitor for signs of infection.
   4. Reposition the tubing.

F. Next-Generation NCLEX® Examination-Style Questions

A 64-year-old African American male client presents to his primary care provider (PCP) with difficulty urinating. The nurse reviews the past medical history, physician's progress notes, and vital signs.

Medical History:
Diabetes
Tobacco use
Hypertension

Physician's Progress Notes:
A 64-year-old African-American male client presents with complaints of hesitancy, weak urinary stream, and straining when voiding. He states that his father was diagnosed with benign prostatic hypertrophy (BPH) when he was 65 years old.

Vital Signs:

Blood Pressure	138/72 mmHg
Pulse	82 beats/minute
Respirations	18 breaths/minute
Temperature	98.8°F

1. Which of the following instructions should be included in the client's teaching plan to decrease urinary symptoms? Select all that apply.
   1. Apply heat via a warm compress to the pelvis
   2. Eat a diet low in green leafy vegetables
   3. Maintain fluid intake of 1500–2000 mL/day
   4. Restrict fluid for 2 hours before bedtime
   5. Avoid caffeine and alcohol
   6. Complete daily bladder training exercises
   7. Take broad-spectrum antibiotics daily

A 60-year-old male client presents to his primary care provider (PCP) for the second time in one month with a urinary tract infection (UTI). The nurse reviews the past medical history, physical assessment, and physician's progress notes.

Past Medical History:
Benign prostatic hypertrophy (BPH)
Gout

Physical Assessment:
The client states, "It feels like I cannot empty my bladder. It is worse than it has ever been." Assessment findings include active bowel sounds to all four quadrants, distended bladder, and clear lung sounds bilaterally.

Physician's Progress Notes:
Results of the digital rectal examination indicate need for prostatectomy. The client appears tearful and states, "Why is this happening to me?" *L. Lawson, MD*

Complete the following sentence by choosing from the list of options below.

2. The nursing diagnosis that requires immediate follow-up includes _____1_____ related to _____2_____.

Options for 1	Options for 2
Fear	Enlarged prostate
Urinary obstruction	Invasive procedure
Ineffective health management	Lack of knowledge

Sexually Transmitted Infections

Go to http://evolve.elsevier.com/Linton/medsurg/ for additional activities and exercises.

NCLEX CATEGORIES

Safe and Effective Care Environment: Safety and Infection Control

Health Promotion and Maintenance

Physiological Integrity: Pharmacological Therapies, Reduction of Risk Potential, Physiological Adaptation

PART I: MASTERING THE BASICS

A. Key Terms

Match the definition in the numbered column with the most appropriate term in the lettered column. Answers may be used more than once.

1. _____ Infections that thrive when the immune system is impaired

2. _____ Conditions that can be transmitted during intimate contact

3. _____ An infection of the ovaries, fallopian tubes, and pelvic area

4. _____ During this period of a disease, there are no signs or symptoms of the disease

5. _____ Lesion that is the first sign of syphilis

A. Chancre
B. Latent
C. Opportunistic infections
D. Pelvic inflammatory disease (PID)
E. Sexually transmitted infections (STIs)

PART II: PUTTING IT ALL TOGETHER

B. Multiple Choice/Multiple Response

Choose the most appropriate answer or select all that apply.

1. What percentage of all cases of STIs involve people between the ages of 15 and 24?
   1. 50%
   2. 65%
   3. 75%
   4. 85%

2. Serologic tests for STIs are designed to detect infectious diseases by measuring:
   1. white blood cells.
   2. red blood cells.
   3. clotting factors.
   4. antigens or antibodies.

3. Patients with gonococcal, chlamydial, HSV, *Trichomonas*, or yeast infections often have:
   1. vaginal or penile discharge.
   2. increased temperature or tachycardia.
   3. generalized infection and rash.
   4. mouth sores and pharyngitis.

4. If males have a whitish- or greenish-colored discharge from the penis and complain of a burning sensation during urination, this is suggestive of:
   1. HSV infection.
   2. chlamydia.
   3. gonorrhea.
   4. syphilis.

5. Female patients with gonorrhea are likely to have vaginal discharge, a burning sensation during urination, abnormal menstruation, and:
   1. dyspnea.
   2. abdominal pain.
   3. hypotension.
   4. edema.

6. Paralysis, mental illness, blindness, and heart disease may occur as complications of:
   1. HSV infection.
   2. cervicitis.
   3. syphilis.
   4. gonorrhea.

7. Two screening tests for syphilis include the rapid plasma reagin (RPR) and the:
   1. VDRL.
   2. RBC.
   3. WBC.
   4. BUN.

8. The treatment of choice for syphilis is:
   1. doxycycline calcium (Vibramycin).
   2. erythromycin.
   3. tetracycline.
   4. penicillin.

9. After completing treatment for primary or secondary syphilis, the patient is advised not to engage in sexual activity for:
   1. 5 days.
   2. 2 weeks.
   3. 1 month.
   4. 6 months.

10. If untreated, sterility, prostatitis in males, and pelvic inflammatory disease in females may result from:
    1. syphilis.
    2. gonorrhea.
    3. HSV infection.
    4. genital warts.

11. Which STI can be transmitted through the placenta, causing an infant to be born with the disease?
    1. HSV infection
    2. Gonorrhea
    3. Syphilis
    4. Chlamydia

12. With an STI, common reasons that patients give for seeking medical care include pain, fever, lesions, or genital:
    1. itching.
    2. edema.
    3. bleeding.
    4. discharge.

13. Specimens collected during a pelvic exam are handled as:
    1. infective material.
    2. clean specimens.
    3. sterile specimens.
    4. chemically unstable material.

14. Untreated STIs can lead to serious complications such as PID and:
    1. edema.
    2. sterility.
    3. shock.
    4. kidney failure.

15. Which emergency drugs for possible hypersensitivity reactions need to be kept on hand when administering drug therapy to patients with STIs? Select all that apply.
    1. Acyclovir (Zovirax)
    2. Diphenhydramine hydrochloride (Benadryl)
    3. Didanosine (Videx)
    4. Pentamidine isethionate (Pentam)
    5. Epinephrine
    6. Corticosteroids

16. Females with HSV infections are advised to have annual Papanicolaou smears because they are at increased risk of:
    1. pyelonephritis.
    2. cervical cancer.
    3. kidney failure.
    4. AIDS.

17. How is HSV transmitted? Select all that apply.
    1. Air droplets
    2. Mouth-to-nose contact
    3. Fecal contamination
    4. Hand contact
    5. Sexual contact

18. Which is the drug of choice for treating HSV?
    1. Penicillin G
    2. Tetracycline hydrochloride (Achromycin)
    3. Acyclovir (Zovirax)
    4. Metronidazole (Flagyl)

19. Which STI has symptoms similar to those of gonorrhea?
    1. Syphilis
    2. Herpes simplex
    3. Chlamydia
    4. HIV

20. Gonorrhea can be found in the pharynx, urethra, uterus, and:
    1. kidney.
    2. rectum.
    3. heart.
    4. lungs.

21. Gonorrhea is transmitted most often by:
    1. infected mothers to newborn infants.
    2. direct sexual contact.
    3. skin lacerations of medical personnel.
    4. toilet seats and doorknobs.

22. The heart, joints, skin, and meninges may become involved with which systemic infection?
    1. Gonorrhea
    2. Syphilis
    3. Chlamydia
    4. Genital warts

23. The treatment for gonorrhea is a single dose of IM ceftriaxone sodium (Rocephin) and:
    1. azithromycin.
    2. doxycycline.
    3. penicillin.
    4. tetracycline.

24. What is the treatment of choice for a patient who has trichomoniasis?
    1. Penicillin
    2. Tinidazole (Tindamax)
    3. Acyclovir
    4. Tetracycline

25. Which is the cause of genital warts?
    1. Human papillomavirus (HPV)
    2. HSV
    3. *Chlamydia trachomatis*
    4. *Neisseria gonorrhoeae*

26. What do Papanicolaou smears detect?
    1. Syphilis
    2. Gonorrhea
    3. Cancer of the cervix
    4. HSV infection

27. Which is the most common bacterial STI because people have no symptoms?
    1. Syphilis
    2. Gonorrhea
    3. Venereal warts
    4. Chlamydia

28. Some STIs are painless, but patients may have pain associated with oral lesions, rectal lesions, or:
    1. vaginal bleeding.
    2. genital edema.
    3. nerve irritation.
    4. pelvic infection.

29. Which statements are related to syphilis? Select all that apply.
    1. Characterized by a papule that becomes a painless red ulcer within a week.
    2. Patients are cured when the chancre disappears.
    3. The first sign of this infection is a chancre.
    4. During the secondary stage, pustules, fever, sore throat, and aching are symptoms that occur.
    5. Disease leaves the patient unable to resist opportunistic infections.

30. Which statements are related to *Chlamydia trachomatis*? Select all that apply.
    1. An infection that is transmitted by contact with the mucous membranes in the mouth, eyes, urethra, vagina, or rectum
    2. Characterized by genital irritation; a thin, gray discharge, and a fishy odor
    3. Treatment consists of antiviral drugs
    4. Characterized by a cauliflower-like mass
    5. Symptoms include a penile discharge that is initially thin and then creamy, accompanied by painful urination
    6. The most common STI in the United States

31. A patient with gonorrhea is being treated with Rocephin. Which side effects would the nurse expect to see? Select all that apply.
    1. Discoloration of teeth
    2. Allergic reactions in patients allergic to cephalosporins or penicillin
    3. Nephrotoxicity
    4. Superinfections
    5. Tachycardia

32. Which STIs can be cured with antimicrobial drug therapy? Select all that apply.
    1. Herpes simplex (HSV-2)
    2. Chlamydia
    3. Genital warts
    4. Gonorrhea
    5. Syphilis

33. Which are signs and symptoms of chlamydia infection? Select all that apply.
    1. Greenish-yellow urethral discharge
    2. May be no signs or symptoms
    3. Painful, frequent urination in males
    4. Lower abdominal pain in females
    5. Enlarged lymph nodes

34. Which are signs and symptoms of syphilis? Select all that apply.
    1. Round ulcer with well-defined margin (chancre) present
    2. Sore throat
    3. Regional lymphadenopathy
    4. Profuse, watery vaginal discharge
    5. Presence of genital warts

35. Which drugs are used to treat gonorrhea? Select all that apply.
    1. Cipro
    2. Bactrim
    3. Penicillin G
    4. Erythromycin
    5. Rocephin
    6. Azithromycin
    7. Flagyl
    8. Acyclovir

36. Which group of drugs is used to treat genital herpes infections?
    1. Antibacterials
    2. Tetracyclines
    3. Sulfonamides
    4. Antivirals

37. Which STIs involve a vaginal or penile discharge for which smears and cultures are taken for diagnosis? Select all that apply.
    1. Chlamydial infection
    2. HSV
    3. Trichomoniasis
    4. Syphilis
    5. Venereal warts
    6. HIV infection

38. Which is a low-risk type of HPV?
    1. Cervical cancer
    2. Anal cancer
    3. Genital warts; condylomata acuminata
    4. Enlarged lymph nodes

PART III: CHALLENGE YOURSELF!

C. Getting Ready for NCLEX
Choose the most appropriate answer or select all that apply.

1. The nurse is taking care of a patient with syphilis who is being treated with penicillin G. Which manifestations may occur during the first 24 hours in patients with syphilis who are treated with penicillin? Select all that apply.
   1. Numbness of the extremities
   2. Sore throat
   3. Headache
   4. Fever
   5. Muscle aches

2. The nurse is taking care of a patient with genital warts. Which medical treatments would the nurse expect to be used for a patient with genital warts? Select all that apply.
   1. Administration of penicillin
   2. Cryotherapy
   3. Surgical removal
   4. Injection of interferon into the lesions
   5. Use of spermicidal gel

3. The nurse is taking care of a patient with gonorrhea and is implementing a discharge teaching plan. Which are ways to reduce the risk of gonorrhea that the nurse would explain to this patient? Select all that apply.
   1. Have all sexual partners treated.
   2. Take the complete prescription of Cipro or tetracycline, even if symptoms disappear.
   3. Avoid unprotected sex until patient and sexual partners have been treated.
   4. Ensure that VDRL blood studies are done.
   5. Encourage douching before and after each sexual contact.

4. The nurse is presenting an education program to a school district advisory council meeting about prevention of STIs. Which are considered unsafe sexual practices in preventing transmission of infection that the nurse would include in the presentation? Select all that apply.
   1. Oral sex without condom
   2. Mutual masturbation
   3. Vaginal or anal intercourse with properly used condom
   4. Ingestion of urine or semen
   5. Open-mouthed kissing

5. Which are common problems for a patient with an STI? Select all that apply.
   1. Fluid volume deficit related to anorexia
   2. Inadequate nutrition related to vomiting
   3. Altered sexual function related to fear of transmission
   4. Impaired self-concept related to diagnosis
   5. Potential injury related to the disease process
   6. Pain related to lesions and inflammation

6. When collecting a sample of vaginal discharge for culture and sensitivity tests, the nurse or person collecting the sample always wears:
   1. goggles.
   2. a mask.
   3. gloves.
   4. a gown.

7. A discussion of sexual behavior can be awkward for the nurse and the patient. Before nurses can deal with patients' sexuality, they must:
   1. present the patient with written information.
   2. be aware of their own values.
   3. ask the patient to demonstrate understanding of the material presented by stating information in his/her own words.
   4. check the patient's chart to see whether he/she has an STI.

8. A patient problem related to possible effects of STI or partner reaction to the STI is:
   1. pain.
   2. potential injury.
   3. anxiety.
   4. disrupted tissue integrity.

9. What is the most important problem related to the stigma associated with STIs, shame, and anger?
   1. Altered sexual function
   2. Pain
   3. Inadequate coping
   4. Potential infection

10. To identify and treat infected individuals so that transmission of the STI can be slowed, the nurse recognizes that partners may be notified and confirmed cases of certain STIs must be reported to the:
    1. United States Department of Health.
    2. hospital administrator.
    3. Department of Public Safety.
    4. local public health department.

D. Next-Generation NCLEX® Examination-Style Questions

A 23-year-old woman comes to the health care provider's office with painful urination, abdominal pain, and vaginal discharge of 3 days duration. The nurse reviews the provider's progress notes and vital signs.

Progress Notes:

7/18/21 0900: A 23-year-old female presents with complaints of painful urination, abdominal pain, and vaginal discharge of 3 days duration. Client has had no serious illnesses or injuries. She reports that she has had two sexual partners in the past 6 months, with her most recent contact 2 weeks ago, when a condom was not used. The patient is concerned about HIV and STIs. She states that she cannot believe she was "so stupid" and is very embarrassed about these symptoms. Physical exam findings are normal except for the genital and pelvic examination. Her vaginal tissues are red and edematous, with a whitish discharge. A smear was taken for examination. Results indicate gonorrhea. A single dose of IM Rocephin was ordered. The client was provided with a prescription for 7 days of Vibramycin due to possible risk of chlamydia. E. Jacobson, FNP.

Vital Signs:

Blood Pressure	130/82 mm Hg
Pulse	84 beats/minute
Respirations	14 breaths/minute

1. Based on the client information provided, what are risk factors for this patient who has gonorrhea? Select all that apply.
    1. Complaints of vaginal discharge
    2. Painful urination
    3. History of no serious illness or injury
    4. Two recent sexual partners
    5. Vaginal tissues are red and edematous
    6. Unprotected sex 2 weeks ago
    7. Client states that she cannot believe she was "so stupid"

An 18-year-old female client presents to her primary care provider for her pap smear. The nurse reviews the provider's progress notes.

Progress Notes:

08/20/21 0800: An 18-year-old female presents with three Condylomata warts located on the vulva and vagina. Warts are pink and soft, with a cauliflower-like appearance. The client states she has been sexually active for 1 year and does not use condoms. Based on observation, the client appears to have genital warts. Biopsy ordered. Nurse to provide further patient teaching. *Sally Joe, MD*.

---

2. Based on the client information provided, which patient teaching would the nurse need to provide? Select all that apply.
    1. "You will need annual Papanicolaou tests to screen for cervical cancer."
    2. "Antibiotics will treat the warts."
    3. "You may resume sexual activity in 1 week."
    4. "Latex condoms may help reduce the risk of spreading genital warts."
    5. "Sexual contact should be avoided while warts are present."
    6. "Your sexual partners should be notified."

Integumentary System Introduction

chapter

56

Go to http://evolve.elsevier.com/Linton/medsurg/ for additional activities and exercises.

NCLEX CATEGORIES

Physiological Integrity: Reduction of Risk Potential

Physiological Integrity: Physiological Adaptation

PART I: MASTERING THE BASICS

A. Key Terms
Match the definition in the numbered column with the term in the lettered column.

1. _____ Benign tumors filled with blood vessels

2. _____ Topical drug capable of dissolving keratin

3. _____ Mole

A. Angiomas
B. Nevi
C. Keratolytics

B. Diagnostic Tests
Match the description or definition in the numbered column with the most appropriate term in the lettered column. Some terms may be used more than once, and some terms may not be used.

1. _____ A test used to diagnose viral skin infections

2. _____ Used to diagnose fungal infections by studying a skin specimen

3. _____ An examination in which the patient's skin is inspected under a black light in a darkened room

4. _____ A test used to identify allergens in which common irritants are applied to the skin

5. _____ The removal of tissue for microscopic examination

6. _____ A specimen no deeper than the dermis is obtained with a scalpel

7. _____ The type of biopsy in which a circular tool cuts around the lesion, which is then lifted and severed

8. _____ The type of biopsy indicated for deep specimens in which sutures are required to close the site

9. _____ Used to detect mites

A. Biopsy
B. Punch biopsy
C. Wood's light
D. Shave biopsy
E. Surgical excision
F. Tzanck test
G. Patch testing
H. Scabies scraping
I. KOH examination

C. Skin Lesions

Match the characteristics and examples of common skin lesions in the numbered column with the letters in Figure 56.2 from the book. Some answers are used more than once and some are not used.

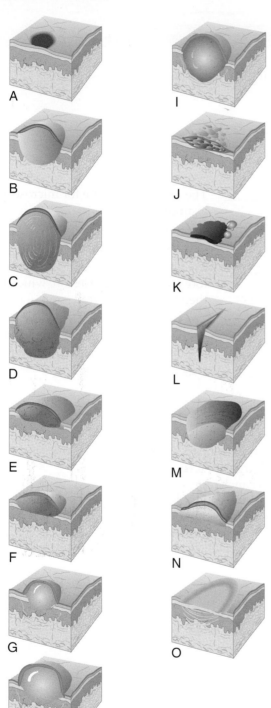

1. _____ Type of lesion in patients with pressure sores and chancres

2. _____ Superficial, irregular swelling caused by fluid accumulation

3. _____ Example is a blister

4. _____ Characterized by dry or greasy skin flakes

5. _____ Distinct flat area with color different from surrounding tissue

6. _____ Raised, solid lesion that may be hard or soft and may extend deeper into dermis than papule

7. _____ Thick, dried exudate remaining after vesicles rupture

8. _____ Any raised, fluid-filled cavity, small in diameter

9. _____ Raised, solid lesion > 1 cm in diameter

10. _____ Any raised, solid lesion with clearly defined margins

11. _____ Distinct linear crack extending into dermis

12. _____ Depression deeper than erosion that may bleed

Match the example or description in the numbered column with the appropriate type of lesion in the lettered column.

13. _____ Freckle, petechia, hypopigmentation

14. _____ Mole, wart

15. _____ Herpes simplex, herpes zoster

16. _____ Acne, impetigo

17. _____ Vitiligo

18. _____ Psoriasis

19. _____ Fibroma

20. _____ Allergic response, insect bite, hives

A. Plaque
B. Wheal
C. Papule
D. Patch
E. Pustule
F. Vesicle
G. Nodule
H. Macule

D. Parts of the Skin

Using Figure 56.1 from the book, label the parts of the skin (A–I) from the terms provided (1–9).

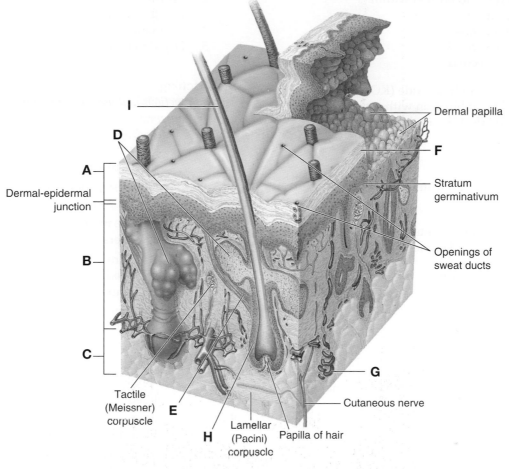

1. _____ Sebaceous gland
2. _____ Hair follicle
3. _____ Dermis
4. _____ Hair shaft
5. _____ Stratum corneum

6. _____ Epidermis
7. _____ Arrector pili muscle
8. _____ Sweat gland
9. _____ Subcutaneous tissue

PART II: PUTTING IT ALL TOGETHER

E. Multiple Choice/Multiple Response

Choose the most appropriate answer or select all that apply.

1. Which are changes that occur in older adults? Select all that apply.
   1. Increased elastic tissue
   2. Increased facial hair
   3. Increased subcutaneous tissue
   4. Thickening of capillaries
   5. Thinning of scalp hair

2. Nevi (moles) are carefully inspected for pigmentation, ulcerations, changes in surrounding skin, and:
   1. vascular irregularities.
   2. amount of edema.
   3. amount of pus.
   4. irregularities in shape.

3. When assessing capillary refill, after applying pressure to cause blanching and then releasing the pressure, the nurse should observe that the color returns to normal within:
   1. 1–2 minutes.
   2. 3–5 seconds.
   3. 30–40 seconds.
   4. 50–60 seconds.

4. The potassium hydroxide (KOH) examination is used in combination with a culture to diagnose infections of the skin, hair, or nails that are:
   1. viral.
   2. bacterial.
   3. caused by parasites.
   4. fungal.

5. Which are assessments of the fingernails and toenails that nurses monitor? Select all that apply.
   1. Capillary refill
   2. Edema
   3. Hemorrhage
   4. Mobility
   5. Color of nail bed

6. A type of therapy used in the treatment of psoriasis, vitiligo, and chronic eczema is:
   1. phototherapy.
   2. soaks.
   3. wet wraps.
   4. débridement.

7. Vitamin A is essential for:
   1. blood clotting.
   2. bone formation.
   3. wound healing.
   4. healthy skin.

8. Food allergies can cause:
   1. scabies.
   2. basal cell carcinoma.
   3. psoriasis.
   4. atopic dermatitis.

9. Which is a topical herbal preparation used as an emollient?
   1. Aloe
   2. Angelica
   3. Balm of Gilead
   4. Ginseg

10. Which of the following skin changes are related to malnutrition? Select all that apply.
    1. Hives
    2. Pruritus
    3. Cracked skin
    4. Dermatitis
    5. Dry skin (xerosis)

A. Matching

Match the actions and uses in the numbered column with the appropriate drug classification in the lettered column (example drugs shown in parentheses).

1. _____ Interfere with viral replication
2. _____ Decrease proliferation of epidermal cells in psoriasis
3. _____ Reduce inflammation in various skin disorders
4. _____ Kill parasites and their eggs; used to treat pediculosis (lice) and scabies (mite) infestations
5. _____ Dissolve keratin and slow bacterial growth; used to treat acne and psoriasis
6. _____ Effective against fungi; used to treat fungal infections
7. _____ Used to treat psoriasis
8. _____ Destroy microorganisms; used to treat skin infections
9. _____ Reduce formation of comedones; increase mitosis of epithelial cells; used to treat acne

A. Keratolytics (coal tar)
B. Topical antibacterials (bacitracin)
C. Antiviral agents (acyclovir)
D. Photosensitivity drugs (methoxsalen)
E. Topical antifungal agents (nystatin)
F. Topical antiinflammatories (hydrocortisone)
G. Vitamin A derivatives [tretinoin (Retin-A)]
H. Pediculicides and scabicides [crotamiton (Eurax)]
I. Antipsoriatics (anthralin)

PART III: CHALLENGE YOURSELF!

G. Getting Ready for NCLEX

Choose the most appropriate answer or select all that apply.

1. The nurse is taking care of a patient who has a skin biopsy scheduled. When a skin biopsy is scheduled, the provider may advise the patient to avoid which drug before the procedure to reduce bleeding?
   1. Diphenhydramine
   2. Tetracycline
   3. Aminophylline
   4. Aspirin

2. Which foods contain nutrients that are vital for healthy skin? Select all that apply.
   1. Liver
   2. Sweet potato
   3. Bananas
   4. Cantaloupe
   5. Spinach
   6. Carrots

3. A nurse is teaching a class about the functions of skin. What would be the correct teaching about how the skin protects the body?
   1. Shields underlying tissues from trauma and pathogens and prevents excess loss of fluids from those tissues
   2. Alters the diameter of surface blood vessels and cools the body through sweating
   3. Creates an oily barrier (sebum) that holds in water
   4. Contains an extensive blood vessel network that can store as much as 10% of the body's total blood volume

4. When completing an assessment of an older patient's skin, what are some of the age-related changes the nurse may expect to see? Select all that apply.
   1. Thinning of skin layers resulting in wrinkling
   2. Increased sebum production by sebaceous glands
   3. Dryness and itching increase
   4. Development of skin lesions including lentigines, acrochordons, and angiomas
   5. Size and number of sweat glands decreased

Skin Disorders

Go to http://evolve.elsevier.com/Linton/medsurg/ for additional activities and exercises.

NCLEX CATEGORIES

Health Promotion and Maintenance

Physiological Integrity: Pharmacological Therapies, Reduction of Risk Potential, Physiological Adaptation

PART I: MASTERING THE BASICS

A. Key Terms

1. _____   Inflammation of the skin where two skin surfaces touch

2. _____   Removal of debris and necrotic (dead) tissue from a wound

3. _____   One of several disorders referred to as *eczema*

A. Débridement
B. Dermatitis
C. Intertrigo

B. Skin Cancers

Match the statement in the numbered column with the most appropriate term in the lettered column. Answers may be used more than once.

1. _____   Type of carcinomas, unlike basal cell carcinomas, that grow rapidly and metastasize

2. _____   A chronic autoimmune condition in which bullae (blisters) develop on the face, back, chest, groin, and umbilicus

3. _____   A condition with painless, nodular lesions that have a pearly appearance

4. _____   Disorder that arises from the pigment-producing cells in the skin

5. _____   Characterized by scaly ulcers or raised lesions

6. _____   Carcinomas that grow slowly and rarely metastasize, but they should be removed because they can cause local tissue destruction

7. _____   Usually caused by overuse of alcohol and tobacco

8. _____   Treatment used is Mohs surgery to determine margins of malignancy

A. Melanoma
B. Squamous cell carcinoma
C. Pemphigus
D. Basal cell carcinoma

C. Burn Depth

Match the description in the numbered column with the type of burn in the lettered column. Answers may be used more than once.

1. _____   Pink to red and painful, like a sunburn

2. _____   Large, thick-walled blisters or edema

3. _____   Burned tissue lacking sensation

4. _____   Burn affecting only the epidermis

5. _____   Burn involving the epidermis, dermis, and underlying tissues, including fat, muscle, and bone

6. _____   Burned tissue is painful and sensitive to cold air

7. _____   Blistered, weepy, and pale to red or pink

8. _____   Dry, leathery, and sometimes red, white, brown, or black

9. _____   Weeping, cherry-red, exposed dermis

10. _____   A severe sunburn

A. Superficial burn
B. Superficial partial-thickness burn
C. Deep partial-thickness burn
D. Full-thickness burn

D. Burns

Match the appearance characteristics in the numbered column with the sensations experienced (in the same depth of burn) in the lettered column.

1. _____ Large, thick-walled blisters covering extensive areas (vesiculation); edema; mottled red base; broken epidermis; wet, shiny, weeping surface

2. _____ Variable, for example, deep red, black, white, brown; dry surface; edema; fat exposed; tissue disrupted

3. _____ Usually appears blistered or weepy and pale to red or pink

A. Little pain, insensate
B. Painful, sensitive to cold air
C. Typically very painful

Match the definition or description in the numbered column with the most appropriate term in the lettered column. Some terms may be used more than once.

4. _____ Removal of necrotic tissue from a wound

5. _____ Covering a wound with skin

6. _____ Can be reduced by the use of pressure dressings in the early stages of care

7. _____ May be accomplished by mechanical means, surgical excision, or enzymes

8. _____ Can be reduced by the use of custom-fitted garments that apply continuous pressure 24 hours a day

A. Skin grafting
B. Scarring
C. Débridement

E. Plastic Surgery

Match the conditions treated with plastic surgery in the numbered column with the type of surgery used in the lettered column. Answers may be used more than once.

1. _____ Birthmarks

2. _____ Excess tissue around the eyes

3. _____ Developmental defects

4. _____ Disfiguring scars

5. _____ Receding chin

6. _____ Facial wrinkles

A. Aesthetic surgery
B. Reconstructive surgery

F. Skin Infestations

Match the signs and symptoms of skin infestations in the numbered column with infestation in the lettered column.

1. _____ Thin, red lines on skin; itching

2. _____ Itching of hairy areas of body (head, pubis); nits (eggs) seen as tiny white particles attached to hair shafts

A. Lice
B. Scabies

PART II: PUTTING IT ALL TOGETHER

G. Multiple Choice/Multiple Response

Choose the most appropriate answer or select all that apply.

1. The most common problem for patients with pruritus is potential for skin breakdown related to:
   1. excessive dryness.
   2. scratching.
   3. moist environment.
   4. inadequate circulation.

2. A nursing problem for the patient with atopic dermatitis may include the potential for infection related to:
   1. soap or skin lotion allergies.
   2. self-care practices.
   3. poor peripheral circulation.
   4. breaks in skin.

3. The assessment of patients with seborrheic dermatitis includes inspecting affected areas for:
   1. bleeding and exudate.
   2. edema and redness.
   3. scales and crusts.
   4. yellow skin and ascites.

4. A common risk factor for developing candidiasis is:
   1. hypertension.
   2. antibiotic therapy.
   3. emotional stress.
   4. tachycardia.

5. The nurse advises the patient with shingles that the condition is communicable to people who have never been exposed to:
   1. measles.
   2. pertussis.
   3. chickenpox.
   4. mumps.

6. The most serious form of skin cancer is:
   1. basal cell carcinoma.
   2. melanoma.
   3. squamous cell carcinoma.
   4. cutaneous T-cell lymphoma.

7. Following a burn injury, plasma leaks into the tissue due to increased capillary:
   1. constriction.
   2. dilation.
   3. production.
   4. permeability.

8. After a burn injury, shifts in fluids and electrolytes cause local edema and a decrease in:
   1. respiratory rate.
   2. CNS stimulation.
   3. cardiac output.
   4. red blood cell production.

9. A patient with a burn experiences a shift of plasma proteins from the capillaries. This is likely to result in:
   1. hypoproteinemia.
   2. increased blood volume.
   3. dehydration.
   4. increased urine output.

10. Which is a complication of untreated fluid shifts in burn patients?
    1. Hypovolemic shock
    2. Kidney failure
    3. Pneumonia
    4. Convulsions

11. What should be included in the teaching plan for a patient with atopic dermatitis? Select all that apply.
    1. Avoid constrictive clothing.
    2. Use sunscreens and moisturizers.
    3. Topical corticosteroids provide the best control of inflammation.
    4. It is helpful to take nystatin for itching.
    5. Malaise, chills, and fever may occur with local tenderness and redness.

12. Acne lesions develop when there is:
    1. increased fatty food intake.
    2. increased sebum production.
    3. increased chocolate intake.
    4. poor hygiene.

13. Which drug used to remove heavy scales in patients with psoriasis can stain normal skin and hair?
    1. Tazarotene (Tazorac)
    2. Glucocorticoids
    3. Methotrexate sodium
    4. Anthralin (Anthra-Derm)

14. Which skin disorder characterized by irritation and redness in body folds is common among patients in long-term care facilities?
    1. Intertrigo
    2. Impetigo
    3. Candidiasis
    4. Pemphigus

15. Which should not be used in patients with intertrigo because it supports the growth of *C. albicans*?
    1. Topical corticosteroid
    2. Cornstarch
    3. Anthralin (Anthra-Derm)
    4. Moisturizer

16. Who is at greatest risk for skin cancer?
    1. Caucasians
    2. African Americans
    3. Native Americans
    4. Hispanics

17. A prominent symptom of psoriasis, dermatitis, eczema, and insect bites is:
    1. fever.
    2. pain.
    3. pruritus.
    4. edema.

18. If one arm and one leg are burned, what is the estimated burn size, according to the rule of nines?
    1. 18%
    2. 27%
    3. 36%
    4. 54%

19. The burn patient is at great risk for:
    1. hyperthermia.
    2. paralysis.
    3. edema.
    4. infection.

20. A patient has just been prescribed isotretinoin (Accutane) for resistant acne. Which are teaching points for this patient? Select all that apply.
    1. A serious adverse effect of isotretinoin (Accutane) is fetal deformities.
    2. Isotretinoin (Accutane) can cause mental depression, possibly leading to suicidal ideation.
    3. Do not apply to eyes, mouth, or angles of the nose.
    4. Avoid sun exposure and use sunscreen.
    5. A common side effect is candidiasis.

21. Which are true statements about acne skin disorders? Select all that apply.
    1. Mild cases of acne respond well to acyclovir (Zovirax).
    2. Comedones (whiteheads and blackheads), pustules, and cysts are characteristics of acne.
    3. Two oral antibiotics that are frequently given for acne are tetracycline and erythromycin.
    4. A drug prescribed for patients if acne is severe and unresponsive to antibiotics is isotretinoin (Accutane).
    5. Acne is a condition in which androgenic hormones cause increased sebum production and bacteria proliferation, causing hair follicles to block and become inflamed.

22. Which are true statements about herpes zoster virus? Select all that apply.
    1. Older adults are especially susceptible to complications, including ophthalmic involvement, from herpes zoster virus.
    2. Patients with herpes zoster virus exhibit early symptoms of heightened sensitivity along a nerve pathway, pain, and itching.
    3. Cold sores or fever blisters are oral lesions caused by herpes zoster virus.
    4. The sites most often infected by herpes zoster virus are the nose, lips, cheeks, ears, and genitalia.
    5. Wet dressings soaked in Burow's solution may be used to treat lesions associated with herpes zoster virus.
    6. Herpes zoster infection is commonly called *shingles*.

23. Which are true statements about candidiasis? Select all that apply.
    1. Candidiasis infections, which are manifested as red lesions with white plaques, are found on the mucous membranes.
    2. Three common sites for candidiasis include the mouth, skin, and vagina.
    3. Candidiasis is a bacterial infection caused by herpes simplex.
    4. Oral candidiasis is treated with nystatin.
    5. One area that is susceptible to candidiasis, owing to the constant moisture found there, is an ostomy site.

24. Which are true statements about impetigo? Select all that apply.
    1. Vesicle or pustule that ruptures, leaving a thick crust
    2. Inflamed hair follicles with white pustules
    3. Inflamed skin and subcutaneous tissue with deep, inflamed nodules
    4. Treated with antibiotic therapy: erythromycin or dicloxacillin
    5. Characterized by scaly ulcers or raised lesions

25. Which are true statements about cellulitis? Select all that apply.
    1. Local tenderness and redness at first, then malaise, chills, and fever
    2. At first, small shiny lesions, then they enlarge and become rough
    3. Treated with electrical current to destroy lesion followed by removal with curette, cryotherapy (freezing), and topical medications
    4. Site becomes more erythematous; nodules and vesicles may form; vesicles may rupture, releasing purulent material
    5. Skin is blistered, weepy, and pale to red or pink

PART III: CHALLENGE YOURSELF!

H. Getting Ready for NCLEX

Choose the most appropriate answer or select all that apply.

1. The nurse is teaching a patient with burns and his family about the different stages of burns. Which problems are most likely to occur in the emergent stage of patients with burns? Select all that apply.
    1. Potential infection
    2. Inadequate nutrition
    3. Impaired tissue perfusion
    4. Fluid imbalance related to fluid volume excess
    5. Pain

2. The nurse is assisting with teaching a community health program about patients with burns. Which problems are related to patients with burns? Select all that apply.
    1. Pain related to tissue trauma
    2. Potential infection related to loss of protective skin barrier
    3. Potential skin breakdown related to scratching
    4. Hypothermia related to impaired heat-regulating ability of injured skin
    5. Impaired mobility related to contractures, pain
    6. Potential skin breakdown related to inflammation

3. The nurse is taking care of a patient with shingles at an outpatient clinic. The nurse will monitor this patient for which problem?
    1. Potential skin breakdown related to excessive dryness, scratching
    2. Potential infection related to moist environment, broken skin
    3. Altered self-concept related to comedones, pustules, and cysts
    4. Pain related to lesions or postherpetic neuralgia

4. The nurse is taking care of a patient with psoriasis in the hospital. The nurse recognizes that which are problems for the patient with psoriasis? Select all that apply.
    1. Potential injury related to improper nail trimming, poor peripheral circulation
    2. Impaired tissue perfusion related to hypovolemia secondary to shift of fluid from vascular to extracellular compartment
    3. Altered self-concept related to lesions and scales on skin
    4. Fluid imbalance related to changes in capillary permeability and accumulation of fluid in body tissues
    5. Decreased socialization related to embarrassment about flaky skin lesions

I. Next-Generation NCLEX® Examination-Style Questions

A 45-year-old police officer came to the provider's office because of a "rash" on his trunk. The nurse reviews the physical assessment progress notes and vital signs.

> 0800: Assumed care of the client. Assessment completed at this time. Client alert and oriented and mildly anxious. He states "I am afraid it might spread and that it might be something serious." Skin on the face, arms, and legs within normal limits. Bright-red lesions with silvery scales are distributed over the anterior and posterior chest, abdomen, buttocks, and hands.

Vital Signs:

Blood Pressure	144/88 mm Hg
Pulse	84 beats/minute
Respirations	16 breaths/minute

1. Complete the diagram by dragging from the choices below to specify one potential condition the client is most likely experiencing, two actions the nurse would take to address that condition, and two parameters the nurse would monitor to assess the client's progress.

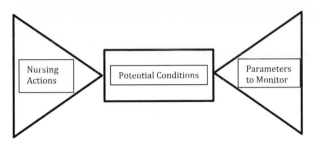

The nurse is caring for a client who presents with seborrheic dermatitis. The nurse reviews the previous shift's nurses' notes.

> Nurse's Notes:
> 1600: A 32-year-old female client presents with fine, powdery scales with redness to the forehead, external ears, and sternal area. Client reports itching to areas. Client states symptoms began 2 weeks ago. Provider notified. James Jonson, RN

2. Which physician orders would the nurse anticipate being prescribed? Select All That Apply.
   1. IV infusion NS at 100 mL/h
   2. Topical ketoconazole (Nizoral) Q 8H
   3. Topical hydrocortisone Q6H PRN
   4. Morphine 1 mg Q2H
   5. Accutane 0.5 mg/kg once daily
   6. Topical zelaic acid (Azelex)

Actions to Take	Potential Conditions	Parameters to Monitor
Demonstrate acceptance of the patient's appearance	Psoriasis	Assess for Fever
Document joint pain or stiffness	Pruritis	Assess for purulent discharge
Encourage the patient to keep the room temperature at 78–95°F with 75%–100% humidity	Atopic dermatitis	Assess for increased redness
Recommend cotton fabric and tight clothing.	Seborrheic dermatitis	Inspect the affected areas for lesions and scales
Encourage use of appropriate shampoos that contain selenium sulfide		Point of care glucose level

Special Senses: Hearing and Vision Introduction

chapter

58

Go to http://evolve.elsevier.com/Linton/medsurg/ for additional activities and exercises.

NCLEX CATEGORIES

Health Promotion and Maintenance

Physiological Integrity: Reduction of Risk Potential, Physiological Adaptation

PART I: MASTERING THE BASICS

A. Key Terms
Match the description in the numbered column with the term in the lettered column.

1. _____ Measurement of the pressure in the anterior chamber of the eye
2. _____ Earwax
3. _____ Medications placed directly in the ear canal
4. _____ Pain in the ear
5. _____ The state of balance needed for walking, standing, and sitting
6. _____ Blind spots in the visual field

A. Cerumen
B. Equilibrium
C. Otalgia
D. Otic
E. Scotomata
F. Tonometry

B. Diseases of the Eye
Match the disease in the numbered column with the effect on the eyes in the lettered column. Some answers may be used more than once.

1. _____ Elevated blood glucose in patients with diabetes
2. _____ Changes in retina due to diabetes

3. _____ Vision problem in neurologic disorders (brain tumors, head injuries, and strokes)
4. _____ Hyperthyroidism
5. _____ Changes in blood vessels of the eye in patients with hypertension

A. May cause bulging eyes (exophthalmos)
B. Causes temporary blurring of vision
C. May cause blindness
D. May be impaired, blurred, diplopia, and loss of part of visual fields
E. May lead to vision loss

C. Eye Structures
Match the descriptions in the numbered columns with the terms in the lettered columns.

1. _____ Located between the lens and the cornea, filled with aqueous humor
2. _____ Middle layer located between the sclera and the retina
3. _____ The colored part of the eye in front of the choroid and behind the cornea
4. _____ The large compartment behind the lens filled with vitreous humor
5. _____ Relaxes and contracts to change the shape of the lens
6. _____ A protective membrane covering the cornea
7. _____ Inner lining of the eyeball

8. _____ Part of the eye that allows light to enter for vision and provides approximately 65%–75% of the focusing power of the eye

9. _____ A transparent structure behind the iris attached to the ciliary muscle

10. _____ Refers to the part of the optic nerve that can be seen when examining the eye with an ophthalmoscope

11. _____ The tough, white outer covering of the eyeball

12. _____ The hole in the center of the iris

13. _____ The clear, gelatinous material that helps to hold the retina in place

14. _____ Enters the back of the eyeball and sends visual images to the brain for interpretation

A. Anterior chamber
B. Choroid
C. Ciliary muscle
D. Conjunctiva
E. Cornea
F. Iris
G. Lens
H. Optic disc
I. Vitreous humor
J. Optic nerve
K. Posterior chamber
L. Pupil
M. Retina
N. Sclera

D. Ear Structures
Match the descriptions in the numbered columns with the terms in the lettered columns.

1. _____ A coiled tube in the inner ear that looks like a snail

2. _____ The outer ear, also called the *pinna*

3. _____ The bony structure behind the auricle filled with air cells and connected to the middle ear

4. _____ Receptors in this part of the inner ear monitor changes in rate or direction of movement to maintain balance during movement

5. _____ Ossicles that conduct the sound waves transmitted by the tympanic membrane to the inner ear

6. _____ The receptor end organ of hearing located in the cochlea

7. _____ Extends from the opening of the ear to the tympanic membrane

8. _____ Consists of the membranous labyrinth and the bony labyrinth

9. _____ Extends from the middle ear to the nasopharynx in the middle ear

10. _____ Receptors in this segment of the inner ear monitor the position of the head to maintain posture balance

A. Auricle
B. External auditory canal
C. Malleus, incus, and stapes
D. Eustachian
E. Mastoid process
F. Inner ear
G. Organ of Corti
H. Cochlea
I. Vestibule
J. Semicircular canal

PART II: PUTTING IT ALL TOGETHER

E. Multiple Choice/Multiple Response
Choose the most appropriate answer or select all that apply.

1. As light enters the eye, it passes through the transparent cornea, aqueous humor, lens, and:
   1. conjunctiva.
   2. sclera.
   3. vitreous humor.
   4. lacrimal glands.

2. Dark spots that are bits of debris in the vitreous humor are called:
   1. flashes.
   2. floaters.
   3. blind spots.
   4. cataracts.

3. If a patient has sensitivity to light, the nurse would document this as:
   1. photophobia.
   2. presbyopia.
   3. myopia.
   4. hyperopia.

4. When the nurse is performing a physical assessment of the eyes, the lids should cover the eyeball completely when closed; when the eyes are open, the lower lid should be at the level of the:
   1. conjunctiva.
   2. retina.
   3. iris.
   4. lacrimal gland.

5. The nurse is reviewing the medical history of a patient with a vision disorder. In addition to eye problems, which are medical conditions that may cause vision disorders? Select all that apply.
   1. Cardiac disorders
   2. Diabetes
   3. Kidney disease
   4. Thyroid disease
   5. Neurologic disorders
   6. Hypertension

6. The pupils are assessed for size, equality, and reaction to light; pupils that are unequal, dilated, or do not respond to light suggest:
   1. diabetes.
   2. liver dysfunction.
   3. inflammation.
   4. neurologic problems.

7. When the nurse asks the patient to focus on the nurse's finger as it moves slowly toward the patient's nose, the nurse is assessing:
   1. presbyopia.
   2. astigmatism.
   3. accommodation.
   4. refraction.

8. Visual acuity is commonly tested using:
   1. the Snellen chart.
   2. the accommodation test.
   3. tonometry.
   4. fluorescein angiography.

9. Following eye surgery, the patient is usually positioned:
   1. flat in bed.
   2. prone.
   3. side-lying on affected side.
   4. with the head of bed elevated.

10. An important aspect of the care of postoperative eye patients is to prevent increased:
    1. blood pressure.
    2. cardiac output.
    3. intraocular pressure.
    4. ocular movement.

11. Which drug has a side effect of vision disturbances?
    1. Digitalis
    2. Lasix
    3. Aspirin
    4. Synthroid

12. A vision of 20/30 on the Snellen chart means that the person can:
    1. read at 20 feet from the left eye and 30 feet from the right eye what a normal person reads at these distances.
    2. read at 20 feet what a normal person reads at 50 feet.
    3. read at 30 feet what a person with normal vision reads at 20 feet.
    4. read at 20 feet what a person with normal vision reads at 30 feet.

13. The measurement of pressure in the anterior chamber of the eye is:
    1. refraction.
    2. electroretinopathy.
    3. tonometry.
    4. angiography.

14. An eye irrigation has been ordered for the patient to remove some chemical irritants in his eye. Place the steps for eye irrigation in the correct order, with 1 the first action and 6 the last action.
    A. _____ Place basin and waterproof pad to collect the fluid.
    B. _____ Gently direct the fluid into the lower conjunctival sac from the inner canthus to the outer canthus.
    C. _____ Wearing gloves, cleanse the eyelids and eyelashes.
    D. _____ Do not touch the eye with the tip of the irrigating syringe.
    E. _____ Position the patient with the affected eye down so that contaminated fluid does not run into the unaffected eye.
    F. _____ Have the patient blink occasionally to move particles toward the lower conjunctival sac.

15. Age-related changes in the inner ear affect sensitivity to sound, understanding of speech, and:
    1. balance.
    2. infection.
    3. cerumen production.
    4. blood pressure.

16. Pain in the ear is called:
    1. otosclerosis.
    2. otitis.
    3. ototoxicity.
    4. otalgia.

17. Ototoxicity means that a drug can damage the eighth cranial nerve or the organs of:
    1. hearing and balance.
    2. vision and sight.
    3. smell and taste.
    4. movement and coordination.

18. When assessing the position of the auricles, the nurse should observe that the top of the auricle normally will be at about the level of the:
    1. nostrils.
    2. forehead.
    3. eye.
    4. mouth.

19. The external auditory canal is inspected for obvious obstructions or:
    1. edema.
    2. cyanosis.
    3. drainage.
    4. jaundice.

20. Which is the only normal secretion in the external auditory canal?
    1. Sebum
    2. Purulent drainage
    3. Cerumen
    4. Mucus

21. People who benefit the most from hearing aids are those with:
    1. sensorineural loss.
    2. mixed hearing loss.
    3. conductive hearing loss.
    4. hearing loss due to Ménière disease.

22. Patients who have had ear surgery may have an inability to communicate effectively as a result of:
    1. dizziness or vertigo.
    2. knowledge deficit.
    3. inadequate self-care.
    4. packing and edema in affected ear.

23. Of all patients with sensory disorders, people who probably suffer the most severe decrease of socialization are those with:
    1. hearing impairment.
    2. sight impairment.
    3. smell impairment.
    4. taste impairment.

24. To prevent one form of congenital hearing impairment, all women of childbearing age should be immunized for:
    1. pertussis.
    2. influenza.
    3. rubella.
    4. hepatitis B.

25. Rinne and Weber tests use a tuning fork to assess the:
    1. ability to hear whispers.
    2. presence of lesions in the vestibule.
    3. conduction of sound by air and bone.
    4. function of the eighth cranial nerve.

26. Which statements are related to sensorineural hearing loss? Select all that apply.
    1. Patients who hear better in noisy settings than in quiet settings have sensorineural hearing loss.
    2. Causes include congenital problems, noise trauma, aging, Ménière disease, ototoxicity, diabetes, and syphilis.
    3. A condition in which the stapes in the middle ear does not vibrate.
    4. A disturbance of the neural structures in the inner ear or the nerve pathways to the brain.
    5. Sometimes called *nerve deafness*.
    6. Patients can hear sounds but have difficulty understanding speech.

PART III: CHALLENGE YOURSELF!

F. Getting Ready for NCLEX
Choose the most appropriate answer or select all that apply.

1. The nurse is assisting with teaching an in-service program about patients having eye surgery. Match the most appropriate problem for patients following eye surgery in the numbered column with the "related to" statement in the lettered column.
   1. _____ Potential for infection
   2. _____ Anxiety
   3. _____ Potential injury
   4. _____ Inability to manage treatment regimen
   A. Surgical procedure
   B. Temporary vision impairment
   C. Lack of understanding of self-care measures

   D. Pressure or trauma

2. The home health nurse is assessing the home of a patient who has had eye surgery. Which of the following are appropriate interventions that relate to lighting for patients who are partially sighted? Select all that apply.
   1. Reduce glare because it interferes with vision.
   2. Make sure the furniture is of a distinctly different color from the floors and walls.
   3. Use dishes and cups with a solid, single color to facilitate self-feeding and reduce spills.
   4. Use handrails when going up and down stairs.
   5. Remove small throw rugs from the patient's home.

3. Which are the most common problems for patients with impaired vision? Select all that apply.
   1. Anxiety related to uncertain outcome
   2. Inadequate coping related to decreased independence
   3. Inadequate knowledge related to altered reception, transmission, and interpretation of visual stimuli
   4. Impaired ADLs (feeding, hygiene, grooming) related to visual impairment
   5. Inadequate circulation

4. What are the goals/patient outcomes related to potential injury for a postoperative patient who has had eye surgery? Select all that apply.
   1. Patient states pain is relieved.
   2. Patient avoids rubbing eyes.
   3. Patient is careful not to bend forward.
   4. Patient demonstrates self-care activities.
   5. Patient avoids lifting.

5. The school nurse is teaching a group of parents about how people can care for their eyes to protect their vision. Which statement should the nurse include in the presentation?
   1. Burning sensations in the eyes should be reported to the health care provider.
   2. Watching too much television or sitting too close to the television injures the eyes.
   3. Eating foods with high vitamin A content will improve vision.
   4. Eyes need to be rinsed regularly to protect vision.

6. The nurse should treat nausea promptly in the postoperative eye surgery patient to prevent:
   1. infection.
   2. hemorrhage.
   3. pain.
   4. increased intraocular pressure.

7. The nurse is assisting with teaching a community health program about care for the person with a visual impairment. Which is the correct teaching regarding measures to support the person with impaired vision and ways to prevent injury?
   1. Raise your voice when talking to the visually impaired.
   2. Advise the person what to expect during procedures.
   3. Keep doors to the person's room partially closed.
   4. To lead a visually impaired person, take the arm of the person and lead him or her.

8. What is the priority consideration of the patient with visual impairment?
   1. Safety
   2. Infection
   3. Hemorrhage
   4. Nutrition

9. If more than one eye medication is being given, the nurse must wait how long between each medication?
   1. 60 seconds
   2. 5 minutes
   3. 30 minutes
   4. 60 minutes

10. A patient who has a hearing and speech impairment comes to the community health clinic. The nurse recognizes which of the following as a priority intervention for patients with an inability to communicate effectively?
    1. Provide adequate lighting toward the patient's face.
    2. Raise the tone of your voice.
    3. If the patient has a good ear, speak to that side.
    4. Avoid using body language when speaking to the patient.

Eye and Vision Disorders

chapter

59

Go to http://evolve.elsevier.com/Linton/medsurg/ for additional activities and exercises.

NCLEX CATEGORIES

Safe and Effective Care Environment: Safety and Infection Control

Physiological Integrity: Pharmacological Therapies, Reduction of Risk Potential

PART I: MASTERING THE BASICS

A. Key Terms

Match the definition in the numbered column with the most appropriate term in the lettered column. Some terms may be used more than once, and some terms may not be used.

1. _____ Inflammation, infection, or both, of the cornea

2. _____ Agent that causes the pupil to constrict

3. _____ Error of refraction occurs when refractive media do not bend light rays correctly

4. _____ Removal of the eyeball

5. _____ Inflammation of the membrane lining the eyelids and the eyeball

6. _____ Clouding or opacity of the normally transparent lens within the eye; causes blurred vision and spots

7. _____ Agent that paralyzes the ciliary muscle so that the eye does not accommodate

8. _____ Bending of light rays

9. _____ The lens is too close to the retina, causing difficulty focusing on close objects (farsightedness)

10. _____ Agent that causes the pupil to dilate

11. _____ Poor accommodation that is due to loss of elasticity of the ciliary muscles; more common in older patients

12. _____ The lens is situated too far from the retina causing difficulty seeing distant objects (nearsightedness)

13. _____ An inflammation of the hair follicles along the eyelid margin

14. _____ A condition in which the lower lid droops and turns outward

15. _____ A common acute staphylococcal infection of the eyelid margin that originates in an eyelash follicle

16. _____ A condition in which the lower lid turns inward

17. _____ An inflammation of the glands in the eyelids

A. Astigmatism
B. Blepharitis
C. Cataract
D. Chalazion
E. Conjunctivitis
F. Cycloplegic
G. Ectropion
H. Entropion
I. Enucleation
J. Hordeolum
K. Hyperopia
L. Keratitis
M. Miotic
N. Mydriatic
O. Myopia
P. Presbyopia
Q. Refraction

B. Matching

Match the actions and uses in the numbered column with the classification of drugs used to treat glaucoma in the lettered column. Some classifications may be used more than once.

1. _____ Initial treatment of acute and chronic glaucoma

2. _____ Increases aqueous outflow

3. _____ Treatment of chronic open-angle glaucoma

4. _____ Action of these topical drugs is to lower intraocular pressure by decreasing the production of aqueous humor

5. _____ Action of drugs is to constrict the pupil, facilitating the outflow of aqueous humor

6. _____ Action of drugs is to decrease intraocular pressure by decreasing the formation of aqueous humor

A. Cholinergic miotics
B. Rho kinase inhibitors
C. Beta-adrenergic blockers
D. Adrenergics

Match the actions and uses in the numbered column with the most appropriate drug classification in the lettered column. Some terms may be used more than once.

7. _____ Used to treat or prevent eye infections

8. _____ Used to treat keratitis

9. _____ Used in open-angle glaucoma treatment; decreases formation of aqueous humor

10. _____ Prevent or reduce inflammation in the eye

11. _____ Used to treat angle-closure glaucoma

12. _____ Treats eye infections caused by HSV-1

13. _____ Used in the treatment of common acute staphylococcal infection of the eyelid margin that originates in a lash follicle

14. _____ Can be ordered with or without antihistamines for long-term management of allergic conjunctivitis

A. Antibacterials
B. NSAIDs
C. Miotics
D. Ophthalmic antibiotics
E. Idoxuridine
F. Mast cell stabilizers
G. Antivirals
H. Adrenergics

PART II: PUTTING IT ALL TOGETHER

C. Multiple Choice/Multiple Response

Choose the most appropriate answer or select all that apply.

1. Medications prescribed after cataract surgery usually include antibiotics and:
   1. miotics.
   2. antihistamines.
   3. anticholinergics.
   4. corticosteroids.

2. One of the leading causes of blindness in the United States is:
   1. conjunctivitis.
   2. retinal detachment.
   3. glaucoma.
   4. cataracts.

3. Which is an inflammation of hair follicles along the eyelid?
   1. Hordeolum
   2. Conjunctivitis
   3. Blepharitis
   4. Keratitis

4. Corticosteroids are contraindicated in patients with conjunctivitis caused by:
   1. herpes.
   2. bacteria.
   3. fungi.
   4. chlamydia.

5. Which drug is prescribed before surgery for a patient with cataracts?
   1. An analgesic
   2. A mydriatic
   3. A miotic
   4. An anticholinergic

6. A patient sees floaters and states: "It is like a curtain has come down across my vision." This is a symptom of:
   1. cataracts.
   2. macular degeneration.
   3. retinal detachment.
   4. glaucoma.

7. Which antioxidants are believed by some health care practitioners to slow the progression of age-related macular degeneration? Select all that apply.
   1. Vitamin A
   2. Vitamin B
   3. Vitamin E
   4. Vitamin K
   5. Vitamin C
   6. Beta-carotene
   7. Zinc

8. Which are the signs and symptoms of cataracts? Select all that apply.
   1. Tunnel vision
   2. Loss of peripheral vision
   3. Cloudy vision
   4. Seeing spots
   5. Floaters in eyes

9. Which are true statements about glaucoma? Select all that apply.
   1. Failure to control intraocular pressure can result in permanent blindness.
   2. A late sign of glaucoma is intraocular pressure that is decreased below normal.
   3. Excess pressure impairs blood flow to the optic nerve and retina, resulting in vision impairment.
   4. An early sign of glaucoma is pain.
   5. Glaucoma usually occurs in one eye only.

10. Which medications are used in the treatment of glaucoma? Select all that apply.
    1. Anticholinergics
    2. Beta-adrenergic blockers
    3. Adrenergics
    4. Cholinergics
    5. Carbonic anhydrase inhibitors
    6. Hyperosmotic agents

PART III: CHALLENGE YOURSELF!

D. Getting Ready for NCLEX

Choose the most appropriate answer or select all that apply.

1. Which are problems for patients with glaucoma? Select all that apply.
   1. Disturbed sensory perception related to vision changes caused by the rejection of transplanted tissue
   2. Anxiety related to fear of actual or potential loss of vision
   3. Pain related to acute increased intraocular pressure
   4. Potential infection related to inflammation of the eye
   5. Inadequate nutrition

2. A patient has had cataract surgery. Following cataract surgery, the nurse should:
   1. advise the patient to sleep on the unaffected side.
   2. have the patient cough and deep breathe.
   3. administer mydriatic agents.
   4. keep the bed in a low position.

3. What are some the infectious and inflammatory eye disorders that a clinic or long-term care nurse may see in patients they interact with in outpatient settings? Select all that apply.
   1. Blepharitis
   2. Hordeolum
   3. Glaucoma
   4. Chalazion
   5. Retinal detachment
   6. Conjunctivitis
   7. Keratitis

4. What are the possible problems for a patient who has had a keratoplasty? Select all that apply.
   1. Potential injury
   2. Pain
   3. Knowledge deficit
   4. Impaired visual acuity
   5. Anxiety
   6. Inadequate self-care

5. A patient has a foreign object embedded in his eye. Who should be responsible for removing the object?
   1. Nurse
   2. Nursing assistant
   3. Health care provider
   4. Optician

E. Next-Generation NCLEX® Examination-Style Questions

A 72-year-old retired welder is seeking medical care because of cloudy vision that has become increasingly worse. The nurse reviews the health history and nurse's notes.

Health History:

A 72-year-old client reports cloudy vision that has become increasingly worse. He reports spots moving across his field of vision. Cataracts were diagnosed, with the right lens affected more severely than the left. He had a right extracapsular cataract extraction under local anesthesia this morning in the outpatient surgery department.

Nurse's Notes:

10/3/21 1200: The client reports mild pain in the eye area at this time. He is alert, oriented, and in the semi-Fowler position. An eye pad is in place over the right eye, protected with a metal shield. A small amount of clear drainage is noted seeping below the dressing. *Jacob Richardson, RN*

---

1. Based on the client health history, which nursing interventions can be implemented to prevent increased intraocular pressure? Select all that apply.
   1. Keep the bed in low position.
   2. Keep the head of bed elevated.
   3. Instruct the patient not to rub the operative eye, strain, or lean forward.
   4. Instruct the patient to lie on the affected side.
   5. Administer stool softeners as prescribed to prevent constipation.
   6. Acknowledge fear of vision loss common with eye surgery.

A 67-year-old male client presents to his healthcare provider with complaints of visual impairment. The nurse reviews the provider's progress notes.

Progress Notes:

10/1/21 0900: A 67-year-old male client states his field of vision appears more narrow and reports worsening over the past year. The client states, "It seems as if I am looking through a tube. Everything is smaller." Intraocular pressure 45 mm Hg. Peripheral vision impaired bilaterally. Rates pain 7/10 to both eyes.

Vital Signs:

Blood Pressure	122/66 mm Hg
Temperature	98.9 F
Pulse	88 beats/minute

---

2. Complete the diagram by dragging from the choices below to specify one potential condition the client is most likely experiencing, two actions the nurse would take to address that condition, and two parameters the nurse would monitor to assess the client's progress.

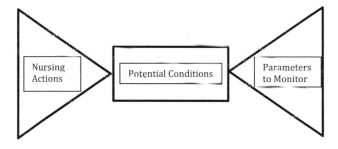

Actions to Take	Potential Conditions	Parameters to Monitor
Encourage client to wear a medical alert tag	Cataracts	Monitor intraocular pressure (IOP)
Administer analgesics PRN	Glaucoma	Monitor temperature
Encourage use of herbal supplements	Conjunctivitis	Monitor pain rating
Educate the client that any drugs that dilate the pupil are contraindicated	Chalazion	Monitor blood pressure
Encourage the use of vitamins C and E		Monitor apical pulse

Ear and Hearing Disorders

Go to http://evolve.elsevier.com/Linton/medsurg/ for additional activities and exercises.

NCLEX CATEGORIES

Health Promotion and Maintenance

Physiological Integrity: Pharmacological Therapies, Reduction of Risk Potential

PART I: MASTERING THE BASICS

A. Key Terms
Match the definition in the numbered column with the most appropriate term in the lettered column.

1. _____ Eardrum
2. _____ Ringing, buzzing, or roaring noise in the ears
3. _____ Sensation of movement that causes dizziness or nausea
4. _____ Capable of injuring the eighth cranial nerve (acoustic) of hearing and balance structures in the ear
5. _____ Hearing loss associated with age

A. Ototoxic
B. Presbycusis
C. Tinnitus
D. Tympanic membrane
E. Vertigo

B. External Ear Infections

1. Which are true statements about otitis externa? Select all that apply.
   1. It is also called *swimmer's ear*.
   2. Treatment of otitis externa includes topical corticosteroids and diuretics.
   3. Drainage in otitis externa may be blood-tinged or purulent.
   4. May be caused by scratching or cleaning the ear with sharp objects.
   5. The most characteristic symptom of otitis externa is itching.

C. Ototoxic Drugs
Match the ototoxic drugs in the numbered column with their most appropriate classification in the lettered column. Some classifications may be used more than once, and some classifications may not be used.

1. _____ Aspirin
2. _____ Erythromycin estolate (Ilosone)
3. _____ Furosemide (Lasix)
4. _____ Cisplatin (Platinol-AQ)
5. _____ Indomethacin (Indocin)
6. _____ Streptomycin sulfate
7. _____ Ethacrynic acid (Edecrin)
8. _____ Quinidine
9. _____ Tetracycline
10. _____ Bleomycin (Blenoxane)

A. Antidysrhythmic
B. Antibiotics/aminoglycosides
C. Antineoplastics/chemotherapy drugs
D. Antihistamines
E. Salicylates
F. Diuretics
G. Antiinflammatories/analgesics

PART II: PUTTING IT ALL TOGETHER

D. Multiple Choice/Multiple Response

Choose the most appropriate answer or select all that apply.

1. The use of a solution to cleanse the external ear canal or to remove something from the canal is called:
   1. audiometry.
   2. irrigation.
   3. débridement.
   4. electronystagmography.

2. Postoperative dizziness or vertigo following ear surgery may give the patient potential for:
   1. injury.
   2. skin breakdown.
   3. infection.
   4. pain.

3. Presbycusis is the result of changes in one or more parts of the:
   1. middle ear.
   2. external auditory canal.
   3. eustachian tube.
   4. cochlea.

4. Patients with impacted cerumen may complain of hearing loss or:
   1. sharp pain.
   2. tinnitus.
   3. bloody discharge.
   4. headache.

5. A very common problem after mastoidectomy or middle ear surgery is:
   1. nausea.
   2. constipation.
   3. oliguria.
   4. seizures.

6. Slow progressive hearing loss in the absence of infection is the primary symptom of:
   1. acute otitis media.
   2. labyrinthitis.
   3. perforated eardrum.
   4. otosclerosis.

7. The most common treatment for otosclerosis is a surgical procedure called:
   1. myringotomy.
   2. stapedectomy.
   3. mastoidectomy.
   4. incision and drainage.

8. A hereditary condition in which an abnormal growth causes the footplate of the stapes to become fixed is:
   1. cholesteatoma.
   2. otosclerosis.
   3. labyrinthitis.
   4. conductive hearing loss.

9. Because the fixed stapes cannot vibrate in patients with otosclerosis, sound waves cannot be transmitted to the:
   1. middle ear.
   2. tympanic membrane.
   3. inner ear.
   4. external auditory canal.

10. An inner ear infection that usually follows an upper respiratory infection and that may lead to Ménière disease is:
    1. otitis media.
    2. otosclerosis.
    3. mastoiditis.
    4. labyrinthitis.

11. The treatment for nausea and vomiting associated with labyrinthitis is:
    1. antiemetics.
    2. analgesics.
    3. corticosteroids.
    4. beta blockers.

12. Which is one of the first signs of ototoxicity with salicylates?
    1. Vertigo
    2. Tinnitus
    3. Dizziness
    4. Anorexia

13. A high-pitched buzzing sound that sometimes becomes a roar often accompanies an acute attack of Ménière disease. It is documented as:
    1. vertigo.
    2. tinnitus.
    3. dizziness.
    4. otitis.

14. When the caloric test or electronystagmography is done in patients with Ménière disease, they will experience severe:
    1. vertigo.
    2. seizures.
    3. headache.
    4. flushing.

15. Following surgery for Ménière disease, the nurse needs to assess the patient for:
    1. facial nerve damage.
    2. fluid volume excess.
    3. inadequate circulation.
    4. difficulty voiding.

16. A labyrinth disorder in which there is an accumulation of fluid in the inner ear is:
    1. otosclerosis.
    2. otitis media.
    3. Ménière disease.
    4. presbycusis.

17. Drugs that can cause permanent hearing loss are: Select all that apply.
    1. antihypertensives.
    2. aminoglycosides (antibiotics).
    3. anticholinergics.
    4. diuretics.

18. Patients who are at special risk of developing ototoxicity because their bodies excrete drugs more slowly are those with:
    1. poor renal or liver function.
    2. pneumonia.
    3. myocardial infarction.
    4. high blood pressure.

19. Which diet may be recommended for patients with Ménière disease?
    1. Increased calcium
    2. Increased vitamin K
    3. Increased potassium
    4. Low sodium

20. Which are potential complications of surgery for Ménière disease? Select all that apply.
    1. Tinnitus
    2. Infection
    3. Hearing loss
    4. Ataxia
    5. Loss of cerebrospinal fluid
    6. Damage to cranial nerve VII (facial nerve)

PART III: CHALLENGE YOURSELF!

E. Getting Ready for NCLEX

Choose the most appropriate answer or select all that apply.

1. A patient with rheumatoid arthritis is taking aspirin. The nurse will monitor the patient for which signs and symptoms of ototoxicity? Select all that apply.
    1. Hearing loss
    2. Ataxia
    3. Infection
    4. Tinnitus
    5. Dizziness
    6. Drainage

2. The nurse is taking care of a patient with Ménière disease. What are the possible problems for this patient? Select all that apply.
    1. Potential injury related to vertigo
    2. Potential dehydration related to vomiting
    3. Decreased socialization related to inability to communicate verbally
    4. Inadequate coping related to change in social interaction
    5. Anxiety related to acute illness
    6. Inadequate self-care related to lack of knowledge about management of the disease

3. The nurse is taking care of a patient who has had a stapedectomy and is explaining to the patient the care that will follow the surgery. Which is appropriate teaching for this patient? Select all that apply.
    1. Unless the health care provider designates a different position, the patient can lie on his back or the unaffected side
    2. Instruct patient to not do anything to increase pressure to the ear.
    3. Increase vitamin K and protein intake in the diet.
    4. Keep ear dry for 2 weeks.
    5. Remind the patient that hearing will return gradually over a 6-week period.

4. The nurse is taking care of a patient who had surgery for Ménière disease 2 days ago. The patient is receiving an antiemetic medication to control nausea and vomiting. Which is a priority collaborative intervention for the patient at this time?
   1. Ambulate the patient 3 times a day.
   2. Offer the patient a soft diet.
   3. Delay nonessential care until the patient tolerates movement.
   4. Assist the patient with taking a shower in the bathroom.

5. The patient who had surgery for Ménière disease 2 days ago asks the nurse how long the dizziness and unsteadiness will last. The nurse responds that:
   1. the patient may feel dizzy for several days and unsteady for several weeks.
   2. usually patients can resume normal activities within a week.
   3. with medication, the dizziness may go away in 24 hours and unsteadiness will go away in 3 days.
   4. when the anesthesia wears off, the patient will probably not experience dizziness or unsteadiness.

6. The nurse asks the patient who has had surgery for Ménière disease 1 day ago to smile and show her teeth. The reason for this is to observe the patient for:
   1. possible transient ischemic attack (TIA).
   2. hemorrhage in the facial area around the mouth.
   3. infection of brain tissue.
   4. facial nerve damage.

7. A male patient at the clinic with labyrinthitis tells the nurse that he is taking some herbal products at home. The nurse should caution this patient that many herbal products can cause dizziness, nausea, vomiting, and drowsiness. Dehydration may be increased if the patient is taking which medications at home for nausea?
   1. Aspirin
   2. Steroids
   3. Diuretics
   4. Antiemetics

F. Next-Generation NCLEX® Examination-Style Questions

A 62-year-old man has had repeated episodes of nausea, hearing loss, and vertigo over the past year. The nurse reviews the health history and physical examination.

Health History:
A 62-year-old male client reports repeated episodes of nausea, hearing loss, and vertigo over the past year. The client reports that attacks last 2–3 hours, during which he is completely incapacitated.

Physical Examination:
10/2/21 0800: The client presents to the ED today after vomiting repeatedly. He is very weak with mild hearing loss. The client appears acutely ill and is unable to sit or stand. Based on the symptoms, client diagnosis is probable Ménière disease.
E. Thomas, MD

1. Highlight the data collected during the health history and physical examination that indicate the presence of Ménière disease.

Review the physical assessment and vital signs below to answer question #2.

Physical Assessment
3/2/21 0900: A 45-year-old female client presents with complaints of dizziness and nausea with movement. She states, "I feel like I am spinning." The client reports recent acute upper respiratory infection that resolved 1 week ago.

Vital signs:

Blood Pressure	112/62 mm Hg
Pulse	88 beats/minute
Respirations	16 breaths/minute
Temperature	98.7°F

2. Based on the client's symptoms, what education can the nurse anticipate that the client will need? Select all that apply
   1. Lie in a dark room if you feel very dizzy
   2. Avoid noise and bright lights during attacks
   3. Avoid sudden movements or position changes
   4. Get enough sleep, tiredness can make symptoms worse
   5. Stay indoors to prevent injury
   6. Slowly resume activity
   7. Drink plenty of water
   8. It is ok to drink alcohol in moderation

Psychobiologic Disorders

Go to http://evolve.elsevier.com/Linton/medsurg/ for additional activities and exercises.

NCLEX CATEGORIES

Psychosocial Integrity

Physiological Integrity: Pharmacological Therapies

PART I: MASTERING THE BASICS

A. Key Terms

Match the definition or description in the numbered column with the most appropriate term in the lettered column.

1. _____ Frequently irreversible side effect of antipsychotic medication that develops after years of use; symptoms include involuntary movements of face, jaw, and tongue, leading to grimacing; jerky movements of upper extremities; and tonic contractions of neck and back

2. _____ A state in which a person has a distorted perception of reality interfering with the capacity to function and relate to others

3. _____ Assumes that mental disorders are related to physiologic changes within the central nervous system

4. _____ A condition that may occur after 1–2 weeks of treatment with antipsychotic medications consisting of masklike face, rigid posture, shuffling gait, and resting tremor

5. _____ Based on the theory that people function at different levels of awareness (conscious to unconscious) and that ego defense mechanisms, such as denial and repression, are used to prevent anxiety

6. _____ An individual may have impaired occupational functioning, restricted social contact, and difficulties with self-care

7. _____ A term used to refer to a group of very serious, usually chronic thought disorders in which psychotic symptoms primarily impair the affected person's ability to interpret the world accurately

8. _____ Side effects of antipsychotic drugs on the portion of the central nervous system controlling involuntary movements

9. _____ Components from this approach include: (1) anxiety is often communicated interpersonally, (2) the patient learns new ways of coping or maturing in a therapeutic relationship, and (3) the establishment of trust is an important first step in working with patients

10. _____ A state of feeling outside of oneself; that is, watching what is happening as if it were happening to someone else

11. _____ Key ideas from this theoretical approach to mental disorders are (1) behavior is learned, (2) behavior increases because of response to that behavior from the environment (i.e., reinforcement), and (3) the way a person thinks about things (his or her thoughts) influences emotional states and behavior

12. _____ Orientation in terms of time, date, place, person, and self, as well as the situation or circumstance the patient finds him- or herself in

A. Biologic approach
B. Cognitive-behavioral approach
C. Depersonalization
D. Extrapyramidal side effects (EPS)
E. Interpersonal approach
F. Parkinsonian syndrome
G. Psychodynamic approach
H. Psychosis
I. Schizoaffective disorder
J. Schizophrenia
K. Sensorium
L. Tardive dyskinesia

B. Types of Psychiatric Disorders

Match the definition or description in the numbered column with the most appropriate term in the lettered column.

1. _____ Major or mild neurocognitive disorders that involve deficits in orientation, memory, language comprehension, and judgment

2. _____ A mental disorder that involves a change in identity, memory, or consciousness that enables patients to remove themselves from anxiety-provoking situations

3. _____ Patient experiences cycles of significantly elevated (or very irritable) or depressed moods

4. _____ A pattern of instability in interpersonal relationships, self-image, and affect, as well as marked impulsivity

5. _____ Patient experiences a marked, persistent fear that is excessive or unreasonable and works hard to avoid the feared object or situation

6. _____ Patient experiences intense fear or discomfort reaching a peak within a few minutes

7. _____ Disorders that involve deficits in orientation, memory, language comprehension, and judgment and are usually reversible with rapid onset

A. Dissociative disorder
B. Dementia
C. Delirium
D. Borderline personality disorder
E. Bipolar disorder
F. Panic disorder
G. Specific phobia

Match the definition or description in the numbered column with the most appropriate term in the lettered column.

8. _____ Person exhibits two or more distinct personalities

9. _____ Loss of body function (e.g., paralysis) without physiologic cause

10. _____ A disorder that is characterized by the patient experiencing one or more physical symptoms which they experience as distressing and/or result in significant disruption in their daily life

11. _____ Pervasive, chronic, and maladaptive personality characteristics that interfere with normal functioning

12. _____ A cluster of symptoms after a distressing event in which the person experiences intense fears, helplessness, horror, or a combination of those feelings

13. _____ Difficulty establishing and sustaining close relationships associated with a pattern of preoccupation with orderliness, perfectionism, and control to the extent that the major part of the activity is lost

14. _____ Preoccupation with having or acquiring a serious illness when medical findings are absent

15. _____ Persistent depressed mood experienced most of the day, most days of the week that lasts for more than 2 weeks

16. _____ Disorder that occurs after exposure to a recent distressing event that is characterized by detachment, derealization, depersonalization, and dissociative amnesia

A. Posttraumatic stress disorder
B. Major depressive disorder
C. Dissociative identity disorder
D. Illness anxiety disorder
E. Somatic symptom disorder
F. Personality disorder
G. Obsessive-compulsive disorder
H. Conversion disorder (functional neurologic symptom disorder)
I. Acute stress disorder

C. Mental Status Examination

1. Which features are assessed during the mental status examination? Select all that apply.
   1. Heart rate
   2. Blood pressure
   3. Appearance
   4. Mood and affect
   5. Speech and language
   6. Thought content
   7. Respirations
   8. Perceptual disturbances
   9. Insight and judgment
   10. Sensorium
   11. Emotional responses
   12. Memory and attention

D. Therapeutic Relationship

Match the description in the numbered column with (A) therapeutic or (B) social relationship.

1. _____ May or may not have clear boundaries and a clear ending.

2. _____ Focus is on personal and emotional needs of the patient.

3. _____ Purpose is to benefit both participants in the relationship.

4. _____ Participants are not formally responsible for evaluating their interaction.

5. _____ The helper has responsibility for evaluating the interaction and the changing behavior.

6. _____ Relationship has some boundaries (purpose, place, time) and clear ending.

7. _____ Relationship develops spontaneously.

8. Which are interpersonal strategies of a therapeutic relationship? Select all that apply.
   1. Sharing observations
   2. Responsibility
   3. Accepting silence
   4. Listening
   5. Professionalism
   6. Clarifying
   7. Being available
   8. Giving advice

E. Drug Therapy

Refer to Table 61.5 in the book. Match the descriptions in the numbered column with the drug classification in the lettered column. Answers may be used more than once.

1. _____ Antidepressant drug that affects serotonin and epinephrine/norepinephrine; may cause cardiac complications

2. _____ Used in the treatment of bipolar disorders with narrow therapeutic range; may cause toxicity signs, including tremors

3. _____ Antidepressants that can be taken once a day without being cardiotoxic; useful in treatment of panic disorder and obsessive-compulsive disorder

4. _____ Antipsychotic agents that treat both positive and negative symptoms of schizophrenia; examples are Clozaril, Zyprexa, and Seroquel

5. _____ Important to maintain hydration and monitor renal function and serum blood levels of drug

6. _____ Antidepressant drugs that require strict diet restriction to avoid hypertensive crisis

7. _____ Mood stabilizer used in the treatment of bipolar disorders

A. Atypical neuroleptics
B. Selective serotonin reuptake inhibitors (SSRIs)
C. Tricyclic antidepressants (TCAs)
D. Monoamine oxidase inhibitors (MAOIs)
E. Lithium
F. Divalproex sodium (Depakote)

PART II: PUTTING IT ALL TOGETHER

F. Multiple Choice/Multiple Response

Choose the most appropriate answer or select all that apply.

1. Repeated checking to see whether the door is locked is an example of:
   1. obsession.
   2. hallucination.
   3. delusion.
   4. compulsion.

2. Many people with obsessive-compulsive disorders have considerably reduced their symptoms once therapeutic levels of which type of drug have been reached?
   1. Analgesics
   2. Antihistamines
   3. Antidepressants
   4. Anticonvulsants

3. Conversion disorders and illness anxiety disorders (hypochondriasis) are examples of:
   1. mood disorders.
   2. somatic symptom disorders.
   3. panic disorders.
   4. obsessive-compulsive disorders.

4. Amnesia and dissociative identity disorder are examples of:
   1. somatic symptom disorders.
   2. dissociative disorders.
   3. panic disorders.
   4. posttraumatic stress disorders.

5. A symptom of dissociative disorders is:
   1. depersonalization.
   2. hypochondriasis.
   3. agitation.
   4. hallucinations.

6. Most patients with dissociative identity disorder report severe:
   1. agoraphobia.
   2. hallucinations.
   3. delusions.
   4. childhood abuse.

7. The primary antianxiety medications are the:
   1. benzodiazepines.
   2. antihistamines.
   3. thiazides.
   4. salicylates.

8. Withdrawal from antianxiety medications should be medically supervised because of the effect(s) of:
   1. amnesia and confusion.
   2. negative feedback.
   3. hormones and histamines.
   4. physical and psychologic dependence.

9. One of the most common psychiatric disorders is:
   1. bipolar disorder.
   2. major depression.
   3. posttraumatic stress disorder.
   4. conversion disorder.

10. As patients respond to antidepressant medications and their energy level increases, what risk may increase?
    1. Mutism
    2. Panic
    3. Suicide
    4. Hypertension

11. What symptoms can major depression include? Select all that apply.
    1. Appetite disturbance
    2. Weight issues
    3. Sleep problems
    4. Amnesia
    5. Loss of interest in activities
    6. Fatigue
    7. Hypertension

12. In its most severe form, major depression can also include what symptoms?
    1. Orthostatic hypotension
    2. Psychosis
    3. Tardive dyskinesia
    4. Parkinsonian syndrome

13. Which are active signs of major depression in a patient? Select all that apply.
    1. Psychomotor retardation
    2. Agoraphobia
    3. No spontaneous movements
    4. Posttraumatic stress syndrome
    5. Downcast gaze
    6. Agitated movements of hand wringing

14. Frequently assessing a patient's suicidal potential and maintaining continuous one-to-one contact, if indicated, are interventions for depressed patients who are at risk for:
    1. sleep disturbance.
    2. anxiety.
    3. harm to self.
    4. low self-esteem.

15. Learning to limit self-criticism and to give and receive compliments are interventions for patients who are experiencing:
    1. risk for harm to self.
    2. low self-esteem.
    3. anxiety.
    4. unresolved grief.

16. The most common medication for patients with manic episodes is:
    1. alprazolam (Xanax).
    2. fluoxetine hydrochloride (Prozac).
    3. lithium and divalproex.
    4. benztropine mesylate (Cogentin).

17. The major problems for people with neurocognitive disorders stem from:
    1. speech and language impairments.
    2. anxiety disorders.
    3. conversion disorders.
    4. cognition and memory.

18. Which herbal preparation is used by many people to relieve depression?
    1. Ephedra
    2. Ginkgo
    3. Ginseng
    4. St. John's wort

19. Which are common physical signs and symptoms of anxiety? Select all that apply.
    1. Decreased heart rate
    2. Elevated blood pressure
    3. Increased pulse
    4. Drowsiness
    5. Trembling
    6. Nausea
    7. Ataxia
    8. Chest pain
    9. Shortness of breath
    10. Confusion

20. What are side effects of antianxiety medications that are associated with sedation? Select all that apply.
    1. Nausea
    2. Drowsiness
    3. Fatigue
    4. Dizziness
    5. Confusion
    6. Fever

21. Which are typical symptoms of schizophrenia? Select all that apply.
    1. Feelings of panic
    2. Disturbed thought processes
    3. Delusions
    4. Distorted perceptions of reality
    5. Abnormal motor behavior
    6. Disturbed emotional responses

22. Which are side effects of drug therapy (antipsychotic and antiparkinsonian medications) used for patients with schizophrenia? Select all that apply.
    1. Agitation
    2. Akathisia (restlessness and inability to sit still)
    3. Orthostatic hypotension
    4. EPS
    5. Neuroleptic syndrome
    6. Hypertensive crisis
    7. Agranulocytosis

23. Which are some probable causal factors of mood disorders? Select all that apply.
    1. Childhood trauma
    2. Neuroendocrine dysfunction
    3. Genetic factors
    4. Learned helplessness
    5. Loss of significant others

24. Which are types of antidepressant medications used for mood disorders? Select all that apply.
    1. Benzodiazepines
    2. TCAs
    3. SSRIs
    4. MAOIs
    5. Antihistamines

25. Which are four levels of consciousness? Select all that apply.
    1. Sluggish
    2. Comatose
    3. Drowsy
    4. Alert
    5. Stuporous

26. The nurse asks the patient, "What do you mean when you say, 'The world is falling apart'?" Which strategy in a therapeutic relationship does this represent?
    1. Sharing observations
    2. Listening
    3. Clarifying
    4. Being available

27. The nurse says, "You are saying that your life is falling apart, and you are also smiling." This is an example of which therapeutic communication intervention?
    1. Sharing observations
    2. Listening
    3. Clarifying
    4. Being available

28. Which are the main elements of suicide risk assessment that are part of data collection in the mental status examination? Select all that apply.
    1. Suicidal ideation (thoughts)
    2. General intellectual level
    3. Plans for committing suicide
    4. Intention to carry out suicide
    5. Memory and attention capabilities

29. Why are benzodiazepines typically used at the initial phase of treatment for a patient with anxiety?
    1. They are the fastest-acting drugs.
    2. They reduce symptoms until other medications can take effect.
    3. They work well with patients who have depression as well as anxiety.
    4. They depress the central nervous system.

30. Which are correct interventions for a patient who is experiencing impaired personal identity? Select all that apply.
    1. Encourage involvement in activities.
    2. Focus on reality.
    3. Make brief, frequent contacts with the patient to interrupt hallucinatory experiences.
    4. Let the patient know that the nurse does not share the delusion.
    5. Connect delusions with anxiety-provoking situations.
    6. Encourage the patient to pay attention to what is occurring in the environment (instead of internal stimuli).
    7. Inform the patient that hallucinations are part of the disease process.
    8. Encourage the patient to express feelings and anxiety.

PART III: CHALLENGE YOURSELF!

G. Getting Ready for NCLEX

Choose the most appropriate answer or select all that apply.

1. In addition to counseling the patient, what are ways to prevent and manage increasing anxiety? Select all that apply.
   1. Rise slowly from a sitting position
   2. Relaxation techniques
   3. Warm baths
   4. Positive self-talk
   5. Physical exercise

2. The nurse is caring for a patient with manic episodes. Which patient problems would the nurse expect to see in this patient? Select all that apply.
   1. Potential injury
   2. Inadequate nutrition
   3. Inadequate coping related to dissociation
   4. Potential for violence toward others related to low frustration tolerance
   5. Disturbed mood

3. The nurse is taking care of a patient with major depression. Which problems would the nurse expect to see in this patient? Select all that apply.
   1. Risk for self-harm
   2. Impaired sleep
   3. Impaired personal identity related to splitting
   4. Impaired self-concept related to negative feelings about self
   5. Inadequate nutrition

4. A patient with depression tells the nurse that he is thinking about killing himself. Which is the best therapeutic response of the nurse? Select all that apply.
   1. "Have you had any past suicide attempts?"
   2. "Have you made any plans to kill yourself?"
   3. "What has happened to you to make you want to kill yourself?"
   4. "Do you intend to carry out your plan to kill yourself?"
   5. "Have you told your family about your thoughts of killing yourself?"

H. Next-Generation NCLEX® Examination-Style Questions

Patrick was admitted to the psychiatric inpatient unit with the diagnosis of posttraumatic stress disorder. The nurse reviews the Health History.

Health History:
Two months ago, the client and his coworker friend were in a truck accident on an overpass. The client reports watching in horror as his friend fell out of the truck which was hanging over the edge. The fall killed his friend instantly. The client was able to climb out of the passenger side and sustained injuries to his back and legs. He received physical therapy for his injuries. For the past 2 weeks, client reports being continually preoccupied by the event, has had persistent insomnia and nightmares, and repeatedly says that he should have been the one to die. He becomes easily irritable, does not show feelings when with others, and jumps whenever he hears a loud noise or someone touches him unexpectedly.

1. Which patient problems were immediately relevant for Patrick? Select all that apply.
   1. Anxiety
   2. Impaired sleep
   3. Impaired personal identity
   4. Inadequate self-care
   5. Posttrauma syndrome
   6. Unresolved grief

A 53-year-old woman is admitted to a psychiatric hospital with a diagnosis of major depression. The nurse reviews the Health History and Physical Examination.

Health History:
During the past few weeks, the client has become increasingly listless, apathetic, and uninterested in anyone or anything. She cries frequently and says that her life has not seemed to be worth living. She complains that she cannot sleep and has no appetite. She frequently talks about wanting to commit suicide. She was referred to a psychiatrist, who recommended that she be admitted to the hospital for treatment.

Physical Examination:
Blood pressure 110/70 mm Hg; pulse 78 beats/minute; respiration 22 breaths/minute; temperature 98.8°F measured orally. Appears apathetic, sad, and cries frequently. Somewhat disheveled. Gaunt and tired-looking.

2. Which are nursing interventions related to the client's problem, risk for self-harm related to suicidal feelings? Select all that apply.
   1. Encourage patient to improve hygiene.
   2. Provide sleep-producing measures such as small snacks, warm baths, and relaxation exercises before going to bed.
   3. Establish a no-harm contract.
   4. Take necessary suicide precautions.
   5. Remove dangerous objects from the environment.
   6. Maintain continuous one-to-one contact.
   7. Assist in identifying symbols of hope in this patient's life.
   8. Involve dietitian in planning an adequate diet.

Substance-Related and Addictive Disorders

Go to http://evolve.elsevier.com/Linton/medsurg/ for additional activities and exercises.

NCLEX CATEGORIES

Psychosocial Integrity

Physiological Integrity: Pharmacological Therapies, Reduction of Risk Potential

PART I: MASTERING THE BASICS

A. Key Terms
Match the definition in the numbered column with the most appropriate term in the lettered column.

1. _____ Chronic, relapsing brain disease characterized by compulsive drug-seeking and use, despite harmful consequences

2. _____ Self-help support process outlining steps to overcoming dependence on something outside oneself, such as alcohol. Part of the Alcoholics the Anonymous process

3. _____ Situation in which two disorders or illnesses occur in the same person at the same time or when one follows the other

4. _____ Unpleasant and sometimes life-threatening physical substance-specific syndrome occurring after stopping or reducing the habitual dose or frequency of a used substance

5. _____ Occurs when blood and tissue levels of the substance decline after prolonged use

6. _____ Need for increasing amounts of a substance to achieve the same effect brought about by the original amount

7. _____ Behavior is highly structured around managing and adapting to the alcoholic's dysfunctional behavior

A. Addiction
B. Delirium tremens
C. Codependent
D. Comorbidity and dual diagnosis
E. Tolerance
F. Withdrawal
G. 12-step program

B. Diagnostic Tests
Complete the statement in the numbered column with the most appropriate term in the lettered column. Some terms may be used more than once.

1. _____ A recent addition to the methods for the detection of used substances; tool used in the diagnosis and follow-up of substance use disorders

2. _____ The preferred way of screening for the recent use of an unknown drug

3. _____ Requires sensitive technology and can detect drug use for up to 90 days after only 2 or 3 days of use

4. _____ Method to identify the presence of amphetamines, barbiturates, marijuana, narcotics, and benzodiazepines

5. _____ The most accurate type of test available to measure the degree of intoxication on initiation of treatment for alcohol use disorder

A. Urine drug screening
B. Hair analysis
C. Blood alcohol study

C. Complications of Substance Use Disorders

Complete the statement in the numbered column with the most appropriate term in the lettered column.

1. _____   A complication of chronic alcoholism that is due to thiamine and niacin deficiencies, which contribute to the degeneration of the cerebrum and the peripheral nervous system

2. _____   Occurs when alcohol becomes integrated into physiologic processes at the cellular level

3. _____   Term used to describe the condition of patients who commonly visualize or describe seeing bugs, snakes, and rats

4. _____   A critical sign of withdrawal in persons with substance use disorders

5. _____   A medical complication that may cause low birth weight and heart defects in newborn babies

6. _____   Condition due to vitamin B_1 (thiamine) deficiency with delirium, altered levels of consciousness that may lead to coma

A. Hypertension
B. Wernicke encephalopathy
C. Fetal alcohol syndrome
D. Hallucinations
E. Physical addiction
F. Korsakoff psychosis

D. Drug Therapy

Match the description in the numbered column with the drug in the lettered column. Answers may be used more than once.

1. _____   Synthetic opioid analgesic that is sometimes prescribed for chronic severe pain

2. _____   Used for opioid detoxification

3. _____   Opioid antagonist

4. _____   Counteracts respiratory depressant effects of heroin and other opioid overdoses

5. _____   Controversial substance as it constitutes substituting another addictive drug for the one misused by the patient

6. _____   Side effects include constipation and sweating

7. _____   Nonopiate antihypertensive drug that partially blocks withdrawal symptoms

A. Methadone
B. Clonidine
C. Naloxone (Narcan)

PART II: PUTTING IT ALL TOGETHER

E. Multiple Choice/Multiple Response

Choose the most appropriate answer or select all that apply.

1. The least likely way to alienate an already defensive patient is to use a manner that is matter of fact and:
   1. nonjudgmental.
   2. assertive.
   3. reassuring.
   4. positive.

2. It is believed that the cause of hangover symptoms is related to the buildup of acetaldehyde and lactic acid in the blood, dehydration, and:
   1. hyperkalemia.
   2. hyponatremia.
   3. hypoglycemia.
   4. hyperthyroidism.

3. Which defense mechanism is used when people addicted to alcohol shift the blame for their behavior onto their spouse?
   1. Rationalization
   2. Intellectualization
   3. Denial
   4. Projection

4. The biggest issue for a patient with a substance use disorder to be addressed at first during rehabilitation is:
   1. rationalization.
   2. sublimation.
   3. denial.
   4. compensation.

5. Which are behaviors that often lead to relapse for a person with a substance use disorder? Select all that apply.
   1. Overtiredness
   2. Detoxification
   3. Withdrawal
   4. Argumentativeness
   5. Depression
   6. Self-pity
   7. Decreased participation in AA meetings

6. Older individuals who have substance use disorders over an extended period of time may experience significant medical problems as a result of decreased ability to:
   1. circulate and absorb drugs.
   2. utilize and react to drugs.
   3. metabolize and eliminate drugs.
   4. transport and detoxify drugs.

7. Patients taking antianxiety or antidepressant agents with alcohol may risk accidental overdose due to:
   1. antagonist effects.
   2. idiosyncratic effects.
   3. stimulant effects.
   4. additive effects.

8. Program developed for health professionals addicted to a substance to prevent having their licenses revoked are called:
   1. Alcoholics Anonymous.
   2. peer assistance program.
   3. Codependents Anonymous.
   4. Al-Anon.

9. Which are characteristics that people with substance use disorders frequently have? Select all that apply.
   1. Damaged relationships
   2. Decreased activity levels
   3. Dysfunctional grieving
   4. Erratic and unprovoked mood swings
   5. Blackouts
   6. Significant problems at work

10. Which findings should be reported to the health care provider because they may indicate the patient is entering physical withdrawal from alcohol abuse?
    1. Mental status changes
    2. High blood pressure
    3. Tachycardia
    4. Nausea and vomiting

11. A patient who has abused alcohol or a benzodiazepine must be monitored for signs of physical withdrawal because the patient may be at risk for:
    1. paranoia.
    2. seizures.
    3. violence.
    4. euphoria.

12. Which supplements may be given to individuals with chronic alcoholism?
    1. Beta carotene and vitamin E
    2. Iron and vitamin C
    3. Folate and vitamin B_6
    4. Calcium and vitamin D

13. Which are symptoms of patients with an overdose of depressants? Select all that apply.
    1. Irritability
    2. Oversedation
    3. Respiratory depression
    4. Impaired coordination
    5. Hyperactivity
    6. Brain damage

14. Which are stimulants? Select all that apply.
    1. Amphetamines
    2. Cocaine
    3. Barbiturates
    4. Hypnotics
    5. Benzodiazepines

15. A patient is dependent on barbiturates. What may happen if the patient abruptly stops taking these drugs?
    1. Rebound sedation
    2. Oversedation
    3. Psychosis
    4. Depression

16. Which are signs and symptoms of chronic inhalation of cocaine? Select all that apply.
    1. Runny nose
    2. Weight gain
    3. Hyperactivity
    4. Hypotension
    5. Damage to the nasal mucosa

17. Hyperactivity, irritability, combativeness, and paranoia are symptoms of the use of:
    1. opioids.
    2. depressants.
    3. anxiolytics.
    4. amphetamines.

18. Which are identified by the DSM-V as drugs associated with substance-related disorders? Select all that apply.
    1. Caffeine
    2. Opioids
    3. Tobacco
    4. Chocolate
    5. Steroids
    6. NSAIDs

19. Which is a common effect of caffeine and nicotine?
    1. Euphoria
    2. Poor judgment
    3. Alters mood
    4. Relaxation

20. Which substance produces euphoria?
    1. Alcohol
    2. Caffeine
    3. Nicotine
    4. Amphetamine

21. Which signs are related to an older patient with alcohol use disorder? Select all that apply.
    1. Malnutrition
    2. Constipation
    3. Cirrhosis
    4. Bone thinning
    5. Poor memory
    6. Dysrhythmias

22. Which defense mechanism do addicts use when trying to justify the reasons or "make an excuse" for their addiction?
    1. Rationalization
    2. Intellectualization
    3. Denial
    4. Projection

23. A few patients may not experience any physical withdrawal symptoms despite a history of prolonged, frequent, and heavy substance abuse. Which factors may affect the incidence of withdrawal effects? Select all that apply.
    1. Weight of the patient
    2. Stage of addiction
    3. Baseline physical status of the patient
    4. Type of drugs being misused
    5. Defense mechanisms used

24. Which are physical characteristics of the appearance of the person with a substance use disorder? Select all that apply.
    1. Obese
    2. Malnourished
    3. Poorly cared for
    4. Evidence of physical trauma
    5. Peripheral neuropathy

25. Which is a correct statement about persons with a gambling addiction?
    1. Prevalence is high in Caucasian females.
    2. Twenty-five percent of those with a gambling addiction seek treatment.
    3. Incidence of gambling addiction is more common in older adults than younger adults.
    4. Involves risking something of value in hopes of gaining something of greater value.

PART III: CHALLENGE YOURSELF!

F. Getting Ready for NCLEX

Choose the most appropriate answer or select all that apply.

1. Which are the goals of an intervention for an impaired nurse? Select all that apply.
   1. Assist the impaired nurse to receive treatment.
   2. Protect the public from an untreated nurse.
   3. Terminate employment of the impaired nurse.
   4. Help the recovering nurse reenter nursing in a planned, safe way.
   5. Assist in monitoring the continued recovery of the nurse for a period of time.

2. Usually there is a 2-year time period after intervention for an impaired nurse to comply with the peer assistance process. Which are steps to be accomplished by the impaired nurse in this 2-year period? Select all that apply.
   1. The nurse is required to attend AA or NA groups regularly.
   2. The nurse participates in peer support groups.
   3. The nurse meets routinely with an identified support person representing the peer assistance program.
   4. The nurse must report how substance abuse impaired his/her practice to the state board of nursing.
   5. The nurse submits random urine drug screens to ensure that no relapse has occurred.

3. Which problems of a patient with a substance use disorder may increase the potential for injury? Select all that apply.
    1. Inadequate problem solving and series of self-perpetuating crises
    2. Refusal to acknowledge actual consequences of substance abuse
    3. Excessive use of the drug and risk for relapse
    4. Driving while under the influence
    5. Returning to places where one used drugs
    6. Using substances to deal with anxiety, emotional discomfort, and stress

4. When patients abusing alcohol state that they can quit easily and that they do not have a problem, they may be experiencing:
    1. inadequate coping.
    2. denial.
    3. potential injury.
    4. inability to communicate effectively.

5. A person with a substance use disorder who has driven under the influence of drugs and who engages in excessive drug use is increasing the potential for:
    1. infection.
    2. injury.
    3. aspiration.
    4. inadequate self-care.

6. Which are significant neurologic signs that may be associated with nutritional deficits in the patient with a substance use disorder? Select all that apply.
    1. Paranoia
    2. Euphoria
    3. Confusion
    4. Memory loss
    5. Tremors
    6. Lack of coordination

7. Which are typical stressors of aging that may cause older adults to use alcohol or experience alcohol use disorder for the first time? Select all that apply.
    1. Cognitive decline
    2. Retirement
    3. Losses of significant others
    4. Confusion related to alcohol use
    5. Family conflict
    6. Health problems
    7. Social isolation
    8. Loss of self-worth

G. Next-Generation NCLEX® Examination-Style Questions

A 37-year-old man was admitted to the hospital for alcohol detoxification. The nurse reviews the health history and physical assessment.

Health History:
A 37-year-old man was admitted to the hospital for alcohol detoxification. He was found lying on the floor at home, unconscious, and appeared to have vomited and been incontinent of urine and feces. He has a long history of alcohol use but claims he does not have a problem because he drinks only beer. He recently lost his job because he was not reporting for work on time, and his wife has threatened to leave him if he does not stop drinking. His two children, ages 8 and 10 years old, are afraid of him when he drinks. His usual intake of alcohol is two six-packs of beer a day. He has been detoxified in the hospital and is now ready for the rehabilitation phase of this treatment.

Physical Examination:
The client's skin and eyes have slight yellowish tinge. There is a cast on his left arm from below the elbow to the fingers. He appears thin and wasted. Client height 5' 10"; weight 160 pounds.

Vital Signs:

Blood Pressure	128/72 mm Hg
Pulse	80 beats/minute
Respirations	20 breaths/minute
Temperature	97.6°F oral

1. Which physical characteristics of this patient show evidence of substance use disorder? Select all that apply.
    1. Malnourished
    2. Lost his job due to tardiness
    3. Evidence of physical trauma
    4. Jaundice
    5. Blood pressure of 128/72
    6. Temperature 97.6°F oral
    7. 37-year-old male

A 48-year-old male client with a history of alcohol abuse presents to the Emergency Department. The nurse reviews the Physician's Progress Notes and Vital Signs.

Physician's Progress Notes:

3/2/21 2100: A 48-year-old male client presents to the ED with anxiety, confusion, irritability, and vomiting. His wife reports that the client has a 15-year history of alcohol abuse but recently attempted to quit. She states that the client occasionally uses cocaine, but has not used in over a month. The client appears to have tremors and lack of coordination. The client weighs 165 lbs, Height 6'0". Ascites noted. *Jean Lewis, MD*

Vital Signs:

Blood Pressure	190/92 mm Hg
Pulse	110 beats/minute
Respirations	24/min
Temperature	98.9°F

---

2. Which physician orders would the nurse anticipate being prescribed? Select all that apply.
   1. Urine drug screen
   2. Blood alcohol study
   3. Methadone
   4. Liver function tests
   5. CIWA protocol
   6. Vitamin replacement
   7. Narcan

First Aid, Emergency Care, and Disaster Management

chapter
63

Go to http://evolve.elsevier.com/Linton/medsurg/ for additional activities and exercises.

NCLEX CATEGORIES

Physiological Integrity: Reduction of Risk Potential, Physiological Adaptation

PART I: MASTERING THE BASICS

A. Key Terms

Match the definition in the numbered column with the most appropriate term in the lettered column.

1. _____ Decrease in body core temperature below 95°F

2. _____ An injury to a ligament

3. _____ Loss of a large amount of blood

4. _____ An injury to muscle tissue or the tendons that attach them to bones, or both

5. _____ Any substance that, in small quantities, is capable of causing illness or harm following ingestion, inhalation, injection, or contact with the skin

6. _____ Presence of blood in the pleural cavity causing the lung on the affected side to collapse

7. _____ Elevation of body core temperature above 99° F

8. _____ Blood in the pericardial sac that causes diminished cardiac productivity

9. _____ All or part of the auricle is torn loose

A. Avulsion
B. Cardiac tamponade
C. Hemorrhage
D. Hemothorax
E. Hyperthermia
F. Hypothermia
G. Poison
H. Sprain
I. Strain

B. Emergency Care and First Aid

1. List, in sequence, the six steps in the initial assessment and immediate intervention in emergency care.

   A. _____ Look for uncontrolled bleeding and apply pressure.

   B. _____ Assess level of consciousness.

   C. _____ Initiate CPR or rescue breathing as needed.

   D. _____ Allow family to be close and look for medical alert tag.

   E. _____ Assess the ABCs: airway, breathing, and circulation.

   F. _____ To assess exposure, remove clothes and observe the injury.

2. What are general guidelines for first-aid treatment of emergency patients? Select all that apply.
   1. Splint injured parts in the position they are found.
   2. Prevent chilling and do not add excessive heat.
   3. Remove any penetrating objects.
   4. Give the unconscious person sips of water.
   5. Stay with the injured person until help arrives.

C. Cardiopulmonary Arrest

1. Which are problems for patients in cardiopulmonary arrest? Select all that apply.
   1. Potential injury
   2. Inadequate peripheral circulation
   3. Adequate tissue perfusion
   4. Inadequate ventilation
   5. Potential inadequate oxygenation

D. Burns
Match the type of burn in the numbered column with the emergency intervention in the lettered column.

1. _____ Superficial, minor burn
2. _____ Sunburn
3. _____ Extensive burns
4. _____ Chemical burns

A. Cover burns with a clean, dry dressing or cloth.
B. Immerse the injured body part in cool water for 2–5 minutes.
C. Remove contaminated clothing and then flush skin with water for 30 minutes.
D. Apply topical preparations with benzocaine.

E. Bites
Match the intervention in the numbered column with the type of bite in the lettered column. Answers may be used more than once.

1. _____ Immobilize the body part with the bite and keep it at or below the heart to minimize absorption of venom.
2. _____ Clean thoroughly and apply a dressing. Seek medical attention for antibiotic therapy.
3. _____ Clean the wound thoroughly and apply a bulky dressing.
4. _____ Calamine lotion or a paste of baking soda or meat tenderizer is soothing.
5. _____ The patient with severe allergies may be given epinephrine, Benadryl, aminophylline, or hydrocortisone.
6. _____ Try to keep the patient still.
7. _____ Advise the patient to have a tetanus booster if immunizations are not current.
8. _____ Remove the stinger with a scraping motion.

A. Snake bite
B. Insect bite or sting
C. Animal bite
D. Human bite

F. Fractures
Match the definition in the numbered column with the appropriate term in the lettered column.

1. _____ A fracture that does not break the skin
2. _____ A fracture in which the ends of the broken bone protrude through the skin
3. _____ A fracture in which the broken ends are separated
4. _____ A fracture in which the bone ends are not separated

A. Complete
B. Incomplete
C. Simple
D. Compound

PART II: PUTTING IT ALL TOGETHER

G. Multiple Choice/Multiple Response
Choose the most appropriate answer or select all that apply.

1. General guidelines for first-aid treatment of emergency patients include:
   1. cover with wool blanket to prevent chills.
   2. remove penetrating objects.
   3. splint injured parts in the position they are found.
   4. give orange juice with sugar if unconscious.

2. The first assessment priorities for first-aid treatment of emergency patients must be:
   1. observation of uncontrolled bleeding or shock and open airway.
   2. systematic head-to-toe assessment and level of consciousness.
   3. evaluate airway, breathing, and circulation and immobilize cervical spine.
   4. palpation of carotid and peripheral pulses.

3. In most cases, the brain begins to die after 4 minutes without oxygen due to hypoxia of:
   1. heart tissue.
   2. nerve tissue.
   3. lung tissue.
   4. blood vessels.

4. Prompt recognition and treatment of cardiopulmonary arrest are important due to the need to maintain the oxygen supply to the:
   1. heart.
   2. brain.
   3. lungs.
   4. blood vessels.

5. Grabbing the throat with one or both hands is the universal sign for:
   1. heart attack.
   2. choking.
   3. danger.
   4. loss of consciousness.

6. If the choking victim is conscious or unconscious, the rescuer performs:
   1. abdominal thrusts
   2. CPR.
   3. 15 chest compressions.
   4. assessment of breathing.

7. If a choking victim is conscious, what is the appropriate intervention?
   1. Perform CPR
   2. Perform abdominal thrusts
   3. Slap back repeatedly
   4. Administer oxygen

8. Choking deaths can be prevented by:
   1. not talking while chewing.
   2. lowering blood pressure.
   3. decreasing weight.
   4. increasing exercise.

9. In an adult, what amount of blood loss may result in hypovolemic shock?
   1. 30 mL or more
   2. 1 pint or more
   3. 1 L or more
   4. 10 L or more

10. Immediate treatment for external bleeding is:
    1. application of ice.
    2. elevate the site of bleeding.
    3. direct, continuous pressure.
    4. check vital signs.

11. The primary symptom of fracture is:
    1. numbness.
    2. tingling.
    3. pain.
    4. hemorrhages.

12. The key to emergency management of fractures is:
    1. application of cold.
    2. elevation of injury.
    3. immobilization.
    4. application of heat.

13. Emergency treatment for sprains and strains includes:
    1. direct wound pressure.
    2. immobilization.
    3. application of heat.
    4. application of splint.

14. Change in behavior, increased blood pressure, and unequal pupils are signs of:
    1. anaphylactic shock.
    2. altered breathing.
    3. increased intracranial pressure.
    4. spinal cord injury.

15. When there is a neck or spinal injury, the nurse first assesses:
    1. blood loss and level of consciousness.
    2. breathing and circulation.
    3. movement of extremities.
    4. sensation in extremities.

16. After a diving injury, while removing the victim from the water, efforts are made to:
    1. immobilize the extremities.
    2. immobilize the neck and back.
    3. turn the victim in a prone position.
    4. turn the victim in a supine position.

17. The primary goals and outcome criteria for the patient with a neck or spinal injury is to:
    1. provide adequate ventilation.
    2. increase tissue perfusion.
    3. reduce anxiety.
    4. decrease potential for additional injury.

18. When chemicals come in contact with the eye, the nurse should:
    1. cover the eye with a loose dressing.
    2. flush with water to irrigate the eye for at least 20 minutes.
    3. apply pressure with a sterile cloth.
    4. place patient in the shower under cold water.

19. The abnormal chest wall movement in flail chest would be described as what sort of motion?
    1. Sawing
    2. Paradoxical
    3. Pulsating
    4. Sucking

20. The abnormal chest wall action in flail chest causes:
    1. inadequate circulation.
    2. increased tissue perfusion.
    3. increased pulse strength.
    4. impaired gas exchange.

21. Interventions for care of the patient with an abdominal wound include:
    1. protection of injured (eviscerated) tissue.
    2. control of bleeding.
    3. restoration of a strong pulse.
    4. reduction of anxiety.

22. When a large body surface area is burned, or any area is severely burned, the nurse should FIRST:
    1. apply medications to the burn.
    2. cover the burn with a clean, dry dressing or cloth.
    3. cover the burn with a cool, wet dressing or cloth.
    4. apply cool water until the burned area is cool.

23. Heat exhaustion is treated by:
    1. pushing fluids with caffeine.
    2. ambulating the victim.
    3. cooling and hydrating the victim.
    4. placing victim in ice.

24. Which are important teaching points to prevent heat exhaustion? Select all that apply.
    1. Avoid strenuous activities in high temperatures or humidity.
    2. Increase fluid intake.
    3. Wear heavy clothing to absorb perspiration.
    4. Take frequent rest breaks.

25. The skin is red, hot, and dry and perspiration is absent in:
    1. heat stroke.
    2. heat exhaustion.
    3. hyperthermia.
    4. hypothermia.

26. The immediate treatment of mild hypothermia is:
    1. wrapping victim in warm, dry clothing and blankets.
    2. massaging to increase circulation.
    3. covering with dressing.
    4. immersing in tepid water.

27. Carbon monoxide poisoning occurs because carbon monoxide:
    1. is blown off too rapidly during exhalation.
    2. binds to hemoglobin and occupies sites needed to transport oxygen to the cells.
    3. binds to white blood cells and causes infection.
    4. is retained and prevents oxygen from being inhaled in adequate amounts.

28. The primary patient problem for a victim of carbon monoxide poisoning is:
    1. inadequate oxygenation.
    2. inadequate circulation.
    3. potential for aspiration.
    4. anxiety related to inadequate oxygenation.

29. The primary patient problem for the victim of drug or chemical poisoning is:
    1. confusion related to effects of the drug or chemical.
    2. potential infection.
    3. potential injury.
    4. potential inadequate oxygenation.

30. Influenza-like symptoms, with or without a "bull's-eye lesion," following a tick bite may be symptoms of:
    1. poisoning.
    2. Lyme disease.
    3. staph infection.
    4. hypersensitivity.

31. What is the danger of too-rapid rewarming as the treatment for a patient with severe hypothermia?
    1. Cardiac dysrhythmias
    2. Heat stroke
    3. Tingling and numbness of extremities
    4. Muscle cramps

PART III: CHALLENGE YOURSELF!

H. Getting Ready for NCLEX

Choose the most appropriate answer or select all that apply.

1. The nurse is teaching a community health class about heat exhaustion. Which common signs and symptoms of heat exhaustion should be included in the presentation? Select all that apply.
   1. Dizziness
   2. Muscle cramps
   3. Pale, damp skin
   4. Hot, dry skin
   5. Absent perspiration
   6. Seizures

2. A patient comes to the clinic following a severe allergic reaction to an insect bite. Which drugs are indicated to prevent anaphylaxis? Select all that apply.
   1. Demerol
   2. Epinephrine
   3. Corticosteroids
   4. Ibuprofen
   5. Benadryl

3. A patient arrives at the clinic reporting a snake bite on his right leg. Which are local effects of snake bites? Select all that apply.
   1. Local itching
   2. Pain
   3. Mild to severe edema
   4. Urticaria
   5. Discoloration

4. Which are goals and outcomes for a patient with cardiopulmonary arrest? Select all that apply.
   1. Decreased coughing
   2. Improving skin color
   3. Spontaneous respirations
   4. Active bowel sounds
   5. Palpable pulse

5. Which is a common problem for a patient with hemorrhage?
   1. Impaired tissue perfusion
   2. Inadequate circulation
   3. Potential electrolyte imbalance
   4. Inadequate oxygenation

6. Which represents a goal for a patient with hemorrhage?
   1. Skin warm and dry
   2. Patent airway with normal respirations
   3. Adequate oxygenation
   4. Decreased blood pressure

7. Which are symptoms that will aid in the prompt recognition of a patient with a head injury? Select all that apply.
   1. Numbness and tingling
   2. Unequal pupils
   3. Changes in behavior, agitation, and confusion
   4. Pain
   5. Abnormal response of pupils to light

8. Problems that might apply to the patient with a head injury during the emergency phase of treatment include:
   1. inadequate circulation related to hypovolemia and anxiety related to possible impending death.
   2. impaired tissue perfusion related to the cessation of heartbeat and inadequate circulation.
   3. inadequate oxygenation related to neurologic trauma and potential injury related to increasing intracranial pressure.
   4. potential injury related to improper movement of the spine.

9. Nursing goals and outcomes for the patient with a neck or spinal injury are based on:
   1. continuous monitoring for signs of increased intracranial pressure and oxygenation.
   2. continuous immobilization of the back and spine and transport for medical care.
   3. prevention of aspiration and maintenance of circulation.
   4. prevention of skin breakdown and shock.

10. If bleeding is under control, the primary patient problem for a traumatic injury to the auricle is:
    1. altered self-concept related to injury.
    2. anemia related to blood loss.
    3. loss of protective barrier: skin related to injury.
    4. inadequate circulation related to blood loss.

11. Which are nursing goals and outcomes for emergency care of the burn victim? Select all that apply.
    1. Adequate oxygenation
    2. Absence of hypertension
    3. Burned areas covered
    4. Skin surfaces free from burning materials
    5. Pain reduced
    6. No symptoms of ileus

12. If a victim of frostbite cannot be transported immediately to a medical facility, what should be done?
    1. Wrap in sterile dressings before warming the affected area.
    2. Perform rapid rewarming.
    3. Rub or massage the affected area.
    4. Immerse frostbitten area in warm water.

13. Which drugs increase the risk of heat stroke by affecting the body's heat-reducing mechanisms?
    1. Adrenergics and bronchodilators
    2. Diuretics and anticholinergics
    3. Steroids and salicylates
    4. Anticoagulants and antihistamines

14. What is the first step in initiating first aid in an emergency situation?
    1. Determine how many are injured.
    2. Determine who is around to help.
    3. Determine if the area is safe for you and the victim(s).
    4. Determine how the victims are injured.

I. Next-Generation NCLEX® Examination-Style Questions

A 55-year-old female client 4 days status post open exploratory laparotomy presents to the Emergency Department with abdominal organs protruding through the wound. The nurse reviews the health history and physician's progress notes.

> Health History:
> A 55-year-old female client presents to the ED with abdominal organs protruding through abdominal wound. The client is 4 days status post open exploratory laparotomy. No significant medical history.
>
> Physician's Progress Notes:
> 1200: The client states, "I was just trying to lift some boxes and this happened". The client is alert and oriented times 4. Bowel sounds hypoactive to all 4 quadrants. The incision to the abdomen has a 1 inch open area. Intestinal organs appear pink in color. *J. James, MD*

1. Which physician orders would the nurse anticipate being prescribed immediately? Select all that apply.
   1. NPO
   2. Reinsert eviscerated organs into the abdomen
   3. Cover eviscerated organs with saline-soaked sterile dressing
   4. Use an abdominal binder to splint the abdomen
   5. Apply topical antibiotic to the incision site
   6. Open the incision for better visualization

A 25-year-old client riding his motorcycle was struck by a speeding vehicle. The client was immobilized and transported to the Emergency Department (ED). Upon admission to the ED, the nurse reviews the pre-hospital documentation.

Pre-Hospital Notes:
A 25-year-old male client riding his motorcycle was struck by a speeding vehicle. The client was thrown into a ditch. The client is alert and oriented x 2, and able to move both arms and legs on the scene. He has abdominal laceration and ecchymosis to the chest. Abdominal distension noted. He lost 600 ML sanguineous fluid from the abdominal wound. Skin is cool, sweaty, and pale; weak, thready pulse. Abrasions are present on all 4 extremities. The client states that his pain is a 10/10 on a 0–10 pain intensity scale.

Vital signs:

Temperature	98.8°F (37.1°C)
Pulse	110 beats/minute
Respirations	24 breaths/minute
Blood Pressure	88/48 mmHg

2. Complete the diagram by dragging from the choices below to specify 1 potential condition the client is most likely experiencing, 2 actions the nurse would take to address that condition, and 2 parameters the nurse would monitor to assess the client's progress.

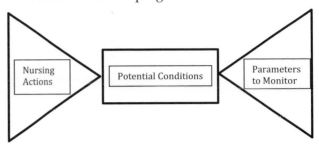

Nursing Actions	Potential Conditions	Parameters to Monitor
Administer packed red blood cells	Hyperthermia	Blood Pressure
Apply direct, continuous pressure	Hemorrhage	Temperature
Administer Tylenol for fever	Hypothermia	Pain level
Appy cold compress skin	Spinal cord injury	Serum albumin
Apply abdominal binder		Hemoglobin and hematocrit